Vocational Rehabilitation

Springer

*Paris
Berlin
Heidelberg
New York
Hong Kong
Londres
Milan
Tokyo*

C. Gobelet, F. Franchignoni

Vocational Rehabilitation

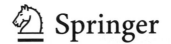 Springer

Charles Gobelet

Clinique romande de réadaptation SuvaCare
Case postale 352
1951 Sion
SUISSE

Franco Franchignoni

"Salvatore Maugeri" Foundation Scientific Institute of Rehabilitation
28010 Veruno
ITALIE

ISBN-10 : 2-287-22609-5 Springer Paris Berlin Heidelberg New York

ISBN-13 : 978-2-287-22609-0 Springer Paris Berlin Heidelberg New York

© Springer-Verlag France 2006
Imprimé en France

Springer-Verlag France est membre du groupe Springer Science + Business Media

SPIN : 149041

Maquette de couverture : Jean-François Montmarché

Members of the European Academy of Rehabilitation Medicine

Pr ALARANTA Hannu
Helsinki (Finlande)

Pr ANDRÉ Jean-Marie
Nancy (France)

Pr BARAT Michel
Bordeaux (France)

Pr BARDOT André
Marseille (France)

Pr BARNES M. Ph.
Newcastle upon Tyne (Grande-Bretagne)

Pr BARNOSELL Francisco
Barcelone (Espagne)

Pr BERTOLINI Carlo
Rome (Italie)

Pr CHAMBERLAIN M. Anne
Leeds (Grande-Bretagne)

Pr CHANTRAINE Alex
Genève (Suisse)

Pr CONRADI Eberhard
Berlin (Allemagne)

Pr DELBRÜCK Hermann
Wuppertal (Allemagne)

Pr DIDIER Jean-Pierre
Dijon (France)

Pr EKHOLM Jan
Stockholm (Suède)

Dr EL MASRY Wagih
Oswestry Shropshire (Grande-Bretagne)

Pr EYSSETTE Michel
Saint Genis-Laval (France)

Pr FIALKA-MOSER Veronika
Vienne (Autriche)

Pr FRANCHIGNONI Franco
Veruno (Italie)

Pr GATCHEVA Jordanka
Sofia (Bulgarie)

Pr GOBELET Charles
Sion (Suisse)

Pr HEILPORN André
Bruxelles (Belgique)

Pr LANKHORST Gustaaf J.
Amsterdam (Pays-Bas)

Pr McLELLAN Lindsay
Hampshire (Grande-Bretagne)

Dr McNAMARA Angela
Dublin (Irlande)

Dr MAIGNE Robert
Paris (France)

Pr MAURITZ Karl-Heinz
Berlin (Allemagne)

Pr MEGNA Gianfranco
Bari (Italie)

Pr MICHAIL Xanthi
Athènes (Grèce)

Dr OELZE Fritz
Hamburg (Allemagne)

Pr RODRIGUEZ Luis-Pablo
Madrid (Espagne)

Pr SJÖLUND Bengt H.
Umea (Suède)

Pr STAM Hendrik Jan
Rotterdam (Pays-Bas)

Pr TONAZZI Amedeo
Saint-Raphaël (France)

Pr VANDERSTRAETEN Guy
Gent (Belgique)

Dr WARD Anthony
Stoke on Trent (Grande-Bretagne)

Dr ZÄCH Guido A.
Nottwil (Suisse)

CONTRIBUTORS

ALARANTA Hannu MD Ph. D.
Specialist in physical medicine and rehabilitation
Associate professor
Käpylä Rehabilitation Centre
Finnish Association of People with Mobility
Disabilities
Nordenskiöldinkatu 18 B
00251 Helsinki
Finland

AL-KHODAIRY Abdul MD
Clinique romande de réadaptation SuvaCare
Service de Paraplégie
Av. de Grand Champsec 90
Case postale 352
1951 Sion
Switzerland

ANDRÉ Jean-Marie Pr
Institut régional de réadaptation
35, rue Lionnois
54000 Nancy Cedex
France

ARNOLD Pierre MD
Clinique romande de réadaptation SuvaCare
Service de réadaptation neurologique
Av. de Grand Champsec 90
Case postale 352
1951 Sion
Switzerland

BAZZINI Giacomo MD
Fondazione Salvatore Maugeri
Clinica del Lavoro e della Riabilitazione IRCCS
Servizio di Fisiatria Occupazionale e Ergonomia
Istituto di Montescano
27040 Montescano (PV)
Italy

BELLMANN Anne Ph. D
Clinique romande de réadaptation SuvaCare
Service de réadaptation neurologique
Unité de neuropsychologie
Av. de Grand Champsec 90
Case postale 352

1951 Sion
Switzerland

BRUSSELMANS Wilfried Ph. D
Centre for Locomotor and Neurological
Rehabilitation
University Hospital Ghent - K7
De Pintelaan 185
9000 Gent
Belgium

CASILLAS Jean-Marie Pr
CHU Dijon
23, rue Gaffarel
21034 Dijon
France

CUXART Fina Amparo MD Ph. D
Hospital Vall d'Hebron
PG. Vall d'Hebron, S/N
08035 Barcelona
Spain

CZAMAY Doris, Mag. (Psychologist)
Berufliches Bildungs – und
Rehabilitationszentrum (BBRZ)
Geiselbergstrasse 26-32
1110 Wien
Austria

DAL POZZO Cristina MD
Medico-Legal Area
INAIL (Worker Compensation Authority)
Via Nancy 2
35134 Padova (PD)
Italy

DELBRÜCK Hermann Pr
Klinik Bergisch-Land
Fachklinik für onkologische Rehabilitation
Im Saalscheid 5
42369 Wuppertal
Germany

DELPLACE Koen Mr
Centre for Locomotor and Neurological
Rehabilitation
University Hospital Ghent - K7
De Pintelaan 185
9000 Gent
Belgium

DIDIER Jean-Pierre Pr
CHU Dijon
23, rue Gaffarel
21034 Dijon
France

DONNER Claudio F. MD
Chief Pulmonary Division
"Salvatore Maugeri" Foundation IRCCS
Scientific Institute of Veruno
Via per Revislate 13
28010 Veruno (No)
Italy

EKHOLM Jan MD
Brostugevägen 1D
756 53 Uppsala
Sweden

EL MASRY WAGIH S. FRCS Ed
Midlands Centre for Spinal Injuries
Robert Jones and Agnes Hunt
Orthopaedic Hospital
Oswestry SY 10 7 AG
Great Britain

FAUCHÈRE Pierre-André MD
Clinique romande de réadaptation SuvaCare
Service de psychosomatique
Av. de Grand Champsec 90
Case postale 352
1951 Sion
Switzerland

FIALKA-MOSER Veronika E. MD Ph. D
Professor and Chairman of Physical Medicine
and Rehabilitation
Univ. Klinik für Physikalische Medicine &
Rehabilitation AKH Wien

Währinger Gürtel 18-20
1090 Wien
Austria

FOURNIER-BUCHS Marie-France Mme
Office AI du Canton du Valais
Av. de la Gare 15
1950 Sion
Switzerland

FRANCHIGNONI Franco Pr
"Salvatore Maugeri" Foundation
Scientific Institute of Rehabilitation IRCCS
Via per Revislate 13
28010 Veruno (No)
Italy

GOBELET Charles Pr
Directeur médical
Clinique romande de réadaptation SuvaCare
Av. de Grand Champsec 90
Case postale 352
1951 Sion
Switzerland

HARTTER Engelbert Pr
Univ Klinik für Physikalische Medicine &
Rehabilitation
AKH Wien
Währinger Gürtel 18-20
1090 Wien
Austria

HERCEG Malvina MD
Universitätsklinik für Physikalische Medizin und
Rehabilitation
Währinger Gürtel 18-20
1090 Wien
Austria

LE CHAPELAIN Cécile MD
Institut Régional de Réadaptation
35, rue Lionnois
54042 Nancy Cedex
France

McNAMARA Angela M. FRCPI. FRCP (Lond)
National Rehabilitation Hospital
Rochestown Ave
Dun Laoghaire
Co. Dublin
Ireland

MICHAIL Xanthi Pr
Diagnostic & Therapeutic Center of
Athens "UGEIA"
Physiotherapy & Rehabilitation Dept
Kifissias aven, & 4, rue Erythrou Stravrou
151 23 Maroussi
Greece Hellas

MILANOVIC Marina Mag. (clinical & health
psychologist)
Berufliches Bildungs – und
Rehabilitationszentrum (BBRZ)
Geiselbergstrasse 26-32
1110 Wien
Austria

MILLER Brian M. Sc B. Comm NDIRS Dip
Counselling
Manager Disability Services
Health Services Executive
NRH
Rochestown Avenue
Dun Laoghaire
Co. Dublin
Ireland

MORGER Willi Dr Jur
Member of Suva's Management Board
Suva
Fluhmattstrasse 1
6002 Lucerne
Switzerland

NIJHUIS Frans Pr
Hoensbroeck Centre for Vocational Rehabilitation
Zandbergsweg 111
6432CC Hoensbroeck
The Netherlands

OLIVERI Michael MD
Unit of Occupational Rehabilitation
and Ergonomics
Rehaklinik Bellikon
5454 Bellikon
Switzerland

PAPPONE Nicola MD
Unit of Rehabilitation Medicine
Occupational Therapy and Ergonomics
Rehabilitation Institute of Telese (BN)
"Salvatore Mauger" Foundation
Clinica del Lavoro e della Riabilitazione,
IRCCS
82037 Telese-Terme
Italy

PAYSANT Jean MD
Institut Régional de Réadaptation
35, rue Lionnois
54042 Nancy Cedex
France

PILET François MD
Av. du Fossau 6
1896 Vouvry
Switzerland

ROTHENBÜHLER Igor Ph. D in progress
Swiss Forum for Migration
and Population Studies (SFM)
Rue St-Honoré 2
2000 Neuchâtel
Switzerland

ROY Christopher W. MBChB, FRCP (Glasg)
Honorary clinical senior lecturer
University of Glasgow
PDRU offices
Southern General Hospital
1345 Govan Road
Glasgow G51 4TF
Scotland/The United Kingdom

SCHIAN Hans Martin MD
IQPR GmbH
Sürther Str. 171
50999 Köln
Germany

SCHÜLDT EKHOLM Kristina MD Ph. D
Brostugevägen 1D
756 53 Uppsala
Sweden

SMOLIK Henri-Jacques Pr
Institut de Médecine du Travail et d'Ergonomie
Faculté de Médecine
7, Bd Jeanne d'Arc
BP 87900
21079 Dijon Cedex
France

STATHI Kyriaki Ph. D
15, rue Zossimadon
185 31 Le Piree
Greece Hellas

TZARA Marianthi MD
14, rue Aggelou Metaxa
166 75 Glyphada
Greece Hellas

VAN LIEROP A.G. Ph. D
Institute for Rehabilitation Research (iRv)
Zandbergsweg 11
6432CC Hoensbroek
The Netherlands

VUADENS Philippe MD
Clinique romande de réadaptation SuvaCare
Service de réadaptation neurologique
Av. de Grand Champsec 90
Case postale 352
1951 Sion
Switzerland

WICHERS Frits B in PH, ing
Heliomare arbeidsintegratie
Verlengde Voorstraat 8
1949 CM Wijk aan Zee
The Nederlands

PREFACE

It gives us great pleasure to write the preface to this book, the second in the series of monographs produced by the European Academy of Rehabilitation Medicine. No part of medicine, no clinical intervention, is complete without thinking about its effect on the person's life and the quality thereof. One of the most powerful determinants of this is work; a source not only of income, but of satisfaction and a sense of purpose and worth.

The Academy, founded in 1969, is composed of senior European doctors specialising in Rehabilitation and Physical Medicine. It meets regularly to discuss matters of importance in the field, including teaching, research and ethical matters. It recognises that the ability of the speciality and of related ones to decrease dependency and increase autonomy and quality of life needs to be better known. Hence the production of these monographs. They will help readers access a vast amount of literature on the practice of rehabilitation and its effectiveness. They should be particularly useful to young doctors preparing for the European Boards certification in Physical and Rehabilitation Medicine as they are authoritative and cover subjects in depth. Topics covered in the series range from basic sciences to the most applied areas.

This book is at the most applied end of the spectrum and, as the authors show, a great deal needs to be done in this area, at a time when the ratio of economically active to dependent members of society is falling. Aside from this, many people define themselves by their work and to many it is enriching, not solely in financial terms.

The first book in the series, entitled "La plasticité de la fonction motrice", edited by Jean-Pierre Didier was published in 2004. Further titles will include the rehabilitation of patients with cancer, and not; the control and function of the sphincters and the rehabilitation of those with musculo-skeletal pain.

Pr M. Anne Chamberlain
President of
European Academy of Rehabilitation Medicine
FRCP, FRCP&CH, OBE
University of Leeds
36, Clarendon Road
Leeds LS2 9NZ
GB

Pr Alex Chantraine
Honorary Secretary

CONTENTS

SECOND PART
SOME EXAMPLES OF VOCATIONAL
REHABILITATION MANAGEMENT IN EUROPE

FIRST PART

VOCATIONAL REHABILITATION: DEFINITION AND APPLICATIONS

Vocational rehabilitation

C. Gobelet and F. Franchignoni

Introduction

Over the last few decades the share of health and social security in total welfare spending has gradually increased in all industrialized countries [1]. Public expenditure for social security in European Union (EU) countries roughly doubled between 1960 and 1985 and since then has slightly increased until now where it represents about 20% of the gross domestic product. The expenses are generally related to three main kinds of benefit: sickness benefits, invalidity benefits (also called disability benefits), and employment injury benefits (including occupational disease benefits). The benefits for work-related injuries and diseases usually have no particular entitlement conditions (apart from that of being employed), waiting periods or time limits, are more munificent and include additional allowances.

There are marked differences among countries in terms of eligibility criteria, specific types of benefit, ease of obtaining the benefits, claims, adjudication and appeal procedures, etc. This is because the organisation of each social security system is affected by economic, socio-cultural and political issues, and is only one element of a broader social framework (including demographic and employment issues, among others).

The different mechanisms and control systems are likely to influence the patterns of utilisation of all these benefits (e.g. certifications, benefit claims, benefits received, etc.) and thus in surveying this material it is difficult to draw general conclusions.

From 1985 to 1994, both sickness and invalidity benefits rose in most European countries (on average by about 20-30% and 15-20%, respectively). In the last few years a dramatic increase in sick leave has been observed in some countries, for example in Sweden since 1997 [2]. In Switzerland (7,500,000 inhabitants) in 2001 the disability compensation insurance, which is responsible for the disability pension payment, paid out 485,000 insurance claims (for physical or psychological disturbances leading to loss of job) for a total of 9.5 billion SFr. The deficit of this insurance was approximately 1 billion SFr for the year 2001: it is explained by an increase of 123% in claims and 165% in total expenditure between 1988 and 2001 [3].

Three main diagnostic groups account for the large majority of sickness and invalidity benefits: musculo-skeletal disorders, mental disorders, and cardio-respiratory disorders. Not all reported work injuries and illnesses are disabling, however and the phychiatrist is most likely to be consulted for conditions associated with prolonged work disability.

In recent years the prevalence of musculo-skeletal disorders producing long-term sick leave (particularly back pain and cumulative trauma disorders of the upper limb) has increased in many industrialized countries [2]. In the USA they constitute about 40% of all compensation claims, with back pain accounting for more than half of these claims [4]. In the UK, musculo-skeletal disorders represent the largest group (28%) of beneficiaries of incapacity benefit, whereas mental and behavioural disorders (milder conditions, in particular) are the second most common reason for being awarded this benefit (20%). In Sweden, psychiatric and stress-related diseases have risen in recent years and this modification has been explained by changes observed in working life conditions (i.e. organizational changes, rationalizations and a labour market not fitted to fully meet these changes) [5]. Similarly, in Switzerland, a 72% increase in invalidity pensions for psychoses and a 239% increase for psychic reactive troubles were observed between 1988 and 2002 [3].

Based on the ICF classification [6] estimates by the European Community Household Panel (ECHP) of the number of people in the EU affected by some form of self-reported disability vary substantially between countries and within the same country compared to previous national surveys (Table 1), and represent on average 14% of the EU working-age population [7]. This percentage concerns all groups of disabled people (with congenital and acquired impairments, with different degrees of disability, with permanent or temporary disabilities).

Table 1 – Mean percentages of disabled persons in the EU, based on the ECHP report and previous national surveys. Legend: A = Austria; B = Belgium; D = Germany; DK = Denmark; E = Spain; F = France; FIN = Finland; GR = Greece; I = Italy; IRL = Ireland; L = Luxembourg; NL = The Netherlands; P = Portugal; S = Sweden; UK = United Kingdom.
In [7]. The employment situation of people with disabilities in the European Union. European Commission. Employment and Social affairs. Study prepared by EIM Business and Policy Research. Directorate-general. Unit EMPL/E.4 August 2001 p 35, National surveys (various years) and ECHP 1996 M.A. Malo, C. Garcia – Serrano, March 2001.

	A	B	D	DK	E	F	FIN	GR	I	IRL	L	NL	P	S	UK
Surveys	29,0	17,0	6,9	7,0	5,8	3,1	5,0	2,2	1,6	–	8,0	16,4	–	17,1	18,8
ECHP	12,5	12,9	17,3	17,4	9,9	15,3	22,9	8,2	7,8	10,9	16,5	18,6	18,4	–	18,8

As for the labour market, the same ECHP data show that in the EU 42.4% of disabled people are employed, 5.6% are unemployed and 52.2% are economically inactive, whereas 64.5% of non-disabled people are employed, 7.4% are unemployed and 28.1% are economically inactive [7]. Thus, participation of people with disabilities in the workforce is lower than that of non-disabled subjects [8,9], and in the last decades the structural changes in the nature of work that have occurred have resulted in a shortage of jobs in which people with disabilities – in particular, the elderly – can remain at work [10].

There are large differences in the percentages of disabled people employed among the EU countries. This is probably due to the discrepancies not only in supporting participation of people with disabilities in working activities, but also in defining disabled people and calculating appropriate participation rates. For example, a more restrictive administrative definition of disability, focussing on people receiving disability benefits, shows that in the Netherlands in 1991 only 18% of disabled people were employed (162,000/900,000): this value represents 2.6% of the workforce in the Netherlands [10]. Similarly, in the UK only 5% of 2.5 million people of working age with disabilities or long-term illness receiving state benefits (incapacity benefit, income support, housing benefit, Council Tax benefit or severe disablement allowance) leave these benefits to resume work each year [11].

Furthermore, employment rates vary greatly between types of disability [7]: people with mental illness, learning disabilities or psychological impairments are less likely to be employed than are people with physical impairments.

The duration of sickness benefits and the point of transition to invalidity benefits or old-age pension vary in each country. In Norway, the dominant predictive factors for the transition from long-term sick leave to disability pension are age and duration of the sickness spells [12]. Nevertheless, both sickness and invalidity benefits have been used in some European countries – easing *de facto* the entitlement conditions – as a better income support than non-employment benefits for workers leaving the labour market before retirement age, particularly during industrial reorganizations or in regions with high unemployment rates [13]. In a few countries, there are also special early-retirement schemes for particular categories of workers. Naturally, when alternatives are available there is an incentive to try to enter into the less restrictive and more generous compensation system.

However, in recent years there has been a clear increase in the interest of policy makers in both containment of public expenditure and social inclusion issues and re-integration policies for people with disabilities. These issues lead to a growing emphasis on review of invalidity status, comprehensive rehabilitation (including workplace adaptations) of those with restoration potential, and return to work in preference to early retirement. A rigorous control of the allocation of the invalidity benefit (that should be assigned only on medical grounds) is always needed as a disincentive for workers with minor problems from leaving the workforce in this way. On the other hand, rehabilitation may strongly contribute to lessen the burden on society of direct and indirect costs related to sick-listed patients and disability pensioners (in terms of reduced sick leave, reduced early retirement, increased productivity, continued payment of taxes, reduced payment of state benefits). Thus Nachemson [14] estimates that the development of comprehensive rehabilitation programs, including vocational rehabilitation interventions, would result in important social and economic gains.

Mention should also be made of the importance of work in our life. Nietzsche considered work as a mean of social control and of "normalization" of behaviours. On the contrary, the sociological and economic approaches judge work as pivotal in the process of social integration [15]. From the late Middle Ages to the 19th century work was an attribute of low social state (the nobility did not work), but in our industrialized society work has progressively gained positive connotations. At the most basic level, earnings from work enable an independent way of life. However for many people work means much more. In our culture the job often reflects a person's identity, social status, and feelings of self-worth, and for many people, losing one's job can be, apart from the financial aspect, a psychologically and socially devastating experience.

In fact, during periods of unemployment or precarious work, psychological problems such as anxiety, loss of self-confidence, and other feelings of psychological distress often appear [16]. For these reasons, although work resumption may not be a goal for all disabled people, it is the aim for the majority of them. Indeed, for many people, return to work is directly related to the quality of life.

While working ability and return to work are critical, the way by which this return is effected is also important. In 1986, the Ottawa chart stated the way by which a society organizes work, work conditions, and free time have to be a source of life and not of illness [17]. In this view, the rapid implementation of rehabilitation programs and especially of vocational rehabilitation could decrease the phenomenon of return to one's job at a reduced level, with lower earnings, or with higher risk for further injury or illness.

Definition of vocational rehabilitation

Many definitions have been proposed for "vocational rehabilitation". In "Vocational Rehabilitation. The Way Forward" vocational rehabilitation is defined as enabling individuals with either temporary or permanent disability to access, return to, or remain in, employment [11]. This definition is similar to that proposed by the International Labour Organisation and based on the objective: "to enable a disabled person to secure and retain suitable employment" [18]. The most complete definition is proposed by Selander [19] : "Medical, psychological, social and occupational activities aiming to re-establish among sick or injured people with previous work history their working capacity and prerequisites for returning to the labour market, i.e. to a job or availability for a job". This last description comprises all the aspects included in a vocational program directed towards the return to work. Vocational rehabilitation deals largely with vocational assessment, work re-training, education and counselling, work guidance and ergonomic modifications, and psycho-social interventions (including vocational orientation and all other forms of preparation for returning to work) [20]. These interventions slightly differ from services to persons with congenital or developmental disabilities who are seeking to enter the labour market for the first time.

According to Selander, where disability remains after medical care, initially the person might undergo medical rehabilitation at primary care level or at a rehabilitation unit, and later people of working age may initiate vocational rehabilitation including both medical and non-medical interventions (functional restoration programs, job counselling, education, etc.) (Table 2).

Table 2 – The normal course from acute care after accident or disease to the return to the labourmarket [from 21] (Taylor and Francis Ltd. http://www.tandf.co.uk/journals).

1	2	3	4 Rehabilitation			5	6
At work	Disease / injury	Medical care	4a Medical rehabilitation	4b Vocational rehabilitation Medical e.g.: functional restoration program	Non medical e.g.: education, work training, modified work	Decision	Return to work ? Disability pension

Although there are differences in the organisation of vocational rehabilitation between countries (and sometimes even between regions within individual countries), the objectives of the vocational rehabilitation are always "to maximise the ability of an individual to return to meaningful employment" [11]. The British Society of Physical Medicine and Rehabilitation states that the best rehabilitation practice for faster and easier return to work improves work and activity tolerance, avoids illness behaviour, prevents deconditioning and chronicity, and reduces pain and the effects of illness or disability.

What is the attitude of the EU Member States towards vocational rehabilitation and reinsertion?

The perception of vocational rehabilitation by the different governments of the EU Member States varies. However, the EU has defined a strategy concerning disabled persons. In November 2000, the Member States undertook to prohibit discrimination against people with disabilities and other categories in the labour market, in the workplace and in vocational rehabilitation [22]. These changes are based both on utilitarian principles (e.g. cost containment in health care and social security benefits, and a better utilisation of the work potential) and on more basic considerations, such as meeting the aspirations of people with disabilities for autonomy and participation in all areas of life [10].

The EU disability strategy is based on three main pillars as defined in the anti-discrimination fundamental social and civil rights society [23]: cooperation between the Commission and the Member States; full participation of people with disabilities; mainstreaming disability in policy development.

To change attitudes towards disabled people in the area of employment is one of the most important aspects of the strategy. This information is available in the Official

Journal of the European Community of December 2000. The aims of this strategy are also reported in the National Action Plans on Employment and in the National Action Plans against Poverty and Social Exclusion [23, 24]. However, if we examine these National Action Plans, we realize that there are great differences among the Member States of the Union in the attitude to disabled persons. For instance, in the National Action Plans on Employment, five countries have a clear and strong position concerning disabled people, whereas the other countries only mention this problem.

The European Commission for Employment and Social Affairs has in this context an important role in:

– "strengthening cooperation with and between the Member States in the disability field;

– promoting the collection, exchange and development of comparable information and statistics and good practice;

– raising awareness of disability issues;

– taking account of disability issues in all policy making and legislative work of the Commission" [23].

An interesting aspect of the EU strategy for disabled persons is the EQUAL programs which test new ways and possibilities of changing discrimination and inequality among people in work or looking for a job. In the EQUAL programs social partners and other key players, such as representatives of discriminated groups in the labour market, are working together to develop and test new ideas in job creation [23].

EQUAL shares information and results through transnational cooperation agreements and transnational cooperation partnerships at regional or national level. The guidelines for the Community Institute EQUAL were published by the Commission of the European Communities on 5th May, 2000 [25]. We would like to mention that among the transnational cooperation agreements, 172 programs target the group of disadvantaged people. Among these 45 concern ethnic minority groups and migrants, 28 people with disabilities, 23 unemployed persons and 76 other disadvantaged groups [25].

What are the factors which affect work ability and return to work?

To establish strategies for reducing sick leave, an understanding of the conditions influencing time off work is crucial. Age, gender, health status, and work experience have traditionally been indicated as playing an important role in both work ability and work resumption [10, 26, 27].

Among sick or injured people, Selander [21] described the following factors as increasing the probability of receiving a disability pension and/or reducing the return to work in musculo-skeletal disorders:

– subject attributes: demographic (older age, foreign origin, low income, low education level, loneliness, etc.) and psycho-social factors (low self-confidence, low health locus of control, low quality of life, depression, etc.);

– medical factors (complex medical history, severe disability, great pain, ADL deficits, etc.) and factors related to treatment/rehabilitation (e.g. type and timing of the rehabilitation);

– factors related to employer and workplace: poor physical work environment (uncomfortable work postures, highly repetitive movements, heavy work, vibrations, etc.), poor psychological and organisational work environment (great time pressure, high work pace, monotonous tasks, stress at the workplace, etc.), etc.;

– socio-economic determinants related to benefit system and labour market (e.g. type and degree of social benefit, regional and national unemployment rates).

The same author described in a dissertation published in 1999 [19] some other factors which are associated with long-term sickness in people undergoing vocational rehabilitation. Again, they are related to socio-professional features (e.g. low social group belonging, earlier sick leave, low belief of vocational return, low job satisfaction, little social support), medical aspects (e.g. low understanding of medical condition, low level of experienced health, back impairments, mental or psychiatric disabilities), family factors (e.g. spouse with disability pension, household composition, personal or family-related problems), and work-related factors.

These findings are in agreement with other recent reports. For example, Niemeyer *et al.* [28] confirmed the role of many psychosocial factors as barriers to workers' recovery and rehabilitation: they include – but are not limited to – dysfunctional emotional states and long-standing behavioural problems (e.g. pain behaviours, history of alcohol abuse, anger and frustration). In addition, many authors observed that long-term sick leave is often associated with work conditions, and insisted on the importance of including the work site in the rehabilitation program for all patients with work-related problems [2, 29, 30]. On the other hand, having belief in vocational return, a positive background for coping successfully (i.e. high sense of coherence) and relatively high educational level [31], as well as job-attachment to the pre-accident employer, availability of modified work, and no compensation/litigation issues [32] have been related to a successful return to work after vocational rehabilitation.

Overall, recent evidence has demonstrated that prolonged work disability is a multifactorial problem that is not only due to biological factors and workers' characteristics, but also closely related to many environmental factors such as the workplace, the health care system, the compensation system (e.g. partial vs. full sickness benefit) and the interactions among stakeholders regarding the disability problem [33-35]. Moreover, the complexity of factors involved in work-related problems and return-to-work, the variability in the patients' medical features, the great difference in type and intensity of vocational treatments (e.g. not always including psycho-social components, ergonomic intervention, and education), and the use of a variety of outcome parameters and follow-up periods account for differential outcome statistics in this field. The problem of migrants and acculturation is another aspect of the complexity of the situation (see chapter by Rothenbühler).

As an example, a very interesting study published by the International Social Security Association Research Program on Back Problems, entitled "Who returns to work and why?", compared the success or failure of work reintegration through medical and vocational rehabilitation in six industrialised countries, with 4 of these being members of the EU (Denmark, The Netherlands, Germany and Sweden) [36]. Subjects (n = 2,752) were studied at the start and after 1 year and 2 years follow up: 77.6% reached the final control and 23.5% dropped out. The return-to-work rate was very different, namely 40% in Denmark and Germany, 60% in Israel, Sweden and United States and over 70% in the Netherlands.

For all these reasons, the need for uniform standards in collection of this kind of outcome data has been strongly suggested [28].

At what time in the course of rehabilitation should vocational rehabilitation be introduced?

The report of the International Social Security Research Program [36] pointed out that the quick start of rehabilitation (within 3 months from the acute onset) is crucial for an effective intervention in lower back patients.

That differs slightly from what is illustrated in the diagram proposed by the Association of British Insurers in their study: "Getting back to work. A rehabilitation discussion paper" [37]. In this diagram (Table 3), the authors consider the injury, the ensuing acute care, the post acute care for inpatients and/or outpatients (and at this time in medical rehabilitation). Functional and vocational rehabilitation are to be started only after a medical plateau is reached.

Our opinion is that, generally speaking, the diagram proposed by Selander [21] (with variable interconnection between medical and vocational rehabilitation) seems to be more realistic and effective. Of course, after severe injuries (e.g. bone fractures, neurological lesions, burns, etc.) the transition from classic medical rehabilitation to intensive vocational rehabilitation can be delayed due to medical factors, but in many patients suffering from subacute musculo-skeletal disorders (and particularly back pain and cumulative trauma disorders) we think that early detection, clinical and ergonomic evaluations, and active treatment (starting 1-3 months after the onset) are the cornerstone of management.

What is the cost-effectiveness of vocational rehabilitation programs?

To prove that the important financial investment made in this area is really cost-effective, the sums invested in vocational rehabilitation programs need to be profitable in terms of

Table 3 – Treatment procedure flowchart as proposed by the Association of British Insurers [37].

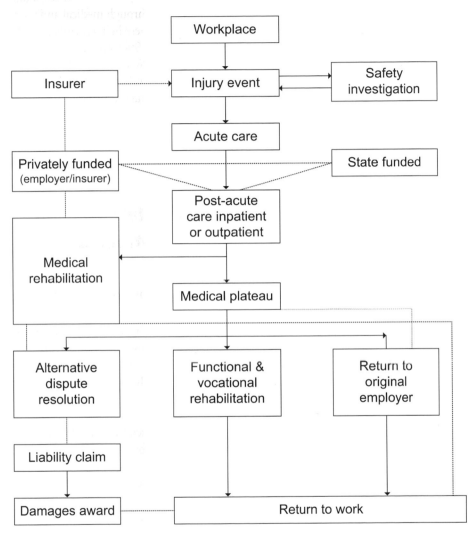

effective return to work and in direct and indirect reductions in disability pensions, sick leave and social payments as well as in increasing the labour force in the market. Moreover, it would be also interesting to know if such programs have a benefit on health-related quality of life.

Unfortunately, there are few scientifically based studies detailing the efficacy of vocational rehabilitation [38]. Furthermore, it is generally difficult to compare such studies because the programs of vocational rehabilitation are different, as are the evaluation methods.

In 1995, Schmidt *et al.* [10] compared the employment success rate of participants in special rehabilitation programs (a cohort of people with disabilities related to 6 different musculo-skeletal or neurological diagnoses) with those in general rehabilitation programs not specifically aimed at work resumption. They investigated to what extent the probability of obtaining work after rehabilitation was predicted by vocational rehabilitation and working on a trial basis, and observed that both variables had a significant impact on employment (odds ratio: 1.96 for vocational rehabilitation, 3.26 for work on trial).

Dean *et al.* published similar considerations in a very important report on the evaluation of vocational rehabilitation programs using longitudinal data [39]. The study presented the analysis of cost-effectiveness of 14 disability cohorts included in a vocational rehabilitation program. The data concerned 28,986 records from clients and represented a 10% random selection of the American vocational rehabilitation case-load. The conclusions were that the vocational rehabilitation program is cost-effective in general, but not universally across specific disabilities, and that based on an 8-year follow up, the long-term earnings gains can be substantial.

Elders *et al.* [40] recently reviewed the literature with the aim of highlighting the effectiveness of intervention programs for return to work after sick leave for back disorders. They found 515 articles, 130 abstracts and 20 reviews. Twelve studies were selected, analysing the effect of ergonomic interventions on return to work (9 randomised controlled trials and 3 prospective cohort studies). The interventions were specially focused on exercises and functional conditioning, education, training in working methods and lifting techniques. The absolute reduction of sick leave and time lost from work ranged from 22-42%. Seven out of eight back school intervention studies (regardless of their program and heterogeneity) showed a significant overall difference in return to work between subjects treated and reference group. Unfortunately, the authors observed that compliance and long term effects were unknown in many studies.

In line with these reports, Linz *et al.* [41] described the effect of a rehabilitation program on 699 subjects suffering from acute work-related musculo-skeletal injuries, in a 1 year study. Using active rather than passive techniques and emphasising patient education and home exercise programs, the number of visits (physical therapy sessions) was 45% less than national benchmark and the programs saved approximately $2,000 per client.

Furthermore, a 6-year follow up study to test the long term cost-benefit and cost-effectiveness of the Canadian Sherbrooke model of management of subacute occupational back pain demonstrated that a fully integrated disability prevention model for occupational back pain (combining an occupational and a clinical rehabilitation intervention) was beneficial for the workers' compensation board and saved more days on benefits than usual care or partial interventions [42].

Finally, last year Schonstein *et al.* [43] performed a Cochrane systematic review of randomized controlled trials of the effectiveness of physical conditioning programs in reducing time lost from work for workers with back and neck pain and stated that these programs for chronic back pain can be effective in reducing the number of workdays lost due to back pain, when compared to usual care. All the trials showing positive results had significant cognitive-behavioural components combined with intensive physical training (for aerobic capacity, muscle strength and endurance, and coordination) and were focused also on evaluation and modification of workplace characteristics.

Conclusion

Disabled people participate less in the labour market than non-disabled people, but in recent years the EU has been developing strategies to raise their employment rates, and European countries are reducing the sizeable differences in their social security systems and pattern of utilization of benefits.

Prolonged work disability results from a complex interaction of characteristics of individuals, the nature of their work, and their environment (including the physical workplace, policies related to work accommodation, and interpersonal relationships) as well as factors related to the benefit system and general labour market.

A number of clinical interventions have been identified as having a potentially positive effect on the outcome of patients with a long-term work-related disability. They primarily include:

– a regimen of physical conditioning (for flexibility, strength, endurance, dexterity, cardiovascular function, etc.), functional activities, and graded work simulation;

– socio-psychological support, addressing the worker's behavioural and vocational needs (e.g. behavioural pain management, individual and family therapy, and vocational counselling);

– ergonomic intervention: workplace accommodations (to minimise acute dynamic overloads, chronic repetitive exertions, and prolonged fixed or constrained postures) and administrative approaches (e.g. modified duties such as job task rotation and modification of worker schedules);

– educational strategies for injury prevention and safe work practice (e.g. proper body mechanics training to minimise the risk of injury) and instruction on a healthy lifestyle.

Vocational rehabilitation may be a positive response to prolonged work disability, accelerating return to meaningful employment, minimising workdays lost, increasing productivity of injured workers, reducing premature retirement, and containing the welfare cost [44]. Early intervention (after sufficient time for healing of injured structures) and the patient's active involvement decrease deconditioning and illness behaviour and foster higher return-to-work rates. Moreover, vocational rehabilitation delivered to patients at risk for job loss (but still employed) can delay job loss [45].

In this way, vocational rehabilitation can provide improvements to quality of life and well-being of patients, as well as having a positive effect on economic and political structures. Indeed, a well-directed vocational rehabilitation program seems to be cost-effective in many different disability situations and have a long-term action, as shown by earnings gains observed 8 years after some programs [39].

Unfortunately, at present we do not know how strongly each factor contributes to outcome compared with the others, and what the best predictors are. Thus questions remain to be answered, for example regarding the intervention components most effective in different subjects and illnesses, the optimal amount and timing for treatment, and the most cost-effective methods of delivering these services. Similarly, it has been pointed out that, at 6 months to 2 years after vocational rehabilitation, only about 20% of subjects had a job, whereas many more were awarded a disability pension [29,46]. This finding demonstrates that there is room for improving the selection criteria for vocational rehabilitation interventions.

Finally, the role of national disability compensation systems in influencing the worker's motivation to return to work should not be overlooked, as well as the importance of specific policies aimed at better (re-)integrating and maintaining disabled people in the labour market.

References

1. Waddell G, Norlund AI (2000) Review of Social Security. In: Nachemson A and Jonsson E (eds). Neck and Back Pain: The scientific evidence of causes, diagnosis and treatment. JB Lippincott: Philadelphia, p427-71
2. Ekberg K, Wildhagen I (1996) Long-term sickness absence due to musculoskeletal disorders: the necessary intervention of work conditions. Scand J Rehab Med 28: 39-47
3. Burri M (2002) Statistiques de la Sécurité Sociale. Statistiques de l'AI 2002. Office Fédéral des Assurances Sociales (OFAS), p2-40
4. Bonfiglio RP, LaBan MM, Taylor RS et al. (1993) Industrial Rehabilitation Medicine management. In: DeLisa ed. Rehabilitation Medicine. Principles and Practice. JB Lippincott: Philadelphia, p169-77
5. Engström LG, Eriksen T (2002) Can difference in benefit levels explain duration and outcome of sickness absence? Disabil Rehabil 24(14): 713-18
6. World Health Organization (2001) International Classification of functioning, disability and health. WHO Library: Geneva
7. Malo MA, Garcia-Serrano The employment situation of people with disabilities in the European Union (2001) Social security and social integration. Employment and Social Affairs. European Communities. EIM Business and Policy Research. Directorate-General Unit EMPL/E.4 p.35 (www.employment-disability.net)
8. Yelin E (1989) Displaced concern: the social context of the work-disability problem. Milbank Q 67 (suppl2): 114-65
9. Walker A, Townsend P (eds) (1981) Disability in Britain a manifest of rights. Martin Robertson: Oxford.
10. Schmidt SH, Oort-Marburger D, Meijman TF (1995) Employment after rehabilitation for musculoskeletal impairments: The impact of vocational rehabilitation and working on a trial basis. Arch Phys Med Rehabil 76: 950-4
11. British Society of Rehabilitation Medicine (2000) Vocational Rehabilitation - the way forward: report of a working party. BSRM: London
12. Gjesdal S, Bratberg E (2002) The role of gender in long-term sickness absence and transition to permanent disability benefits. Results from a multiregister based, prospective study in Norway 1990-1995. Eur J Public Health 12(3): 180-6

13. Blondal S, Scarpetta S (1999) Early retirement in OECD countries: the role of social security systems. OECD Economic Studies No. 29, 1997/II, p7-54

14. Nachemson A (1999) Back pain and causes, diagnosis and treatment updated in 1999. Sweden, SBU. Swedish Council on Technology Assessment in Health Care 108: 1-5

15. Petrusov E. Le rôle du travail comme facteur d'intégration (2000). http: //www.ac grenoble.fr/webcurie/pedagogie/sciences economiques et sociales/cours/ Tem/intra/cours/ changem solida/travail integr/coursw.html

16. Warr PB (1982) Psychological aspects of employment and unemployment. Psychol Med 96(2): 43-47

17. Charte d'Ottawa pour la promotion de la santé (1986). OMS, p1-2

18. International Labour Organization (1998) Vocational rehabilitation and employment of disabled persons. International Labour Conference, 86th Session. ILO: Geneva.

19. Selander J (1999) Unemployed sick-leavers and vocational rehabilitation. A person level study based on a national social insurance material. Dissertation from the Department of Rehabilitation Medicine. Karolinska Institute. Stockholm, Sweden

20. Marnetoft SU, Selander J, Bergroth A, Ekholm J (2001) Factors associated with successfull vocational rehabilitation in a Swedish rural area. J Rehabil Med 33: 71-8

21. Selander J, Marnetoft SU, Bergroth A, Ekholm J (2002) Return to work following vocational rehabilitation for neck, back and shoulder problems: risk factors reviewed. Disabil Rehabil 24(14): 704-12. Taylor and Francis Ltd. http: //www.tandf.co.uk/journals

22. EU anti-discrimination directives (02.12.2000) Council Decision of 27 November 2000 establishing a community action program to combat discrimination (2001 to 2006) (2000/750/EC). Official Journal of the European Communities L 303/23-38

23. Europa. European Commission. Employment and Social Affairs. Disability issues. The European Union Disability Strategy. http://europa.eu.int/comm/employmentsocial/disability/ strategyen.html

24. Europa. European Commission. Employment and Social Affairs. Social Inclusion. http://europa.eu.int/comm/employmentsocial/indexen.html

25. EQUAL (May 5th 2000) Guidelines http://europa.eu.int/comm/employmentsocial/ equal/indexen.html

26. Yelin E (1986) The myth of malingering: why individuals withdraw from work in the presence of illness. Milbank Q 64: 622-49

27. Natvig K (1983) Social, occupational and personal factors related to vocational rehabilitation. Otolaryngol 12: 370-6

28. Niemeyer LO, Jacobs K, Reynolds-Lynch K et al. (1994) Work hardening: past, present, and future-the work programs special interest section national work-hardening outcome study. Am J Occup Ther 48(4): 327-39

29. Tellness G, Bruusgaard D, Sandvik L (1990) Occupational factors in sickness certification. Scand J Prim Health Care 8: 37-44

30. Durand MJ, Loisel P (2001) Therapeutic return to work: rehabilitation in the workplace. Work 17(1): 57-63

31. Melin F, Fugl-Meyer AR (2003) On prediction of vocational rehabilitation outcome at a Swedish employability institute. J Rehabil Med 35: 284-9

32. Voaklander DC, Beaulne AP, Lessard RA (1995) Factors related to outcome following a work hardening program. J Occup Rehabil 5(2): 71-85

33. Durand MJ, Loisel P, Hong Qn *et al.* (2002) Helping clinicians in work disability prevention: the work disability diagnosis interview. J Occup Rehabil 12(3): 191-204
34. Rondinelli RD, Robinson JP, Scheer SJ *et al.* (1997) Industrial rehabilitation medicine. 4. Strategies for disability management. Arch Phys Med Rehabil 78(3 suppl): 21-8. Review
35. Eklund M, Eriksson S, Fugl-Meyer AR (1991) Vocational rehabilitation in northern Sweden. II. Some psycho-socio-demographic predictors. Scand J Rehabil Med 23(2): 73-82
36. International Social Security Association Research Programme (2002) Who returns to work and why? – A summary. ISSA: Geneva, p11
37. Association of British Insurers / Trades Union Congress (2002) Getting back to work. A rehabilitation discussion paper. TUC: London
38. James P, Cunningham I, Dibben P (2003) Job retention and vocational rehabilitation: the development and evaluation of a conceptual framework. Research report 106 – Middlesex University Business School and the University of Strathclyde for the Health and Safety Executive. HSE Books: Sudbury (UK)
39. Dean DH, Dolan RC, Schmidt RM (1999) Evaluating the vocational rehabilitation program using longitudinal data. Evidence for a quasi experimental research design. Eval Rev 23(2): 162-89
40. Elders LA, Van der Beck AJ, Burdorf A (2000) Return to work after sickness absence due to back disorders: a systematic review on intervention strategies. Int Arch Occup Environ Health 73: 339-48
41. Linz DH, Shepherd CD, Ford LF *et al.* (2002) Effectiveness of occupational medicine center-based physical therapy. J Occup Environ Med 44(1): 48-53
42. Loisel P, Lemaire J, Poitras S *et al.* (2002) Cost-benefit and cost-effectiveness analysis of a disability prevention model for back pain management: a six year follow up study. Occup Environ Med 59(12): 807-15
43. Schonstein E, Kenny DT, Keating J *et al.* (2003) Work conditioning, work hardening and functional restoration for work with back and neck pain. Cochrane Database Syst Rev (1) CD001822
44. Disler PB, Pallant JF (2001) Vocational Rehabilitation. BMJ 323(7305): 121-3
45. Allaire SH, Li W, La Valley MP (2003) Reduction of job loss in persons with rheumatic diseases receiving vocational rehabilitation: a randomized controlled trial. Arthritis Rheum 48(11): 3212-8
46. Kvamm J, Nielsen CV (2003) Vocational rehabilitation: a descriptive follow up study. Ugeskr Laeger 165: 2815-1819

The point of view
of the insurance company

W. Morger

Introduction

I would like to preface my contribution on rehabilitation by quoting a few borrowed words, "Despite integration measures, the financial burden for insurance company payments will be for pensions. *However, reintegration measures will gain priority for ethical, socio-political and economic reasons and finally also in the financial interests of the insurance company itself.*"

This quote contains a few central ideas on today's topic:

It sets the principle: Integration before pension.

This principle is simultaneously justified:

– it is in the interests of the accident victim (ethical aspect);

– it is economically meaningful and also takes the financial interests of the insurance company into consideration (financial aspect).

The message behind this quote is right up-to-date. However, it dates back almost 40 years – it is taken from the statement by the Council of Ministers to the Swiss parliament in 1958. This formed the basis for the introduction of disability insurance in Switzerland. It introduced a new approach; previously the task of helping the disabled was primarily seen as ensuring a minimum living income for the disabled by means of public and private welfare.

I would first like to address the principle of "Integration before pension" as it is understood in Switzerland in more specific terms. Then, I will describe how rehabilitation is organized in our country and the role that accident insurance plays in it. I will conclude by describing the effects of rehabilitation on compensation.

General principles

The concept of rehabilitation

In line with the recommendation of the World Health Organization, rehabilitation is comprehensively defined as follows: "Rehabilitation is the coordinated deployment of medical, social, occupational, technical and educational measures to improve functioning, training and retraining as well as to adapt the person affected and their surroundings with the aim of regaining the best possible functioning and an appropriate place in society." It thus has a medical, an occupational and a social dimension. The definition points out the exceptional complexity of rehabilitation. The individual measures overlap and interact. In the final analysis, therefore, the only approach to rehabilitation must be holistic in nature, in other words, one that includes all these measures.

Integration before pension

Integration measures clearly take precedence over mere financial benefits in Switzerland. The maxim of "rehabilitation before compensation" – in Switzerland we usually talk of "integration before pension", which means the same thing – is not expressly mentioned anywhere in legislation. However, it can be deduced from various regulations that list the prerequisites for financial benefits (particularly in the case of disability pensions). It is basically undisputed. The focus is on ethical considerations; but economic aspects must not and cannot be disregarded.

Two conclusions can be drawn from the principle:

– the insured person has a legal right to integration measures;
– the insured person has an obligation to undergo integration measures before being able to claim financial benefits.

The central idea applies to the entire social insurance system and not just to statutory accident insurance. To begin with, it applies wherever compensation for inability to work due to ill-health is under discussion, this means insurance companies that cover disability benefits (accident insurance, disability insurance and occupational pension schemes). However, the same considerations also apply to unemployment insurance. The comprehensive revision of the unemployment insurance law on 1st January 1997 clearly placed the emphasis on the reintegration of the unemployed. To achieve this goal, a wide range of job-market related measures were created.

Principle of appropriateness

The principle of appropriateness as a general constitutional principle pervades all areas of the law. The principle of appropriateness can basically be sub-divided into three aspects:

– the precept of suitability;

– the precept of necessity;
– the balancing of public and private interests.

Attention should also be paid to these limits when interpreting and applying social insurance standards.

In our context, this means that the principle of "integration before pension" does not have absolute importance. In other words, limits are set on the right to integration measures in terms of insurance benefits and on the insured person's obligation to participate in the sense of taking part in the integration measures. These abstract and theoretical sounding statements can be illustrated by two examples:

Medical rehabilitation

Social security is not liable for every conceivable form of treatment. The insured person only has the right to receive suitable treatment whereby this term is interpreted generously in practice to the benefit of the recipient. Conversely, the insured person must not undergo all treatments. Reasonableness – part of the principle of appropriateness – forms the boundary for this obligation to participate and tolerate. According to precedents, arthrodesis in the upper ankle joint is considered reasonable whereas for example, hip arthrodesis is not.

Occupational rehabilitation

The justice system demands that the individual measures are effective for the purposes of integration (a certain degree of success can be anticipated), are lasting (success must be expected to last during the major proportion of the period of activity) and thus be economically appropriate (cost-benefit consideration). For less expensive measures such as finding jobs, therefore, a relatively small degree of health-related difficulties is sufficient as a reason for a claim. In the case of retraining, the guide figure used in practice for support by disability insurance is a 20 percent degree of invalidity. If the insured person fails to participate in a reasonable integration measure – this applies both to medical and occupational measures – the compensation assessment is based on the result of a successfully completed measure.

Whether an insured person has the right to an integration measure or whether, on the other hand, has to submit to an integration measure is finally decided in the individual case on the basis of all circumstances.

Responsibility for rehabilitation measures

Self-integration

Primarily, the insured person is responsible for reintegration efforts. On his own initiative, he must take all reasonable steps to reduce the consequences of disability as much as possible. This includes, for example, finding a job and accepting reasonable work. The principle of "self-integration before claim for integration and before pension" as set out by the highest Federal insurance court, "is a discharge of the insuree's obligation to reduce damage." The question of self-integration is largely an issue in the occupational sector, especially with minor disabilities.

Integration as the task of social security

However, insured persons also have the right to support from social security. In Switzerland, the integration of accident victims is financially supported by two institutions:

- accident insurance is responsible for *medical* integration;
- disability insurance is responsible for *occupational* integration.

I will be going into the details of this responsibility and the tasks of the two branches of insurance – accident and disability – as well as into the demarcation between the two when talking about the various rehabilitation categories.

Medical rehabilitation

Concept

The aim of medical rehabilitation is to eradicate or improve a physical injury caused by an accident. To this end – and this is how medical rehabilitation is generally understood (e.g. in Germany) – the medical rehabilitation chain starts with first aid at the site of the accident and covers all in- and outpatient medical measures (treatment).

In Switzerland, a distinction is usually made between curative medicine and rehabilitation medicine:

The aim of curative medicine is to correct organic damage.

In contrast, rehabilitation medicine deals with the established or chronic consequences of accident and illness. It is not oriented towards the actual injury but the effects on capabilities linked to this that lead to social and occupational restrictions.

Rehabilitation medicine is not an alternative to curative medicine. Quite the opposite, in fact, it is a necessary supplement to it. While in curative medicine the strategy is causal, the patient is fairly passive and the doctor determines what happens, the structures in rehabilitation are different; the methods take a bio-psycho-social approach, with the patient assuming an active role while the doctor assists. Boundaries are fluid.

In the vast majority of cases, medical care amounts to nothing more than curative medicine; in the narrower sense, rehabilitation medicine is restricted to severe cases. In order to gain a comprehensive picture, I will base the following explanations on medical rehabilitation in its broader sense.

Medical care

In Switzerland, medical care is the responsibility of the cantons. They provide this by means of a network of public as well as private hospitals. Outpatient care is handled by independent doctors, both general practitioners and specialists.

This system of medical care applies to all health problems, including accident injuries. Accident care is thus integrated into the public health system. There are no special procedures to follow in the case of accidents. The insured person has a free choice of hospital and doctor (free choice of service provider).

Special clinics are available for the medical rehabilitation of individual types of injuries. The paraplegic centres as well as Suva's own rehabilitation clinics in Bellikon and Sitten are examples of such clinics.

Content and scope of medical treatment

An accident victim has the right to medical treatment appropriate to the consequences of the accident. Therefore, Suva reimburses, in particular, the cost of:

- – outpatient treatment;
- – medicaments and analyses;
- – treatment, care and stay in a hospital;
- – spa and bathing treatment as prescribed by a doctor;
- – means and appliances beneficial for treatment;
- – any rescue and transportation required.

In addition, the accident insurance company also covers the cost of appliances and equipment that compensate for physical injuries or the loss of functions (artificial limbs, orthotics, orthopaedic footwear, hearing aids and spectacles, but also lifts).

Role of the accident insurer

The accident insurer as cost-bearer

The accident insurer must pay for medical treatment insofar as it is appropriate and medically indicated. No limit is set on outpatient treatment in terms of time or cost; there is a right to treatment as long as a significant improvement in the state of health can be anticipated. In the case of inpatient treatment, the accident insurer assumes the cost of a general admission. The accident insurer reimburses the costs to the service provider directly (principle of payment in kind).

Case accompaniment

Medical treatment is in the hands of independent doctors and hospitals. However, accident insurers have the right and obligation to monitor the treatment process and to issue instructions for appropriate treatment. For this purpose, Suva has its own medical service (interdisciplinary team of doctors and occupational doctors at its headquarters in Lucerne as well as district doctors in the local agencies). Their main task is to advise the insurance company in specialist medical matters (causal context, indication, length of treatment, etc.). However, they are also partners and conciliators for the doctor providing treatment in diagnostic and therapeutic issues. These doctors make a decisive contribution to medical quality assurance thanks to their medical assessments based on background files or supported by their own examinations and their scientific activities.

Economical treatment

However, the accident insurance company also has the statutory task of ensuring that accidents are dealt with in an economical way. Alongside the case accompaniment already mentioned, it discharges this responsibility by concluding tariff agreements (doctors' agreements/hospital agreements) with the service providers based on key economic data and monitors treatment costs using modern methods such as management ratios.

Occupational rehabilitation

In the vast majority of cases nowadays, top-quality medical treatment means full restitution or such a good result that the next link in the rehabilitation chain – occupational rehabilitation – is superfluous. The necessity for occupational measures is estimated at less than 5% of cases.

Responsibility

As I mentioned previously in connection with the principles, occupational integration is primarily the task of a special branch of insurance – disability insurance. Occupational integration is its primary aim. Accident victims also have the right to integration measures offered by disability insurance; accident insurance itself has no benefit category of its own termed "occupational measures".

Occupational integration measures

Occupational rehabilitation comprises all measures that are necessary to prepare and implement the rehabilitation of a disabled person into professional life. The following benefits are included:

– job counselling service;
– initial professional training;
– vocational retraining and reintroduction;

– job placement;
– financial assistance.

Insured persons who are unable to continue with previous activities as a result of their disability have the right to *job counselling*. Alongside clarifications about preferences and suitability, this also includes trial placements and practical job trials. Experience has shown that the insured persons with the best chance of successful occupational integration are those who can be given a job with the same employer. The cost of any *reintroductory training* as well as for any adaptation of the workplace is borne by disability insurance. When a change of job location is necessary, daily benefits are paid for 180 days during the period of familiarization or training, so that the employer has no financial obligations. If the previous job can no longer be carried out or there are significant limitations – in practice, this is considered to be a degree of disability of at least 20% – *retraining* for a new job better suited to the disability is examined. Training costs and any additional expenses for travel and overnight accommodation are borne by the insurance company. Disabled persons also have the right to daily benefits during the retraining period. Another possibility is *financial assistance* to start up in business on a self-employed basis.

Counselling services and job placement are carried out by specially trained advisors. They also accompany trial jobs and retraining. Each canton has the relevant departments. In complex cases, a thorough inpatient vocational clarification process is conducted. There are five of these vocational clarification centres (BEFAS) throughout Switzerland. In addition, there are specialized clarification centres for individual types of injuries, for example for the visually impaired and brain damaged.

Occupational appliances and equipment

Disability insurance also covers appliances and equipment that are needed to carry out jobs. In particular, these include:

    – disability-related job equipment, additional appliances for operating apparatus and machinery;
    – individually adapted sitting and standing equipment;
    – individually adapted work surfaces;
    – disability-related structural changes in the workplace;
    – under certain circumstances, the cost of motor vehicles or vehicles for the disabled is also met.

These appliances and items of equipment are listed in an annex to the legislation.

Role of the accident insurance company

As already mentioned, occupational integration is not among the statutory tasks of the accident insurance company. However, it is not possible to simply ignore the matter nor is it indicated; successful occupational rehabilitation is also in the (financial) interests of the accident insurance company. Suva therefore endeavours both on its own behalf and on behalf of the insured person to actively promote the reintegration of its accident victim into professional life in various ways, particularly in the following way:

Medical appraisals as the basis for occupational rehabilitation

If no significant improvement can be anticipated from further medical treatment, the Suva doctors compile a medical progress report (final report). In it, they not only list the residual disabilities but also the remaining abilities. This is therefore of major importance since the aim of occupational rehabilitation is to use these physical functions alongside other skills. This profile of skills forms part of the basis for occupational reorientation for disability insurance.

Close cooperation with disability insurance

As soon as the course of treatment indicates that occupational integration measures will be necessary, Suva has the insured person registered with disability insurance in order to start the relevant clarification steps. In this way, the necessary measures are initiated at an early stage or on time. However, it must be admitted that we have difficulty with the loss of time involved in this transfer of responsibility. In order to achieve a seamless transition, Suva and disability insurance have concluded cooperation agreements.

Reintegration in the former company

I have already mentioned that, as a rule, reintegration with the same employer produces the best results. Our field staff therefore exploits their many years of contact with employers and their knowledge of companies in order to clarify and foster a return to the former workplace or at least arrange another job within the same company. Employers are motivated to further employ their injured employees by the fact that this can have a positive influence on their premiums (bonus/malus system based on risk development).

Own occupational clarification measures in the Suva rehabilitation clinics

Suva offers accident patients a comprehensive system of rehabilitation in its own rehabilitation clinics, i.e. medical measures (physical medicine, neurorehabilitation, orthopedic rehabilitation) are supplemented by occupational clarifications and job counselling. Training workplaces are available for practical work. These measures for occupational clarification are offered on behalf of disability insurance. Thanks to an agreement between disability and accident insurance, the transition from medical to occupational rehabilitation can be coordinated and substantially accelerated.

In this connection, special reference must be made to two concepts: the work-oriented test system "*Evaluation of functional efficiency*" and the ergonomic training program that develops on this "*Work-conditioning*" or "*Work-hardening*". The evaluation of work-related functional efficiency ("Isenhagen system") uses a standardized range of tests covering the most important physical work-related effort such as lifting, carrying, kneeling, etc. The ergonomic training program is a structured, goal-oriented treatment program adapted to individual needs with the aim of reintegrating the patient into the job process.

Taking integration measures into account when determining compensation

If occupational measures are undertaken by the disability pension company, a decision on remuneration by the accident insurance company (particularly disability pension) is suspended. During the integration period, the insured person receives daily benefits from the disability pension company. On the basis of the results, a decision is then taken on any further claims against the accident insurance company.

Social rehabilitation

A further link in the rehabilitation chain is social rehabilitation. This includes all measures for mental, family, social and economic integration. In this connection, occupational rehabilitation can be considered part of social rehabilitation; occupational and social rehabilitation – in many cases also medical rehabilitation – thus frequently go hand in hand.

It is impossible to give a conclusive list of measures that comprise social rehabilitation. Examples might be supporting people's contact with their surroundings, improving their residential situation, assistance with leisure-time activities (particularly sporting activities) and participation in social and cultural life.

In contrast to occupational integration, *social* integration is not the *direct* aim of disability insurance. However, the importance of a person's surroundings on successful and lasting rehabilitation has not been overlooked in this. Nevertheless, the decision has been taken not to promote arrangements for social reintegration via individual benefits but indirectly via contributions to charities. Disability insurance currently supports numerous organizations involved in private disability assistance (specialist and self-help organizations), which advise the disabled person and their relatives, provide further training courses, organize transportation and promote leisure-time activities for the disabled – particularly sports. Disability insurance also supports residential homes and workshops for the disabled by means of contributions to construction costs and extra outlay due to disability requirements.

To supplement this, the disability pension company promotes social integration directly by financing various appliances and items of equipment for self-care or for contact with surroundings, such as electronic communications equipment, tape recorders, environmental control equipment, stairlifts and structural changes to living accommodation generally required due to disability.

Effect of rehabilitation on benefits

The focus of rehabilitation is on ethical considerations. Frequently, rehabilitation measures are costly, take up a great deal of time and require the coordinated deployment of a variety of specialists. Rehabilitation can thus turn into a very expensive undertaking. Whenever it is a question of money, the question of return on investment inevitably crops up. These inconvenient questions multiply when money is scarce.

The yardstick used to measure success depends on the observer's standpoint. Patients, relatives and medical specialists all see success from their own perspectives. Let us take someone with severe brain damage as an example. If, as a result of rehabilitation measures, the patient succeeds in becoming sufficiently independent that he no longer needs institutional care but can return to his family circle, that is undoubtedly a major success, primarily for the person affected but also for medicine. Of course, those who are footing the bill are also interested in cost control. This means the insurance company as well as the premium-payer (employer and – in the case of non-occupational accident insurance – the employee) and the economy in which the money has to be earned – so, in the end, we all foot the bill. In my example, little has changed for those bearing the cost, since the full lack of wages is owed as well as the bills for treatment. From an economist's standpoint, the partial success achieved is viewed positively since the enormous cost of long-term institutional care has been saved. Those who pay the bills are again interested in that.

Even though nobody has any doubts about the ethical sense of rehabilitation, the economic aspects should not and cannot be ignored; they must not, however, be the sole decisive factors.

In order to give a figure for the economic benefits, it would be necessary to do a cost comparison: the cost of rehabilitation and success would have to be compared with the cost of neglected or insufficient rehabilitation. No comprehensive and systematic analyses are available.

The financial success or the financial effect on compensation can be impressively documented in another way, however. The importance of rehabilitation in economic terms can be demonstrated on the basis of regional results, specific cases and general considerations.

Although less than 1% of accidents result in pensions, pensions are responsible for more than one third of insurance costs. The few cases with permanent benefits are therefore tremendously important. Disabilities can be avoided or reduced by means of tailor-made rehabilitation measures. If the degree of invalidity can be reduced by just 1%, this results in savings for Suva of around 10,000 Swiss francs per pension.

Another meaningful comparison is between the financial consequences with and without rehabilitation in individual cases. The following case is just such an example:

Assumption:
35-year-old manual worker
Insured wage: 5,000. -- Swiss francs
Accident with severe injuries to both arms
– 2 years' inability to work, subsequently on a pension.

Costs:

Treatment costs, acute hospital care 50,000. -- Swiss francs
Rehabilitation costs 30,000. -- Swiss francs
Cost of daily benefits 100,000. -- Swiss francs
Pension (premium reserve) *581,000.* -- Swiss francs*
Total costs 761,000. – Swiss francs

* Thanks to medical and occupational rehabilitation, the pension was set 50% lower. Without this support, the insured person would have claimed a full *pension with a premium reserve amounting to 1,162,000.-- Swiss francs. In this case, rehabilitation helps to save costs for the insurance company of more than half a million Swiss francs.

It is obvious that each case is individual and different. This calculation, however, gives a starting point for the amount of benefit to be gained from successful reintegration.

Outcome rehabilitation clinics

Reduction in the degree of invalidity			5% = 50,000.-- Swiss francs
Patient category	Number	Reduction in degree of invalidity in %	Effect (in millions of CHF)
Artificial limbs	50	15	7.5
Brain-damage	330	25	82.5
Loss of function	900	15	135.0
Total			*225.0*

Input	Running costs of clinic	76m Swiss francs
Outcome	Savings in invalidity pensions	225m Swiss francs
Difference in Suva's favour		*149m Swiss francs*

The savings in insurance benefits (outcome) amount to around three times the running costs of the clinic (input).

Rehabilitation does not actually create additional costs but costs are redistributed: short-term and time-limited treatment costs and daily benefits replace expensive long-term costs such as pensions and total dependency benefits. Since the cost of disability due to neglected or insufficient rehabilitation amounts to many times more than integration efforts, the economic benefit of tailor-made rehabilitation is obvious.

Assessment of the current system

It is indisputable that rehabilitation promises the greatest success when it is approached comprehensively. The individual medical, occupational and social measures are interwoven, cannot always be separated and can overlap in terms of time. One may question whether the assignment of tasks to various insurance carriers – as practised in Switzerland – is ideal: it can also be seen as a contradiction to holistic rehabilitation. With responsibility resting with one source, duplication, administrative processes and delays could be avoided that are not only costly but also jeopardize the success of any rehabilitation. It is a well-known fact that the time factor plays a substantial role in rehabilitation; there is a danger of chronification. Sometimes people refer to the "point of no return" in this connection.

If the aim is to have rehabilitation from one source as the "ideal situation", we encounter difficulties in Switzerland because of the country's size or lack of size. Separate, special rehabilitation routes for accident insurees fail due to the limited number of cases. This is further compounded by our multilingual problem.

Looking at the existing system, it is evident that it works well and the level can be described as high. The principle of "rehabilitation before pension" sets the same parameters for both branches of insurance and provides a joint goal that holds everything together.

For any separation, it is essential to know how the links are interwoven. In order to ensure a seamless transition from medical to occupational measures, Suva and the disability insurance have concluded an agreement that provides for, among other things, mutual information, the inspection of files as well as uninterrupted compensation for the insured person. In addition, "boundaries" are shifted where meaningful. For example, disability insurance has transferred occupational clarification to Suva for patients in our rehabilitation clinic, so that occupational integration can be initiated during the predominantly medical stay. A check into where further opportunities for increased cooperation or optimisation are possible still needs to be made.

The mass of legal regulations concerning rehabilitation is extremely dense, perhaps too dense in some areas – particularly in the case of rehabilitation appliances and equipment. In addition, numerous directives issued by the relevant federal offices show cantonal implementation organs the way. This has the advantage that insured persons receive equal treatment irrespective of the canton they happen to live in. In view of the broad spectrum of possible measures, however, it is necessary to grant the decision-makers a large amount of room to manoeuvre if they are to meet the specific conditions of individual cases and treat them properly. For this reason, I do not think that the legal regulations need expanding or that this would provide a solution to existing weak spots.

The main problem in successful occupational reintegration has less to do with the current system as with the current difficult economic situation. Pressure of competition on a national as well as an international basis forces companies to step up productivity even more. Well-trained employees are needed, in particular those who are in possession of their full physical and mental powers and are resilient. As a result, the willingness of companies – as well as the possibility – to support weaker members of society declines.

What this means is that the basic principle of "integration before pension" is not called into question but the possibility of implementing it has become more difficult.

Since equal opportunities for the disabled and non-disabled are at risk in a difficult economic climate, there are calls for companies to be compelled by law to set up workplaces for the disabled. The question of a quota system, as practised by our neighbours in Austria and Germany, has been discussed at various times but, so far, Switzerland has no such regulation. I doubt whether employment for the disabled can be federally enforced; in my opinion, no genuine integration can be achieved in this way. It cannot be imposed. I feel that a better solution is (a) to motivate and convince employers that the further employment and hiring of the disabled is meaningful and also rewarding and (b) to create the corresponding incentives for this. These incentives could, for example, take the form of premium relief if disabled persons continue to be employed, as is the case with the bonus/malus system or in the form of financial support (wage payments) during the training period for new hirings.

Concluding remarks

On 12th October 1995, the Council of Europe accepted the "Charter for the assessment of occupational integration of people with disabilities" as an official recommendation. This charter indicated that people with disabilities should be integrated as much as possible into a normal working environment; any social and occupational discrimination against people with disabilities was to be resisted.

I believe I can state that everyone here is convinced of the ethical sense of rehabilitation. I also believe that nobody doubts its economic benefit. The spirit and funding behind comprehensive rehabilitation are undisputed. The difficulties lie in the implementation of this acknowledged principle in the current economic climate. The disabled find it more difficult to get a job than the non-disabled. Surveys also show that, in most countries, the disabled are more affected by unemployment. Health is an important criterion in the training and hiring of new employees. Rehabilitation and rehabilitation reforms must therefore be discussed in dependency on economic development. Improvements cannot be made by the social insurance companies alone but only in cooperation with employers and with the business world.

I wish to make it quite clear that I am in favour of comprehensive rehabilitation as foreseen by the WHO definition, both from an ethical and an economic point of view. Different paths may lead to the goal, and different countries may choose different solutions, but rehabilitation is not the sole responsibility of insurance companies. Success depends on the environment, both economic and social. Over the past few years, this climate has become harsher, and relief cannot be expected in the near future. External factors such as structural changes in the economy, demographic development and changing values – all of them affecting rehabilitation – are largely beyond the sphere of influence of insurance institutions. However, we should set about convincing the public that rehabilitation is an essential pillar of accident insurance, just as important as prevention while

underlining the cost-benefit advantages derived from rehabilitation. The target of rehabilitation is the best possible integration. This is not only in the interests of the injured
person. It is also in the interests of the insurers, the economy and society at large.
Nevertheless, it is imperative to monitor the efficiency of the measures taken and the
overall results to ensure the rational use of limited financial resources. This is the major
challenge to insurers today. It is one that must be met!

Disability as a process

P.-A. Fauchère

Introduction

The medical world has to give verdicts on disabilities, yet a certain number of patients display inconsistency in the connection between the severity of their organic injuries and their effects on personal and socio-professional performance. It is difficult to understand how some people with minimal somatic injuries can develop towards serious dysfunction while others, much more seriously affected physically, succeed in reassuming a level of total autonomy and a good quality of life. This apparent contradiction leads to a re-examination of the widely held belief that a link of linear and proportionate causality exists between a physical injury and any resultant personal and social handicap. The explanation of this clinical reality extends from the integration of the psychological, professional and social context via a wider concept of a disability process rather than remaining focused on the single somatic deficiency. The biopsychosocial model put forward by Engel [1] seems to be the one that best accounts for the complexity of this disability process. In this chapter, we will be examining several viewpoints in connection with this problem in the context of a theoretical time and model.

Disability process

In a series of articles published in the JAMA [2] in 1963, Hirschfeld and Behan explained the concept of the *accident process* in order to solve the dilemma posed by the lack of proportion between minor somatic injuries and severe and lasting disability. The authors documented a psychological context as the cause of accidents and injuries in the majority of the 300 cases of industrial workers referred to them within the framework of compensation claims. To them, the somatic damage was not isolated to be positioned in the field of a "before" and an "after" in relation to the traumatic event concerned. They put forward the hypothesis of an accompanying psychosocial weakness. These authors felt that the accident represented a solution to the patient's problems, with the development towards chronicity being reinforced by the fact that, and I quote, "The use of illness as a solution to the problems of life is now reinforced by legal factors which make incapacity the cornerstone of continued financial support". This statement of the problem remains a topic of current interest.

Following on from there, Weinstein [3] expanded the concept with the *illness process* leading to *disability process*, the symbolic blow to health being not just initiated by an accident but by an episode of illness. The model presupposes a dysphoric period (drop in self-esteem within the context of psychological difficulties) that runs parallel to a drop in job productivity. It is at that critical moment that the symbolic blow to health occurs (minor accident or episode of illness) that legitimizes the drop in job productivity for the subject himself, for those around him and for society. The disability thus becomes acceptable enough for a medical tag and, as a result, psychosocial and financial support as provided for by society. Self-esteem can be restored since the disability has become legitimate. In fact, this concept of the disability process supports the idea that behavior with a socially accepted illness can be a response to internal and external demands that go beyond the adaptive capabilities of the subject in question. At this stage, there is not much chance of reversing the disability. The process ends in a new balance between the needs of the subject and the internal and external demands made on him. The patient's behavior is, however, well known to clinicians with the setbacks to treatment suggested and the subject's apparent capability to control his own symptoms.

Disease or abnormal behaviour?

Considerations over several years have seen the development of explanatory models of this particular form of behaviour by these patients in the healthcare system and in society in general. There was the idea of *primary and secondary gains* of the illness, based on the theory of neuroses. There was the concept of a *sick role* that highlights obligations but even more the benefits that a given society bestows on the fact of being ill. Mechanic and then Pilowsky [4] developed the idea of *abnormal illness behaviour* for a way of responding that is poorly adapted to the actual state of health, in spite of having been given sufficient and appropriate information by healthcare professionals. Matheson [5] conceptualized the *symptom magnification syndrome* for a disability behaviour model that is worked out and maintained under the influence of social factors and allows the individual to exert control over his environment and over his own mental equilibrium. All these models are of interest in terms of a global or biopsychosocial understanding of a patient and opens doors in terms of clinical psychology and treatment. However, they describe processes or behaviours and do not have any illness value as such.

In the matter of *somatoform disorders*, modern psychiatric nosology wanted diagnostic entities very close to those covering the processes of abnormal illness behaviour or symptom magnification syndrome. The best known example of this is definitely the *persistent somatoform pain disorder*, which bears the number F45.4 in the WHO international classification of diseases. Somatoform disorder is understood to mean a clinical picture of disorders of somatic appearance for which the diagnosis points out the preliminary exclusion of a somatic complaint as well as any other psychiatric complaint that would explain them better. The disorder should again mean significant suffering, personal and social dysfunction and provide, in most cases, support or exclusion from disagreeable tasks that the subject would otherwise be unable to obtain. In fact, this second part of the diagnostic sort out factors in the relational and social dimension of these somatoform disorders. In fact, this nosological concept introduces an operational boundary for certain clinical situations that go beyond the medical field in the strict sense. Seen in this way, these somatoform disorders can only frustrate the conventional biomedical model both at treatment level as well as at their evaluation level in terms of incapacity for work.

Psychodynamic disability factors

It would take too long here to go into the extensive conceptualization work carried out in the field of psychosomatics, in the meaning of the influence of the psyche on the development of symptoms or genuine physical disorders. We will restrict ourselves to quoting a few salient elements that have sometimes been absorbed into current medical parlance.

According to psychoanalytical theory, neurotic disorders result from *primary gains* and can cause *secondary gains*. In the case of somatoform disorders, the primary gains have the role of reducing inner mental conflicts and tensions by producing symptoms that have the appearance of somatic disorders, making use of defense mechanisms such as repression, regression and denial. As a result, they are the basis for somatoform "neurosis". The secondary gains are a consequence of illness. Patients can obtain certain benefits from their state to get added attention from those around them or to avoid a situation or a role that they would otherwise be unable to avoid. These secondary gains can thus contribute towards maintaining the severity or chronicity of the disorder. It should be emphasized that, in psychodynamic theory, these are the result of subconscious mechanisms and are therefore not controlled by willpower.

Universities in Boston, Chicago and Paris have worked out concepts that have progressively made up the coherent core of psychosomatic theory. In this connection, we can mention the *giving up – given up, hopelessness – helplessness syndromes* which are a pre-illness psychological state occurring after a loss in the life of an individual. The classic entities of *alexithymia* and *pensée opératoire*, which are terms for an inability to or difficulty in describing or being aware of emotions or mood, have been conceptualized in parallel. They would explain the propensity for certain subjects to express inner mental conflicts by means of somatic symptoms or disorders. All the work focusing on the problem of *narcissism* should also be mentioned as this is apparently a frequent one among a certain patient category. It should be understood as a lack of self-esteem, forcing the subject to constantly prove that he is worthy of being loved. It is the functional pattern frequently encountered in destructive developments after a minor accident for some workaholics. With work addicts of this type, the triggering traumatic event takes on a disproportionate significance since it reveals the underlying vulnerability.

Value of the triggering traumatic event

The disability process is most frequently based on a triggering traumatic event. This could be severe mental or physical trauma that, in the normal course of things, would go towards disability in a development seen as proportionate. However, there can be a picture of post-traumatic stress disorder (PTSD) that can occasionally remain chronic and seriously disabling. The clinical presentation, however, is typical with intrusive and distressing recollections (flashbacks, nightmares) of the event, the avoidance of clues related to the trauma and increased arousal (difficulty in sleeping, irritability, hypervigilance).

However, the triggering trauma is apparently most frequently of a minor nature. It is nevertheless indispensable to make inquiries into the details, the way it was experienced and the emotions that accompanied it (anger, revolt, shame, feeling of abandonment, extreme fear). Clinical experience has revealed that sometimes one is surprised by the intensity of what happened during the event that a priori was not serious. Current consensus is to award much more importance to the significance of the traumatic event for a subject than to its objective severity evaluated by a neutral observer. Sometimes, it is noted that the avoidance of the workplace as the site of an accident generates behaviour in a disabled person. The genuine causes of this behaviour are often unknown to the caregivers even though they are treatable and the prognosis is not necessarily poor since they are similar to a simple phobia. Therefore the former psychopathological terrain must be taken into account (history of abuse in childhood, personality disorders, affective disorders, etc.) that may become the melting pot for psychiatric comorbidity with is own intrinsic disability value [6].

Cognitive factors of disability

Earlier, we saw that certain types of trauma can generate avoidance behaviour that can severely impede any return to the workplace and contribute to the adoption of invalidity status. Cognitive therapy puts forward that certain psychological difficulties originate in the erroneous *belief* in which the individual is more upset by the view he has of matters than by their objective reality.

In the area of interest to us, it is known that a *fear-avoidance belief can* lead to disability behavior for fear of causing pain or of injuring oneself by certain movements, with subjects setting themselves into a sort of preventive inaction. The same mechanism asserts itself when the patient sees his disorders in such a way that he is convinced that there is a major risk if he uses force or moves in such a way inadvertently. This is the case with certain lumbar trauma patients who live in constant fear of becoming paralyzed and ending up in a wheelchair. Such beliefs obviously carry a high risk of encouraging long-term disability even if certain observations reveal that they could be reversible with the relevant psychotherapy [7].

Certain convictions make up the core beliefs acquired in the course of development and more or less activated at some moment or other in life. The idealization of physical integrity, that is the only capital in the case of some manual laborers, can originate from a belief that "to be somebody good, I must always work harder, more and better than others". Such subjects would obviously have great difficulty in coping with an even minor attack on their physical health.

Socio-cultural factors

Socio-cultural factors can have a decisive impact in some developments towards disability as some of the literature might appear to suggest [8]. The targeted questioning of certain nosologically controversial entities such as chronic fatigue syndrome and fibromyalgia or late whiplash syndrome can create fascinating elements for thought.

Nowadays, our medical practice is confronted by a certain number of controversial nosological entities that have emerged in a variety of contexts, to our knowledge most frequently within the framework of occupational medicine or from a claim for acknowledgement or compensation (Table 1). These diagnostic entities are sometimes in relatively current use, such as chronic fatigue syndrome and fibromyalgia. These can be associated with chronic low back pain, other instances of chronic pain without conclusive organic basis and late whiplash syndrome for disorders attributed to cervical torsion. Other symptomatic pictures are less common such as sick building syndrome, myalgic encephalitis, myofascial pain syndrome and chronic temporomandibular disorder. Some of them take us back to controversies that have mobilized North America such as Gulf war syndrome and silicone breast implant toxicity [9].

Table 1 – List of controversial nosological entities.

Chronic low back pain
Fibromyalgia
Late whiplash syndrome
Chronic fatigue syndrome
Myofascial pain syndrome
Chronic temporomandibular disorder
Repetitive stress (or strain) injuries
Myalgic encephalitis
Sick building syndrome
Multiple chemical sensitivities
Gulf war syndrome
Silicone breast implant toxicity
Somatoform disorders

These diagnostic designations cover clinical situations that have a certain number of characteristics in common. First of all, they give the appearance of a truly organic illness with the patients most frequently rejecting any psychological problem. The etiology of these complaints is poorly known even if countless hypotheses are documented in this connection. The subjects concerned most frequently report a triggering factor (accident, infection). These complaints sometimes take on an epidemic nature (sick building syndrome). The clinical picture is frequently vague and unsystematic. It involves common complaints, picking up on the everyday experience of all and sundry: tiredness, pain, sleep disorders. The symptoms appear to be under the subject's control. There is frequently an enormous discrepancy between clinical presentation and the importance of the alleged disabilities. Diagnostic tools are poor. There are sometimes doubts about the reality of the symptoms and even the existence of the illness in question - something that is nevertheless not normal in the field of medicine. These complaints are, after all, always difficult to treat but remain stable in their relative mildness outside of their incapacitating nature. In themselves, they never call the vital prognosis into play (Table 2).

Table 2 – Common characteristics of these controversial nosological entities.

Appearance of an organic illness without any clear indication of a specific injury
Vague symptoms relating to the everyday experience of all and sundry
Symptoms that appear to be under the control of the subject
Discordance between the clinical organic picture and the importance of the disabilities
Objection to any psychological problem
Difficult treatment but stability and benignity in the long term
Diagnostic tools unsatisfactory
Doubts about even the existence of the illness concerned

In fact, these nosological entities diverge resolutely from the paradigm of a classic biomedical ailment with its etiology, verifiable injuries and its development with or without treatment, documented in the relationship between the clinic and histopathology. In the majority of cases, these situations are definitely positioned as a form of behaviour in keeping with a much wider context than the single somatic incident designated as the starting point. This broader view of the problem has been noticed for countless years.

In this connection, it is interesting to point out that the majority of the controversial nosological entities mentioned above are connected to unfavourable psychological factors, to a high incidence of psychiatric comorbidity, even simply seen as the equivalent of mental problems. Some authors compare chronic fatigue syndrome, for example, to a form of disguised depression. Most frequently, the patients concerned, however, reject psychological problems unless they are those that they admit to as a consequence of their suffering and handicaps caused by their illness which, according to them, is organic in nature. The fact that the doctor first treating them wishes to refer them to a psychiatrist is frequently experienced as a rejection and calls into question the sincerity of the complaints. A psychiatric diagnosis is normally ill received by the patient himself, by those around him, society and probably also the healthcare community.

Sociologists [10, 11, 12] tell us that every culture provides for codes of conduct and defines as far as behavioural constellations that allow a departure from these. In the healthcare sector, any culture would define its *misbehavioural patterns*, that is to say socially acceptable symptoms that are recognized as such by the people around the subject in question, by his professional counterparts and social insurance companies. The illness patterns might be mobilized in important moments of stress, the status of being ill being perhaps one of the most economical solutions of a poorly adapted response authorized by our culture.

In the author's opinion, the clinical palette of these diagnostic labels applicable to acceptable illness patterns makes certain presuppositions. The symptoms must be dependent on the appearance of organicity. The disorder must be recognized as being incapacitating while still remaining benign and never questioning the vital prognosis. The symptoms are apparently under the subject's control at their relational value level. The medical body has then reached its diagnostic and therapeutic limits in terms of evidence-based medicine. In this respect, some nosological entities mentioned above (Table 1) are made to measure for labeling the final outcome of a chronic disability process. They are perhaps an appropriate behavioural pattern rather than a true illness, while a minor medical or surgical event develops into a disproportionate disability both in terms of its length and its severity.

Discussion

Modern diagnostic classifications are credited with having determined a certain number of morbid entities, permitting a common language and remarkable progress in terms of evidence-based medicine. In actual fact, they list scientifically recognized illnesses, i.e. universally accepted as being such in the majority of industrialized countries with their sets of treatment, psychosocial support and acknowledgement by the community. These are biomedical ailments in the strict sense (cancer, infection) and major psychiatric pathologies (psychoses, dementia, uni- and bipolar affective disorders).

Other diagnostic entities remain controversial to avoid being modeled on the biomedical pattern. However, this pattern does pose the question of their reality as a diagnostic entity without the suffering of those who bear these diagnoses being put in question. In our case, this mainly concerns chronic low back pain, fibromyalgia, chronic fatigue syndrome and late whiplash syndrome. The major group of somatoform disorders can be associated with these even if their psychiatric connotation gives a diagnostic label that is far less acceptable socially. This group of illnesses has tailor-made characteristics for becoming the final outcome of a disability process and are often the final diagnostic label of chronicity. They could be a misbehavioural pattern, in the meaning of socially acceptable behaviour in response to excessive internal or external demands. They force the questioning of the widely-held belief that there is a line of linear and proportionate causality between a physical injury and the personal and social handicap that will ensue. We have already seen that, alongside the socio-cultural factors amply explained here, the elements relevant to the person himself (psychodynamic and cognitive factors), the singular impact of trauma and psychosocial terrain also constitute a melting pot for chronic disability.

The biopsychosocial model put forward by Engel [1] is probably the one best able to integrate all the factors involved in the disability process. He suggests that the specific biological disorder of a disease does not necessarily result in its clinical manifestation. It does not explain all the aspects of the illness. It is simply a necessary but insufficient condition. The illness cannot be reduced to its biological component because it mainly manifests itself at psychosocial level. Many evidence-based arguments show that personality type, lifestyle, existential problems and culture affect the way a biological disturbance is expressed. In itself, the biomedical model remains insufficient to explain the long-term disability process.

Conclusion

Not forgetting the countless working hypotheses that explain the disability process in response to excessive internal and external demands, the limitations of a therapeutic approach are immediately apparent (medication, manipulation, surgery) in terms of classic biomedical functioning. Instead, efforts should evidently be concentrated on psychosocial measures in the widest sense of the term, in the knowledge that in the case of chronic low back pain, for example, the efficacy of this early holistic approach has already been demonstrated extending as far as modifications in the workplace. In terms of prevention, we are faced with the question of escape routes that our society must provide for those among us who are less capable at the personal, social and professional level. The label of somatic, psychosomatic or psychiatric illness is not, perhaps, the best of solutions.

Bibliography

1. Engel GL (1977) The need for a new medical model: a challenge for biomedical science. Science 196: 126-36
2. Hirschfeld AH, Behan RC (1963) The accident process. JAMA 186(3): 193-9
3. Weinstein MR (1968) The concept of the disability process. Psychosomatics 19(2): 94-7
4. Pilowsky I (1995) Low back pain and illness behavior. Spine, 20 (13): 1522-4
5. Matheson LN (1988) Symptom magnification syndrome. In: Isernhagen SJ (ed), Work Injury, Gaithersburg, Maryland, Aspen Publishers: 257-82
6. Marshall RD, Olfson M, Hellmann F et al. (2001) Comorbidity, impairment, suicidality in subthreshold PTSD. Am J Psychiatry 158(9) 1467-73
7. Vlayen J, Kole-Snijders A, Boeren R et al. (1995) Fear of movement / (re) injury in chronic low back pain and its relation to behavioral performance. Pain 62: 363-72
8. Schrader H, Obelieniene D, Bovim G et al. (1996) Natural evolution of late whiplash syndrome outside the medicolegal context. Lancet 4; 347(9010): 1207-11
9. Ferrari R, Kwan O (2001) The no-fault flavor of disability syndromes. Medical Hypotheses 56(1): 77-84

10. Linton, R (1936) The study of man: an introduction / by R Linton. – Student's ed. – New York: Appleton-Century-Crofts (The Century social science series)
11. Kirmayer LJ, Young A (1998) Culture and somatisation: clinical, epidemiological and ethnographic perspectives. Psychosomatic Medicine 60: 420-30
12. Perrin E (1996) Douleur et culture. Le point de vue d'une sociologue. Doul et Analg 4: 91-7

Inability to work, disability and vocational rehabilitation: does the general practitioner have a role to play in these processes?

F. Pilet

Introduction

More than 10% of people aged between 15 and 65 who consult a general practitioner leave the practice with a sick note certifying their inability to work [1]. In 20% of cases relating to sickness and 3% relating to accidents, this incapacity will last for more than 3 months. After a period of one year, 4% of these patients are still unable to return to work and, of these 4%, only one in four will ever resume any form of gainful employment [2, 3].

Certifying long-term incapacity is frequently a very heavy burden for a doctor. On the one hand, he must accompany the patient through a difficult physical, psychological and social process and, on the other hand, he is under pressure from employers, private insurance companies and public social institutions.

In fact, everything happens as if the doctor has become responsible for his patient's incapacity because, with his signature, he is the one who has to attest to his patient's objective or subjective unfitness for resuming work! The increasing medicalisation of social suffering, which is a result of the decline in the economic climate, turns doctors into ready-made scapegoats – ideally suited to shouldering the responsibility for exploding costs in social insurance, disability insurance in particular.

The aim of this contribution is to answer the following questions: is a general practitioner a simple bystander in the game played out by employees who are either sick or injured, their employers, insurance companies, social institutions and vocational rehabilitation services? Or is he an actor and, if so, does he hold any trump cards in his hand? If this is the case, when and how can he play them?

Backdrop

Economic and social settings

In order to better understand the position and the role of the general practitioner in the entire process, which ranges from a loss of ability to work through to possible work resumption, some thought must first be given to the economic and social settings in which this process takes place.

During the last quarter of the 20th century, western societies have experienced a profound change in their scale of values since the market economy has put values such as dignity, loyalty, trust, security as well as those derived from the concept of human rights, way behind profit! Even work, which once had an important place in this scale at the turn of the 20th century, has lost its value: in a world dominated by the virtual game of capital traded on the stock exchange, workforces are no longer needed to make a profit. Going concerns are thus disappearing on a daily basis, with full order books and motivated employees, simply because others are playing with the capital needed for their operation. It would be wrong to underestimate this development of values on the health of workers and on the difficulties of vocational rehabilitation when their illness or accident has kept them away from their workplace.

In a society where Man's own humanity is called into question [4], where human beings are reduced to an addition of costs (wages, national insurance contributions, health insurance, disability, etc.) or profits (purchasing power, consumption), people's motivation for work is in a perilous state and is directly threatened by even the least attack on health.

Working conditions

If they are improved in terms of stress on the motor system and in terms of accident prevention, working conditions have suffered severely from the tension that is prevalent in the global economic system. Just-in-time production (reduction of stocks), maximum elimination of downtimes, extremely short-term objectives for production and profitability, permanent job insecurity and the progressive removal of less productive employees (particularly for medical reasons) are all factors that have a substantial effect on health, illness, absenteeism and disability. A recent study conducted in Switzerland showed that, in times of job insecurity the health problems have increased threefold, analgesics consumption 3,5 and sleeping drugs twofold [5]. Several studies on a Swiss and European level have demonstrated that working conditions have a considerable impact on morbidity in general and on disability [6, 7]. What is most disturbing about these studies is that they have all shown a clear increase in this phenomenon over the last ten years. An inquiry conducted in 2003 among general practitioners, internists and psychiatrists in the Canton of Geneva (Switzerland) revealed that more than one in four visits to a doctor by actively employed patients was linked to a problem with working conditions! [8]

Social security system

European countries have a variety of systems of benefits for a long-term loss of earning ability due to illness or accident. But what these systems have in common is their lack of adaptability to developments in the economic world. I will explain this, using the example of the Swiss system.

One element of collateral damage in the modern economic war is the exclusion of a growing number of people who have been written off by the system because their mental or physical capacity has not enabled them to adapt sufficiently to the increasingly difficult pressures imposed on them or because their productivity is too low. As a result, the number of people dependent on the support of social institutions such as unemployment benefit, disability insurance or other minimum allowances will only increase. This leads to the following paradox: the more the system produces disabled people and other "social misfits", the more it accuses them of profiteering and the less inclined it is to finance the outcome of this exclusion!

The evident shortcomings in the social security system include the following:

– lack of funding which will only deteriorate;
– slow reaction and action times which put any chance of vocational rehabilitation at a very severe disadvantage, with this torpidity linked both to the system rules and insufficient funding;
– constant hypocrisy in denying the influence of the job market and in implementing virtual rehabilitation. The specialists in disability insurance in Switzerland always make use of the legal argument, according to which people who lose their ability to work for medical reasons could theoretically work in a specially adapted activity even if everybody knows for a fact that no such activity exists in the job market, in any case not for a partially disabled person. "It is not the responsibility of disability insurance to finance the consequences of the economic recession", is what one hears. Perhaps, but whose responsibility is it? The result of this policy of separate insurance coverage (unemployment, disability insurance) is that countless people find themselves without any financial support either from the one or the other and have to go begging for social assistance from their local authorities whose coffers are also slowly emptying.

This situation is well pointed out by Jean-Claude Guillebaud [4], who makes an analogy with the feudal system.

It is therefore not surprising that, given such a context, efforts aimed at vocational reintegration meet with all sorts of barriers. To believe that the success or failure of rehabilitation depends primarily on the skills of the doctors, physiotherapists, occupational therapists or socio-occupational specialists shows naivety or denial. Of course, these skills are necessary but are by no means enough.

In other words, and to take up the analogy of the game in the introduction, in the game that is played out around vocational reintegration, employees have a few trump cards as do rehabilitation specialists and general practitioners, but the vital cards are in the hands of a business world that dictates the rules and modifies them as the game goes on without consulting the other players!

Let us now take a look at our trump cards as general practitioners. If we do have a few, let us at least try to play them judiciously.

The trump cards held by general practitioners

Treatment

Chronic illnesses

In cases of chronic illness accompanied by a gradual loss of physical or mental abilities (rheumatism, bronchial obstructive syndromes, degenerative neurological diseases, coronary pathologies, chronic depression, etc), general practitioners hold two important cards:

- *long-term relationship;*
- *anticipation.*

Within the framework of a long-term personal relationship, doctors can help patients to *progressively accept their chronic illness*, with all the grieving processes involved. The acceptance of an irreversible pathology is, in fact, the first step and is indispensable for the mobilising of new resources, new faculties of adaptation in daily life, particularly in terms of work and for envisaging a possible change of occupation.

This role of accompanying the sorrow that represents the loss of certain functions needs good skills on the part of a doctor, who must allow the patient to express his anger, his discouragement, his sadness, his feeling of injustice by actively listening and empathising, to enable him in time to accept what has happened.

Anticipation is his second master card: when the doctor foresees that the illness his patient is suffering from will sooner or later lead to the end of his current job, he can – or rather he should – encourage the patient to imagine adapting to this development: changing the type of work he does while remaining in the same profession or even a complete change of occupation by looking into personal resources that have so far not been exploited to the full. The vocational centres for adults are valuable in this respect and the patient can benefit especially well if he takes this step without any pressure, of his own free will, which will also encourage creativity on his part. This ability to imagine and create something new is heavily undermined if one waits until the patient has had to stop working for medical reasons and he is under bureaucratic pressure from unemployment or disability insurance departments.

This anticipation is truly the task of the family doctor, who can, with the help of specialists, establish a sort of prognosis while his patient is not necessarily able to predict the developments to which he will be exposed.

Acute illnesses and accidents

The unexpected occurrence of a serious acute illness or an accident with disabling consequences pose problems of a completely different order: the shock of the event, the possible existence of a third party who is responsible makes acceptance much more difficult and naturally, makes anticipation impossible.

Beyond the differences in personality among patients and beyond the very varied circumstances that might surround the occurrence of an accident, the greatest and most frequent suffering among victims seems to be the lack of recognition: recognition for the upheaval that the event has caused in the patient's life, recognition for the losses sustained, recognition for the pangs of death, the feeling of injustice, the impression of no longer being worth anything, recognition of the immeasurable sorrow of functional limitations.

With an experience of 22 years as general practitioner, this lack of recognition by the medical world and the insurance companies seems to be one of the major factors in an unfavourable course of treatment, particularly after accidents, and of course even more so if a third party was the cause.

In these acute cases, a doctor's empathetic attitude when treating the patient will once again be vital. Above all, doctors must play their validation card: validate the multiple feelings provoked by the event, validate the losses and suffering. However, working with grief is much more difficult in this type of situation and for two reasons:

– Just as with the sudden loss of someone close, the suddenness of an event makes grieving less easy and acceptance more difficult.

– The torpidity of the administrative, legal and medical system of the insurance companies seriously hampers this grieving process, which can become pathological: it frequently takes months or even years for various insurance experts to reach a final decision on the degree of recognition for the losses suffered (generally without having listened to the patient, which reinforces the latter's impression of a totally arbitrary decision).

It is practically impossible to grieve for someone who has disappeared in contrast to someone who has died. In the case of sudden loss following an accident or an acute illness, everything seems as if the injured part of the person has disappeared as long as the insurance company has not issued its final verdict, as long as it has not recognized the loss, as long as it has not made restitution to the patient for the part of his body that is dead. Thus any grieving process is blocked until this recognition has taken place. And if, for various legal reasons, the insurance company refuses to recognize the loss, the lost function will remain so forever and grieving will be impossible. This is the situation for chronic painful cases in which the original injury was not necessarily very serious but for which the suffering had not been recognized.

In such situations, the role of the general practitioner is therefore particularly difficult: how to help the patient grieve for a loss that goes unrecognised, to mourn for something that has disappeared? All the more so since the doctor often also has to indicate with his certificate that the patient is fit to start work again or to take up another type of job, at least part-time.

Mission impossible? After so many years in practice, I might be tempted to believe that.

Identifying the critical moments in the course of symptoms

It is important for a family doctor to identify the signs of unfavourable developments at a very early stage and to actively investigate the work-related causes of suffering. As the team at McGill University in Montreal showed for low back pain, interventions in the workplace are much more effective than any medical measures, which are frequently doomed to failure [9, 10].

Above all, it is once again a matter of recognizing suffering, of putting a name to it and not just denying it by repeating that nothing medically identifiable has been found. Actually, this pain has a name: overwork, excessive stress or responsibilities, conflict with others in the workplace. Just because you cannot measure this type of suffering with a blood test or see it on X-rays does not mean that it does not merit treatment. Some of these measures, in particular personal intervention with employers or social insurance bodies are also the role of the family doctor. This ability to identify workplace problems at a very early stage probably represents one of the major trump cards in the general practitioner's game.

Familiarity with the network

By means of relationships that have progressively developed with the various actors in the professional network, the family doctor can play a very useful role. The specialist doctors, the centres for vocational rehabilitation, the people responsible for unemployment benefit and disability insurance, the social services, the employers are just as much people with their own points of view and who general practitioners end up getting to know. Putting them in contact, creating a synthesis, translating the bureaucratic language for the patient and pointing out the inconsistencies of the system to the professionals involved all constitute just as much the tasks of the family doctor.

The patient's family represents another important network. Inviting a spouse or even the patient's children to an interview provides a better understanding of how the family functions, to see secondary benefits in the illness and to identify certain negative consequences of the medical and occupational situation on the family as a whole [11].

The quadruple agenda

In the teaching of medical consultancy, teachers refer to the notion of the double agenda [12]: that of the patient, with his expectations, his wishes, his anxiety, his family and vocational setting, and that of the doctor, with his preventive and therapeutic objectives, his lack of time and sometimes his different kind of pressure (employer, insurance).

What these two agendas have in common is the fact that they are frequently hidden agendas – not intentionally, but simply because they are not openly expressed or clarified. The result is that consultation can end in a dialogue between the deaf if the doctor, for example, intends to direct the patient's attention to the multiple factors of cardiovascular risks while the patient only wants to talk about his aching feet, his job under threat and his son who smokes cannabis!

Whenever a patient stops working, there are not two but four hidden agendas that clash:

– *that of the patient, of course;*

– that of the doctor;
– that of the employer;
– and finally, that of the insurer.

Sometimes late in the evening after having finished writing up my insurance reports, I dream of getting these three other protagonists into my office with their different agendas and listening to them crossing swords directly rather than through me.

Without going so far as to turn this dream into reality, it would seem vital in any case for doctors to have a clear awareness of the existence of these four rarely explicit agendas

Locus of control

The expression "locus of control" was coined by psychologists to designate the place to which the individual attributes control of his destiny [13, 14].

If the locus of control is external, responsibility for events is attributed to external factors and not to the person himself: he cannot do anything about it, he is in the role of a spectator, or even a victim. If the locus of control is internal, the individual attributes part of the responsibility for what happens to himself, he will tend to make greater use of the experience gained and to take this into account. He sees himself as an actor.

The personality type of a patient can be evaluated with various tests. This personality will influence the behaviour of a person in the choice of his job and certainly his reactions to a temporary or permanent loss of ability to work. In today's business world, the places where decisions are made are increasingly tending to move further away from where the work is done. Employees, even if highly motivated initially, come to realise that there are hardly any links between their commitment to work and the development of their company: after having invested hours and hours of overtime without baulking, after having accepted harder and harder constraints, countless employees in fact are declared redundant for reasons that have nothing to do with the quality of their work. This development in business operations clearly reinforces the feeling of external locus of control, seemingly even more so among those co-workers who already have this personality trait: I have no control over my destiny.

When unable to work because of medical reasons, this phenomenon will play a decisive role: development will depend more on the doctor, the employer, the expert, the lawyer or the insurance company than on the patient.

Can we dream of an ideal system?

I have been asked what I would ideally expect, as a general practitioner, from a social insurance and vocational rehabilitation system.

It is obvious that I would neither be so naive nor presumptuous enough to claim that I could invent the ideal system! I will limit myself to giving a few leads, a few features that such a system should include, in my view, in order to be efficient.

Rehabilitation first and foremost, profitability perhaps

As mentioned before, the social security system has little impact on developments in the business world. However, these developments should be taken into account and physicians should stop making the economic profitability of an injured or sick person their main objective. We are living in a society that is reducing the number of persons economically active by any means possible. No rehabilitation system after illness or accident will be able to reverse this trend. It is vital to be aware of this.

For this reason, the ideal system should, above all, aim to restore a place, a role and dignity to any person excluded for reasons of health – without profitability being the prime objective.

Integrate the various means of social security

The ideal system of a social safety net should integrate all means of support for those excluded – whatever the cause of exclusion (financial reasons, unemployment, difficulties in coping with increasing stress in the working world for physical or mental reasons!). Integration of this type would avoid the multiplicity of bureaucratic processes that just bounce the ball back, with the patient finding himself between two stools, meeting neither the demands of unemployment insurance nor those of disability insurance. This passing back and forth is humiliating and strongly reinforces the impression of an external locus of control. Some countries have partly resolved this difficult problem by creating a minimal reintegration income.

The assumption of responsibility should therefore be based on the simple fact of exclusion with no other prejudices, which would not prevent any subsequent demands towards the person thus helped, for example, by means of contracts for integration and rehabilitation.

Recognition: a priority

Recognising the suffering, recognising the losses suffered by a person as a result of illness or accident should be the primary requirement without prejudging the action to follow. We have all had the paradoxical experience that rehabilitation in a serious disability such as paraplegia or amputation frequently causes fewer problems than where the pathology is less severe but also less visible. The reason appears simple: for the paraplegic or amputee, there is immediate recognition by the society, the medical world, the insurance companies. The case is indisputable, which helps the grieving process. In contrast, a person suffering from chronic pain or depression has nothing to show to those around him, his doctor or the experts, which would allow his suffering to be recognised. The human cost of this despairing fight for recognition is frequently dramatic: after years of vain proceedings, countless patients find themselves completely exhausted, without financial or psychological resources, excluded not only from the working world but also from society, without the support of insurance, forced to beg for minimal social aid from the appropriate authorities.

Looking at the system as a whole, swift financial recognition of the loss suffered as a result of illness or accident would probably not be much more expensive than years of useless proceedings which are profitable to lawyers and to the medical profession and which set enormous and inefficient bureaucratic procedures in motion.

Recognition of this sort, within a short period of time, would definitely benefit the reintegration process.

Personalised follow-up

As a priority, the means available in a rehabilitation system should focus on a personalised follow-up of the patient. In theory, such measures exist within the disability insurance systems but since staffing levels are frequently insufficient, implementation is often too late and contacts so distant that efficacy remains very weak. The majority of patients involved feel neither recognised nor supported and merely wait for a verdict. Unfortunately this is probably one of the best ways to encourage passivity.

Early and regular follow-up by a case-manager who has received special training in support would seem to be an investment with serious added value in a good rehabilitation system.

In this type of support, early contact with the employer – if there still is one – would be indispensable, as would the provision of vocational orientation for cases where a complete change of occupation appears necessary. Some social insurance groups in the European Union are orienting themselves with perspectives such as these.

Personal efforts at reintegration must not be penalised

The rules of social insurance systems do not always support people who try to find work themselves. A person receiving a pension is therefore not necessarily interested in regaining a source of income.

No system, however efficient, can prevent some people abusing it. Some penalties should therefore be devised for those who cheat. However, care should be taken that, in wishing to avoid abuse at all costs, this does not lead to making the system less functional, less encouraging or less effective.

Conclusions

Any reduction in physical or mental capacities as a result of illness or accident and the resultant inability to work represents a loss that can only be accepted after a grieving process if it has been recognised by medical, insurance or administrative bodies. This recognition is the first, indispensable step in any attempt at vocational rehabilitation.

In a business world where Man's own humanity is under serious threat from his lust for profit, it would seem to be the task of the general practitioner, in the first instance, as well as the entire social support system for those excluded, to defend certain human values such as dignity.

In this sometimes perverse game that is played out around the inability to work and rehabilitation measures, we have seen that the general practitioner holds some decisive cards. He has to play his trump cards at the right time, the first being the recognition of the authenticity of physical, mental and social suffering by the individual struck down by illness or accident.

The existence of the general practitioner (family doctor) is under serious threat in modern health systems where care procedures become consumer goods just like a mobile phone or a takeaway pizza, goods that can be obtained from emergency departments or emergency services. If general practitioners disappear, who will be left to defend human dignity?

References

1. Dünner S, Decrey H, Burnand B, Pécoud A (2001) Sickness certification in primary care. Soz-Präventivmed 46: 389-95

2. Société Suisse des Assureurs Accident et grand groupe privé d'assurance en cas de maladie (2004). Données personnelles

3. Gobelet C (2003) Réadaptation professionnelle. Revue Médicale de la Suisse Romande 123: 599-602

4. Guillebaud J-C (2001) Le principe d'Humanité. Edition du Seuil

5. Domenighetti G (2003) Abstract Société Suisse de Médecine Psychosociale, Lugano

6. Conne-Perreard E (2003) Effets des conditions de travail défavorables sur la santé des travailleurs et conséquences économiques. Publication du Service Cantonal de la Santé et Sécurité au Travail, Genève (www.eurofound.ie/working/surveys.htm)

7. Merllié D, Paoli P (2003) Dix ans de conditions de travail dans l'union européenne. Fondation Européenne pour l'amélioration des conditions de vie et de travail. Office des publications officielles des communautés européennes. Luxembourg

8. Conne-Perreard E, Usel M (2003) Enquête auprès des médecins internistes, généralistes et psychiatres du canton de Genève concernant un lien entre conditions de travail et problèmes de santé motivant une consultation médicale. Publication de l'Office cantonal de l'inspection et des relations du travail, Genève

9. Loisel P, Abenhaim L, Durand P, Esdaile J et al. (1997) Population based randomized clinical trial on back pain management. Spine 22(24): 2911-18

10. Durand M-J, Loisel P, Durand P (1998) Le retour thérapeutique au travail: une intervention de réadaptation décentralisée dans le milieu de travail. Description et cadre théorique. Revue Canadienne d'Ergothérapie 65: 72-88

11. Vanotti M (2001) Maladies et Familles. Ed. Médecine et Hygiène, Genève

12. Côté L, Bélanger N, Blais J (2002) L'entrevue centrée sur le patient et ses moyens d'apprentissage. Can Fam Physician 48: 1800-5
13. Ryan RM, Deci EL (2000) Self-determination theory and the facilitation of intrinsic motivation, social development, and well-being, Ann Psychol 55: 68-78
14. Voirol C, Rousson M (1999-2000) Le concept d'intennalité comme outil de prévention et de traitement de l'épuisement professionnel? Université de Neuchâtel, Div. économique et sociale, Mémoire de licence

Cultural aspects
of vocational rehabilitation processes

I. Rothenbühler

Introduction

How do cultural factors intervene in vocational rehabilitation? In the European context, the importance of migrational transitions and the questions of integration and participation of the immigrants in the host societies turns the question towards various areas of health care and social assistance. It is from this migratorial point of view that we shall treat the notion of the cultural dimension within the vocational rehabilitation of immigrants. Nowadays, the socio-professional context presents new stakes and new tensions in job management, within the work teams, in the communication and the quality of that communication. Faced with the methods of exclusion, the professionals of social and medical assistance are facing a situation that is more and more difficult [1]. The difficulty is often due to a growing diversity and greater geographical distances from the original regions and from values and customs from those of today's world. This vision often rests on the intercultural realities drawn from the melting pot of common sense, on the basis of a position without self criticism permitting ready made judgements. It also rests on an ethnocentricity which feeds the distinction and differentiation processes of the different social groups, through depreciation or rather through contempt of other cultures as opposed to one's own [2]. Other than the fact that the term is used to apply to some imaginary and naïve categories for which the reality cannot be proven, this position is nevertheless dangerous when it is the fruit of scientific constructions of which the social and cultural phenomena are the privileged objects. Our theoretical position comes from a way of thinking which is in opposition to these categories based on a substantialist vision of culture. On the contrary, we will be looking at their significances and their values in terms of dynamics, change and reconstructions [3].

This chapter pursues the following objectives: clarifying what we mean when we say cultural factors within the processes and the measures taken in vocational rehabilitation. It certainly will not be a catalogue of values, attitudes and cultural customs of immigrants according to their nationality, race or religion, an intercultural manual for health care professionals. On the contrary, we will put forth evidence of the limits of the cultural variable faced with the potential for creative and fruitful interaction between those in need of care and the carers, defining thus the pragmatic and anthropological stakes involved in this interaction.

The pluriculturality defies social, political and professional practices through integration and participation of immigrants in their host society in terms of social interaction. The migratorial phenomena which question these vocational rehabilitation (VR) practices give us reason to limit our questioning to two problematics that we will treat as two complementary aspects situated on different levels: the interactions between the vocational rehabilitation experts and the patients whose expectations opposing the medical world, and the universe of meanings, of values which refer to themselves. The cultural factors are considered essential to our topic as non substantial, dynamic and relational. Thus, we propose to create a framework of reflection permitting the reader, by the range of the points made here, to note the following questions between the lines of its practice: how do the nursing staff and the doctors treat the diverse meanings, the values, attitudes and behaviour to which they are exposed in their rehabilitation practices? How does one promote access to the offer of social and therapeutic services to each and every person touched by some disability, according to the language spoken, the judicial status, the nationality or the religious affiliation?

After evoking the theoretical aspects of the cultural and intercultural questions in connection with the theme of this book, we will more precisely define the notion behind VR. Then we will present existing data concerning the role of national affiliation in the case of invalidity and rehabilitation, adding to that certain anthropological notions of health and sickness. In the second half of the chapter, we develop a reflection on the experience of sickness and accidents within the refuge and immigrational problematic in Lausanne (in the French-speaking part of Switzerland), through experiences shared by immigrants in precarious situations whom we have had the opportunity to accompany. We elaborate on the anxiety – provoking characteristics of physical and psychological disabilities in the migrational context from which can not be isolated, the acculturation process as a potentially dynamic creator and the challenge presented by the social suffering through the politics, the migratorial practices and health, which includes VR.

The notion of culture referred to as a horizon

We propose from the start a deeper understanding of the use which we shall make of the various derivations of the notion of culture, in order to avoid any misunderstandings concerning its status. First of all, what there is of culture in social dynamics comes from collective and contextual interiorisation of practices and significations through the process of socialization [4], both of enculturation and of acculturation. We separate enculturation, constituted by the forms of interiorisation based on the family and the initial sociocultural context that the individuals encounter, from the acculturation which consists of the interiorisation of values and significations that follow the contact with other social groups presenting an exogenous dimension [2]. The experience of discontinuance within the enculturation group can sometimes bring about important ruptures in identity, conspicuously on the individual level. The cultural factors can in no way be distinguished from the cognitive, affective, social, economical, political, judicial and identity factors. But we insist on the limits and the imprecise contours of the cultural factors, of the heterogeneities belonging to those of the same region or nation and the active role of the individuals who appropriate them through strategies and dynamics which are simultaneously personal, familial and communal.

The intercultural dimension of the professional practices in VR take on a very different connotation as a culturalist approach attributing to the behaviours and specific values of the various populations according to their linguistic and national origins. This position is essential to the theme which holds our attention faced with the omnipresent risk of explaining the unresponsiveness, the communication difficulties, the therapeutic failures and the misunderstandings which benefit from the generalizations about the "muslim culture", the "latin culture", the "fulani culture", etc.... This tendency often goes with an overdetermination of the linguistic, national, religious, ethnic belongings and the prejudice issued by common sense [6] and popular discourse. The values and significations available within a singular and specific acculturation experience are individually and collectively rearranged, according to the migratorial project's criteria, living conditions, individual resources and collective mobility. Above all, that is what is effectively meant to be recognized in the manner in which the immigrant patients affected by temporary invalidities should be handled. The notion of horizon [7] borrowed from the hermeneutics will be useful to us in designing that which reunites in a coherent fashion, for a group or an individual, the whole of the practices, norms, values and significations available. In the domain of vocational rehabilitation, contrary to other types of social intervention, in health or in education, we are missing research work which articulates the experience of the immigrants and the social and identity transformations which rebound on the effective practices. Some ethno-sociological investigations have looked into the displacements and the imaginary communal influences and the refiguration of local identities in their context, permitting one to feel the extreme changes of the cultural boundaries [8, 9], which are far more difficult to recognize than the social boundaries [10] within which the cultural symbols do not allow themselves to be enclosed.

A contextual look at vocational rehabilitation

To study cultural factors in VR we should observe the practices and the discourses within the formal and informal tissue affected by the intervention of a VR process, with the natives and the foreigners in fear of missing an essential part of the cultural dynamics which underlie the interactions within the complex of rehabilitation dispositives and processes. An anthropological approach demands, before interrogating ourselves on the cultural dimension of a practice, that we define what is meant by the term referred in this practice. The semantic universe of the notion of VR can undertake variations from one country to another, from one linguistic area to another. I take the position to define the cultural factors at stake in VR in a constructivist and system perspective, like a socially and culturally constructed phenomenon, from which the forms and the institutions which constitute it vary with the degree of geopolitical and historical contexts. More concretely, in Switzerland for example, it concerns agencies of medical care and assistance devices, provided by the legislation in order to permit some of the subjects with the incapacity to exercise for some physical or mental reason their profession, to be able to reintegrate their professional activity. VR principally aims at an objective of professional reinsertion [11]. The boundaries are relatively susceptible, in the sense where the strategies and the resources used by the subjects outside the circumscribed framework of devices remain difficult to measure and to control by the experts of rehabilitation. It carries with it not only a formal dimension which corresponds to the judicial, political and administrative devices as well as medico-social and paramedical devices and their coordinated network of intervention, but also an informal dimension constituted by the whole of the adopted behaviour by the actors, carers and patients.

We also keep in mind that the stage for rehabilitative process includes a political and sociocultural stage depending of the country conditioning the social and sanitary practices as well as the integration and discrimination processes. Like all dispositives written in a sociopolitical and socioeconomic framework, the VR finds within itself the relevant tensions of immigrant participation and of foreigners in the public space of the host country. The ideology and the strongly political assimilationalist practices [12] have made the object from a recent remonstrance of the European Commission against racism and intolerance [13]. One of the research studies of the Swiss Forum for Migration and Population Studies (SFM) shows that there is no concept of integration elaborated in the Swiss enterprises. But the isolated measures and appropriate solutions [14] demand more on the immigrants' part in terms of adoption of values, norms, and of prescribed behaviour than they favour the development of attitudes and singular conducts based on their own cultural horizons.

VR cannot scientifically be conceived as an organisation of therapeutic means in view of the professional reinsertion through the recovery of physical and psychological capacities without being registered in the defined contexts and the constraints that they impose. The importance of economical factors and on an individual level, of the capacity to remain active as a productive force are important to be considered to avoid the spectrum of progressive exclusion that is unavoidable, with penalizing economic and social sanctions.

We have to consider that VR is a western notion which is exported through the channels of globalisation in a movement of marketing logic implantation, of delocalisation, of technocratisation and of the rapid growth of the world communication network. It has not yet penetrated in the common sense of the regions from which the majority of the immigrants come, no more than the notions of social security or of networks of assistance.

Epidemiological and anthropological contributions

To our knowledge, there exist very few studies concerning VR from the cultural or inter-cultural point of view. Interesting work has been made in Switzerland concerning the pain treatment with immigrants [15].

Another study made in the state of S. Gallen (Switzerland) [16] brings to light an important initial fact: the musculo-skeletal troubles and their psychological consequences are clearly more frequent in the foreign population, contrary to the malignant tumours or the cardio-vascular affection for which the difference is less clear. This observation takes on an important meaning once we place it in correlation with a study by the Suva [17] which shows that if the risk of accident or illness linked to the job is effectively clearly higher for foreigners than it is for the Swiss, the difference is however insignificant when one compares the two categories within the same group of professions, the activities which surround construction for example. Thus being a part of a socio-professional category is a more significant factor than the nationality as far as work related accident risks are concerned. It also just so happens that the non-medical risk factors take on an even more determining part that the various populations are marginalized.

Concerning the therapeutic prognosis, we also have information concerning the psycho-social factors [18] that show that these factors which influence the evolution of back pain towards chronicity are less medically oriented than psychosocially or socio-professionally oriented (depressive tendencies and anxieties, unfavourable self prognostics, personal problems, lower education, dissatisfaction and insecurity on the job, inefficient coping techniques, etc.). The invalidating processes have also been studied in the lumbar trauma field [19] and reveal identical signs concerning their evolution. For example, an investigation centered on the case of Italian immigrants working in Switzerland and suffering from back problems indicates that the predictability of the success of therapeutic programs of retraining is strongly affected by autoprognostics of the evolution and to future perspectives.

In a study of the impact of migration on the immigrants' health [20], it can be observed that the musculo-skeletal troubles are often related to an unfavourable psychological evolution and contributes to the mutual reinforcement of the invalidating processes. Unfortunately, we do not have data on the factors linked to accident prevention, other than the risk linked to the professional activity. Thus, it remains nonetheless difficult to draw more conclusions from the above elements, concerning the influence of cultural horizons of the patients. Nevertheless, Weiss [20] brings, on the basis of Herzer's study [16], the following facts into evidence: the nationality is much less important than the socio-professional category and of the professional activity in the rehabilitative processes.

What can be said then about the cultural factors?

The cultural dimension of the illness and its healing has been treated abundantly in medical anthropology. In regards to VR, taking into consideration the EMIC discourse [21] seems a necessary point of departure. The approach consists of centering oneself on the theories appropriate to the patient and on the collective significations to which it refers. This approach necessitates a moving off centre on the part of the practitioner where he will become conscious of the fact that his status and his function are not straightforward for the patient and the efficiency of the treatment strongly depends on mutual understanding. When leaving experience is over causal explanations, the illness appears in its subjective dimension, such as it manifests itself in the conscience of the patient. Medical anthropology uses the term illness [22] to describe this dimension of the sickness in opposition to the notion of disease which designs the sickness made objective by the biomedical diagnosis. Finally, the explanatory models of the illness [23] are studied by numerous anthropologists, with the goal of favouring the emergence of semantic ensembles to which the illness is reattached and begins to make sense for the patient. In the construction of the cultural epidemiology, the putting together of qualitative interview dispositives constructed on the process of collecting EMIC (Explanatory Model Interview Catalogue) information [24], defines three aspects of discourse from people concerning their illnesses: the patterns of distress, the perceived causes and the search for help. The practitioner can then go deeper into his investigation by distinguishing these three moments in relationship to the suffering.

The population on whom our attention is focused

Until the 1990s, the immigrant population concerned by VR primarily constituted of emigrated workers, previous seasonal workers whose benefit was a temporary or a permanent permit, some naturalized afterwards. Work was their principal reason for emigration. The paths of these workers is heavily marked by the experience of necessary acculturation to their acquired autonomy in a society marked by its assimilation politics. This is the reason why one speaks of nationality in the comparative approaches on invalidity and rehabilitation, without concerning oneself with the specific cultural horizons of the persons studied. Our contribution is to try and turn towards the future of the practice of VR and to carry our interest even more so towards the present immigrant population which is arriving in Europe, because the flight from the native countries towards the West is the last hope of a dignified life, hope that is forged, in part, out of myths in regards to western life. The principal causes of migration were in direct relation with the sole perspective of work and its remuneration now substituted by the necessity of survival and their dignity. The population which dates from recent immigrations remain clearly less present in the statistics of clinical visits for rehabilitation [25]. The psychosocial and politico-judicial problems which emerge between the lines of the actual migratorial politics also preoccupy the actors of health and migration strategy [26].

Explanatory models and the meeting of horizons

Does the nationality itself continue to have little relevance in the predictability of the therapies aimed at being rehabilitating in the case of the newcomers? Studies are lacking on this subject, but new observations are multiplying. It is a matter of keeping in mind the pre-migrational and migrational experiences of these people as well as the conditions of their welcome and installation in the host country. In fact the vicissitudes of living constitute the fragile psychosocial foundation which has a tendency to rapidly bring on somatizations and chronic pain when it is not taken into account in the medical and psychiatric treatment. These aspects cannot be treated separately from the cultural factors which reveal themselves in an inextricable imbrication with some social, political and judicial factors influencing their trajectory. The manner in which the immigrants conceive their problematic is also the fruit of the articulation of all the parameters of their living conditions in an individual, familial, and even a communal construction in which the cultural dimension cannot be isolated in any way. It is recognizable in the significations that the patients give to their pains and in the causes that they attribute to their illness. This construction of meaning is always dynamic and cannot be attributed to a culture abstractly localized outside of the person immigrating and who determines it. Immigration is a paradigmatic situation of the emergence of cultural interpersonal and intergroup reorganizational processes between an affirmation of their own postures and a critical position and a certain distanciation facing them [15].

Faced with an invalidated person and particularly if they are an immigrant, the professional made to take a part in the readaptation process finds themselves with different choices before them. Relative to that which we have evoked earlier, one can interact with the person on the bases of a single vision of the body and the suffering proposed by the dominating concept of the institution, which imposes on him the significations of medical science and the assimilation of the patient within that coherent ensemble that the doctors and nurses master. If not, they can move off centre from this biomedical horizon in order to leave room for the experiences of suffering linked to the accident, its causes, according to the meaning that the patient gives them.

There are no patients who have no knowledge or theory concerning their sufferance [28]. In the stories told by the immigrants that we have met, we notice three sensitive aspects in relationship to health and illness, relevant to this study of rehabilitation processes within the framework of immigration: the suffering linked simultaneously to the invalidity and to the physical and psychological pain, the perspective of healing or of recuperating to a state of health and employability as a consequence of that healing and the conditions of exercising a professional activity. The third aspect is particularly significative in the context which imposes on the immigrants an integration project principally in terms of access to work. This integrational approach is easily interiorised by the male immigrants themselves, who often feel responsible for creating the well-being of their family on their capacity to be able to meet their needs, in their own country as well as in exile. Let us take a detailed, bottom up, look at these three aspects.

Fragments of experiences
of invalidity within immigration

We realized through the interviews for assistance held with several immigrants in precarious situations that the men are significatively more active than the women on the professional level and in the search for employment. In the first generation immigrant family
models, one finds here many dichotomous conceptions of the division of work or the
roles within the family. Quite often, the man, feeling the responsibility for the subsistence
of the family, finds himself dishonoured by the fact that he is unable to meet their needs.
In fact, the precariousness of his rights to remain and of his status means, added to the
linguistic challenge, that the access to formation and to work is almost non existent, just
as recognition of his acquired competences in the host country, and that the accessible
work is the theatre of diverse forms of discrimination [14]. However, the large majority
of male immigrants aspire to work, whatever their status.

For the women, activity often proves to be more determining than the wages in their
motivation to work. The acculturation experience transforms their role of housewife,
lower in value and insufficient for permitting the dynamic equilibrium of the integration
process, in a multiplicity of roles and functions which renders the women more polyvalent. Through the impulsion often given by the women of the host country, with the goal
of permitting the women to play their role in the process of community integration [29],
a number of centres for immigrant women have been opened in Switzerland since the
beginning of the 1990s. Diverse activities going from language courses to activities of
benevolent occupations, right on through to diverse workshops from birth preparations,
sewing, or simply meeting places, permitting the women access to an autonomy more
rapid than the men, the moment the latter are confronted with exclusion from the job
market. In the case of refuge seekers, the proportion of women on the market is 20% to
40% for the men, which represents a third of the persons employed [30]. The number of
women exercising a professional activity outside of the home is then, proportionally to
the men, quite a bit higher than in numerous native countries and it is sometimes the
woman who works whereas the man stays at home in the exile situation. If the preceding
facts are not specifically cultural, it remains none the less a strong attack on the self-
esteem of a number of men for which the conception wants the man to be the bread
winner of the family. The acculturation process of the woman being reinforced by the
experience outside the home and more frequent contacts with her peers, the women
equally have more facility to question the models that ruled the couple before, which
brings about a double problematic. A distance inserts itself between the man and the
woman, through the differentiation of their activities, the woman emancipates herself
more and more from her former positions on the one hand. A second distance is born,
more painful still, from the fact that the man no longer has the same sociocultural and
intellectual resources for elaborating this new concept of the immigrant couple in society
on the other hand, a situation which can only be experienced as a loss and becoming
insecure on the identity level. It appears that the most direct means to put some balance
back into parts of this fragile elaboration consist, for the man, in finding a job [15]. In

the question of rehabilitation, the experience of professional inactivity is central, as a motivational and a non-motivational factor according to the situations: the more the invalidity is experienced as devaluating and dubious, markedly, the more the efforts of the health care professionals, nurses, risk in vain. What comes out, from the sum of the interviews held with the male immigrants in precarious positions, is that rehabilitation is strongly desired, within the immigrant population in general. Thus we take with some reserve the declarations made by some doctors according to whom the immigrant patients often show themselves as being resistant or uncooperative, preferring to consider these declarations from a more interactionist and contextual reader's angle.

Moving beyond employability, an important preoccupation of the immigrants is the recovery of health. In the case of migration, the feeling of security is weakened by social precarity. In this context, the results of an illness or an accident susceptible of becoming invalidating show themselves as being even more anxiety provoking as the necessary resources in professional and social integration are weak. Illness or accident quickly become the perfect opportunity for supplementary moral and psychological fragility which grow from the difficulty of the task. In VR one will win in therapeutic and communicational efficiency to inquire about the manner in which they are perceived by the immigrants, particularly when the linguistic capacity constitutes an obstacle in the formulation of questions on the patients' part. Numerous patients in the acculturation process have the caricatural perception of the biomedical system which limits itself to the doctor being the all powerful; they are often little prepared to seize the complexity of the therapeutical devices and the multiplicity of professional identities of the participants that they meet. For example, the intervention of psychiatrists or psychotherapists, who remain strongly linked with the negative connotations of psychiatric establishments, is often not understood and is often associated with the treatment of madness. Many of the immigrants refuse the psychotherapeutic consultation or have ashamed of it. Taking into consideration the EMIC discourse is then a necessary point of departure in these situations. The professional is then interested in the patient meanings which implies a moving off centre by which one will become conscious of the fact that the efficiency of the treatment depends strongly on the intercomprehension and of the sharing of the meaning of his intervention. The sharing of the significations contribute to restitute to the patient an expert competence about his own situation, to let him or her participate in the dialogue and to seize the potential resources in the manner that he or she has to understand and to explain what has happened to him or her.

To get to the source of the disabling event implies taking into consideration the manner in which the physical and psychological suffering is experienced and interpreted. The construction of the cause and meaning of the suffering and the means available to remedy it necessitates an intersubjective negociation between the person and the individual carers involved in the network. Outside that intersubjectivity, two dangers await: the risk that the sufferance be rationalized into categories of their own reflection in the world of care, or to the subjectivity of the carers, and the risk of enclosing the patient in a culturalized way than the one attributed to their sufferings, in the country or native region of the subject. The works in intercultural research bring into evidence a tendency for the professionals in the social and psychosocial fields to reify the culture of the immigrants [6] and to attribute to them intentions founded on stereotypes. This attitude consists in part of enclosing the person in a rigid and reductive culture and another part of isolating the culture from all other social, political, psychological and identity aspects from the immigrants', experiences.

The negociation has cultural implications, of course, but also social and interpersonal implications. The subjective relation of the patient with his illness is important in the perspective of rehabilitation in order to make room for the experience of the subject as a performative expression in complement to the built meaning in the biomedical model. It is the dimension of the experience of the loss of health, of autonomy which will become the object of the intervention in rehabilitation, in a way in which the subject is able to participate in the project with their willingness and subjective conscience. If one is not able to recognize one's self in the causes and the explanations furnished of their illness by the professionals or if they do not understand them, obviously it will be complicated to obtain their adhesion and their active participation in the treatments. The biomedical and functional aspects of the invalidity are not minimized by these considerations. The technical competences, the medical diagnosis and the physiotherapy work notably keeps all their validity. In fact, the technical nature of biomedicine constitutes a pledge of credibility and is the object of much hope for the majority of the immigrant patients that we have met. It is exactly at this point that the anthropologists and the medical and paramedical personnel must cross ways with their knowledge and approaches in order to prepare the ground on which the rehabilitation can germ and grow. This preparation implies for the patient a cognitive, affective and relational predisposition to enter actively into the therapeutic project and to invest themselves in it with whatever means they have. The defended postulate in this chapter is that this predisposition is reinforced if the meaning of the illness, its gravity, its consequences, the meaning of the interventions and the perspectives of healing are shared between the members of the medical and paramedical personnel and the patient, as difficult as the communication and the construction of common significations may be.

Acculturation

Every immigrant is caught in the movement and the strategies, sometimes contradictory and sometimes complementary, aiming at integrating new semantic and societal universes which conditions the effectuated experience in the host country. They consist, in general and when conditions permit, of maintaining as strong as possible a coherence between the belonging to the multiple horizons built through the experience of immigration and notably those relative to the participation in the sociocultural lifestyle of the host country. The manner in which they are articulated with the values and resources borrowed from the experience of enculturation in the native country influences considerably the success of this process, faced with the challenge of acquiring autonomy of thought, movement and of subsistence in the present situation. According to the pressures exerted by the politics of refuge and of integration on the immigrant populations on a macro-social level, the acculturation can take on different forms which are the results of weighty constraints on the subject and the strategies that these last put to work within their space of mobility to which they dispose. The access to training and to work, the financial precarity, the absence of rights and the insecurity are the factors restraining the acquisition of values, of significations and the adoption of social behaviour permitting evolution in the host society. They generate segregational conditions, even exclusion, when the stabilizing of practices and values borrowed from enculturation first in the "ghettoized"community is not possible [31]. The contextual identities generated have no equivalents which develop simultaneously in the native countries. They are the products of immigration and exile. They have maximum relevance in distress situations in which invalidity due to illness and to accidents is one of the penalizing forms in the migratory project.

The constructed resources by the immigrants within the process of acculturation play a central role in the process of rehabilitation, significantly in respect to the degree of security attained in the host society. The spoken and transmitted languages, the possibility of conserving some cultural and religious practices while acquiring new significations and the stability of the status and the authorization to stay are some of the central elements of the process. For the subject in rehabilitation, the fact that it concerns an ensemble of social and identity dynamics in which the attempts to follow through on one's life project is central. Thus we will be attentive to the manner in which the evolution of identities, the rearranging of the diverse memberships of the patient taking place within the framework of life in general and of the universe of values and of significations which organize them, so as to reduce the anxiety provoking character of the rehabilitation experience and to permit an elaboration of one's meaning, between the patient and the various intervenants of the medical team and the carers.

The doctors and the carers see their difficulties increase further still, when the statutory and political problematic of their patients is not well known or ignored. The intervention of interpreters or of cultural mediators does not resolve the problem, often linked to the disposition of the carers to recognize the personal and subjective universe of the patient as a central element of the therapeutic perspective. What becomes an obstacle in the ethnocentric apprehension of the hard of hearing, is the fact that the sense given by the immigrant subjects to their suffering is interpreted as a deviation [3] faced with the objective vision of the biomedical paradigme. It becomes a therapeutic resource when the carers integrate it in a complementary manner and accept to allow a displacement by a foreign meaning but this is also true for the patient and the medico-social institution, in the condition that the universe of significations of the patient be recognized in what is the coherence of the patient. This comes back to recognition of the person in their entirety and according to the meaning that they give to the events which shape their paths.

Subjectivity and social suffering

The development of local suffering towards more and more globalized forms is a world-wide phenomenon alimented by the consumerist logic of televised information [32]. From where we are, the show is non-threatening, being at once from a point of view geographically distant from the troubles. This brings with it a banalizing of the suffering of others and the dilution of the moral conscience which frees itself of its responsibility, when it meets the victims of these same events, in their country of destination, come to search for protection. They find themselves caught between the denial of the material and historical foundations of their suffering and the suspicion of abuse of hospitality which is more and more conditional. This aspect of the migratory shock makes for a painful experience on an asymmetrical foundation, placing the immigrants in a position of weakness. This distinguishes it from the "cultural shock" in its more generic dimension and founded on an experience of otherness outside all social hierarchies, case of the typically ideal figure extremely rare in the social reports. Between non-recognition of the effective reality of their experience in their homeland and restriction of rights and of autonomy in their host country, the immigrants develop a multitude of psychosomatic troubles as physical reactions to so many unsatisfactory responses to the living conditions imposed on them.

Social suffering engenders a mobilizing resistance to material and symbolic resources, the attitudes and behaviour of the subjects, in view of recreating a coherent system of explanation of their situation and the conditions of a rapid return to health. When the capacities of resistance are too strongly damaged, the chronic pain syndrome becomes the means of abandoning the struggle without losing face. Within the dynamic process of somatization which consists of expressing the moral and psychological pains, the subject avoids the subjective existential crisis and psychological downfall [15]. The physical pain is considered as exterior to oneself and does not affect identity, contrary to psychological pain which gives the sensation of madness and brings on a devaluation of one's self. As to what specifically concerns the practice of VR, the probability of recovering the capacity to work is approached by these strategies of psychological and identity survival. Moreover, the conditions for obtaining a work permit or refuge being more and more restrictive in the majority of the European countries, the medical certificate becomes, for some, the last recourse possible before the definitive return. We are observing now a tendency to research, through the diagnostic bias, the attestation of a legitimacy to remain in the host country, with the hopes of a stable permit sooner or later. For the immigrants for which the access to work is precarious, the VR constitutes even more so the risk of suffering a return more or less close than the perspective of earning their right to stay through the return of stable employment. These strategies drag some immigrants into "the fires of hell" from which they will not come out unharmed, sometimes depressive or even partially handicapped [33]. From the non-attribution of the status of political refugee to the impossibility of return for medical reasons, the recognition, by the doctors, of the objective dimension of the disease becomes the last possible means of obtaining assistance and recognition of the injustice and the pain that accompanies it.

More than the regularities that we might try to isolate in the observation of the person's origins from the diverse regions of the world, which becomes in fact the object of strong individual variability when taking a closer look at it, the situation generates as identity strategies which interest first the anthropologist. The emergence of these new identities of the psychosocial and professional precariousness in the context of immigration and the adaptative methods that they invent are unavoidable, within the challenge that constitutes the VR of the immigrants, victims of illness or accidents, in the normalization process of the practices and of the politics of public health.

Conclusion

It is through the development of resources and of solicited strategies through the structural and conditional aspects of the situations experienced in exile that we have envisioned their impact on the VR process. The therapeutic context precisely defines an ensemble of stakes and assigns the roles and the differentiated functions to the implicated actors. The rehabilitation of the person can only be completely understood in interdependance with the ensemble of social interrelations from which they play themselves out. This remark closes our voyage across the cultural dimension of VR, bringing to light that if immigration emphasizes the importance of communication within the relations, it indicates, in between the lines, that these reflections are valid for all interactions in readaptative situations and that the horizons of expectations of the patients and of the professionals necessitate some adjustments beyond national and linguistic appartenance. The professionals of rehabilitation are the transitional actors operating between the present sufferance of the patient and the recovered autonomy, between the suffering from it and the means not to suffer from it [34], between the inhibition and the action. The health care institutions have a tendency to protect themselves behind an ethnocentric vision of the dispensing of welcome and of aid to the latter [35]. The perspective of an intercession between the social situation and the political authority which decide the laws and of their application is the only form of receivable assistance, at the end of the chain of specialized interventions and the placement within the network. The consideration given to this daily tension and to its significations that the patients accord themselves is the first step necessary to the construction of a therapeutic perspective.

When the normalizing practices and politics of our institutions reject the allophonic persons or the petitioners of refuge in the register of radical otherness, the cultural factors add themselves to other dimensions as a source of insecurity and of supplementary exclusion, depriving the patients of psychological resources and necessary symbolics in the journey to rehabilitation. In treating the manifestation of otherness in their therapeutic care practices, with the requirement of a work of intercomprehension and of moving off centre from their own universe of significations and values, the professionals will opportunely create for themselves an apprenticeship the same as the subjects in rehabilitation.

References

1. Bischoff AN, Tonnerre C *et al.* (2000) Communication interculturelle et accès aux soins, le défi du multilinguisme dans le contexte médical. Les défis migratoires : actes du colloque CLUSE "Les défis migratoires à l'aube du troisième millénaire". P. Centlivres and I. Girod. Neuchâtel, Seismo: 395-401
2. Lombard J (1994) Introduction à l'ethnologie. Armand Colin, Paris
3. Alber J-L (2001) Penser les relations interculturelles : une perspective anthropologique. Normes proposées pour les cours de communication interculturelle, UNESCO Berne
4. Dubar C (1999) La socialisation : construction des identités sociales et professionnelles. Armand Colin, Paris
5. Rothenbühler I (à paraître) L'altérité pour les praticiens des thérapies complémentaires : enjeux de formation. Bulletin de l'ARIC
6. Abdallah-Pretceille M (1997) Du bon usage des malentendus culturels : pour une pragmatique de la culturalité. Revue suisse de sociologie 23(2): 375-388
7. Grondin J (1993) L'horizon herméneutique de la pensée contemporaine. J. Vrin, Paris
8. Rinaudo C (2000) Fêtes de rue, enfants d'immigrés et identité locale : enquête dans la région niçoise. Revue européenne des migrations internationales 16(2): 43-57
9. Simon P (2000) "L'invention de l'authenticité : Belleville, quartier juif tunisien". Revue européenne des migrations internationales 16(2): 9-41
10. Barth F (1969) Ethnic groups and bounderies. Little, Brown and Cie Boston
11. Tack S (1999) La réadaptation professionnelle des invalides pour quels objectifs? L'invalidité en souffrance. R. Darioli. Genève, Médecine & Hygiène: 87-92
12. Dasen PR (2001) Intégration, assimilation et stress acculturatif. Intégrations et migrations : regards pluridisciplinaires. C. Perregaux, T. Ogay, Y. Leanza and P. Dasen. Paris, L'Harmattan: 187-210
13. Swissinfo (2004) Contre le racisme, la Suisse doit faire davantage, Swissinfo
14. Dahinden J, Fibbi R *et al.* (2004) Integration am Arbeitsplatz in der Schweiz. Swiss Forum for Migration and Population Studies: 249, Neuchâtel 4.
15. Sabbioni M, Salis Gross C *et al.* (1999) Le traitement de la douleur chez les patients migrants : perspectives interdisciplinaires. L'invalidité en souffrance. R. Darioli. Genève, Médecine & Hygiène: 41-53
16. Herzer H (2000) Zunehmende Invalidisierung trotz medizinischem Fortschritt bei Schweizern und Ausländern. Schweizerische Ärztezeitung 81(47): 2668-72
17. Molinaro R (1994) Missbrauchen Ausländer die Unfallversicherung der Schweiz(er) ? Medizinische Mitteilungen(67): 12-7
18. Keel P, Perini C *et al.*, Eds. (1996) Chronifizierung von Rückenschmerzen: Hintergründe, Auswege: Schlussbericht des Nationalen Forschungsprogramms Nr. 26B. Eular, Basel
19. Thali A, Stern S *et al.* (2000). Die Rolle psychosozialer Faktorenbei protrahierten und invalidisierendenVerläufne nach Traumatisierungenim unteren Wirbelsäulebereich. Bulletin des médecins suisses 47: 2668-72
20. Weiss R (2003) Macht Migration krank ?: eine transdisziplinäre Analyse der Gesundheit von Migrantinnen und Migranten. Seismo, Zürich
21. Headland TN, Pike KL *et al.* (1990) Emics and etics: the insider – outsider debate. Sage, London

22. Kleinman A (1988) The illness narratives suffering and healing and the human condition. Basic Books, New York

23. Kleinmann A (1995) Pitch, picture, power: the globalization of local suffering and the transformation of social experience. Ethnos 60(3-4): 181-91

24. Weiss, MG (2001) Cultural epidemiology: an introduction and overview. Anthropology & medicine 8(1): 5-29

25. Suva (2001) Rapport annuel. Sion, Suva: 44

26. Chimienti M and Cattacin S (2001) Migration et santé : priorités d'une stratégie d'intervention : rapport de base d'une étude Delphi. Forum suisse pour l'étude des migrations, Neuchâtel

27. Rothenbühler I. (2002) Espace-Hommes. Une pédagogie du passage, du don et de la réciprocité. Regards croisés sur l'interculturalité. La pédagogie interculturelle en question. E. Abdel-Sayed. Chaumont, Initiales: 79-92

28. Young A (1982) The anthropologies of illness and sickness. Annual review of anthropology 11: 257-85

29. Hirsch G, Tschopp N (2002) Camarada, la maison des femmes exilées. SAVI, Genève

30. Piguet E, Ravel J-II (2002) Les demandeurs d'asile sur le marché du travail suisse : 1996 2000. Forum suisse pour l'étude des migrations et de la population, Neuchâtel

31. Berry JW (1989) Acculturation et adaptation psychologique. La recherche interculturelle. J. Retschitzki, Bossel-Lagos M. & Dasen PR. Paris, L'Harmattan: 135-45

32. Kleinmann A (1995) Writing at the margin: discourse between anthropology and medicine. University of California Press, Los Angeles

33. Salis Gross C (2002) Trauma und Medikalisierung : die Flüchtlingserfahrung in der Schweiz. Tsantsa 7: 22-30

34. Caloz-Tschopp M-C (à paraître) Quand la pratique bouscule la théorie ; un apport de la philosophie à la formation et la recherche interculturelle. Les approches interculturelles et interlangagières entre savoirs issus de la recherche et savoirs d'expérience : une interculturalité nécessaire ? C. Perregaux, P. Dasen and Y. Leanza. De Boeck Bruxelles

35. De Jonckheere C, Bercher D (2003) La question de l'altérité dans l'accueil psychosocial des migrants. IES Ed Genève

Functional Capacity Evaluation (FCE)[1]

M. Oliveri

Introduction

In the case of the persistent pain and/or disability due to illness injury, diagnoses often correlate poorly with physical performance capacity. As early as 1959, David Mechanic made the often quoted statement: *"Illness and disability vary independently"* [1]. The cause of different extents of impairment (diagnosis, clinical findings), activity (functional performance) and participation (occupational and social integration) according to ICF classification [2] is to be found in the complex interaction of the processes of physical adaptation and mental habituation as well as the influence of contextual factors. As a result, the judgement of work-related performance capacity mainly based on clinical findings and diagnoses is problematic in many cases. Likewise, self-estimation of physical abilities of patients suffering from chronic pain and disability is often no longer based on reality or is not reliable, in particular if they were absent from work for a longer period. An ergonomic assessment based on work-simulation tests (e.g. lifting and carrying, elevated work, step ladder climbing, etc.) allows a more realistic and reliable judgement of work-related physical performance capacity. Since the 1970s, such assessment systems for work-related functional capacity evaluation (FCE) have been developed. A comprehensive overview can be found in the work by Innes and King [3, 4, 5], guidelines have been described by Hart [6].

Basic aspects of test methods and the significance of evaluated capacity profiles

Psychophysical performance tests

In 1969, Snook described the *psychophysical* evaluation method [7]. The dual notion "psychophysical" expresses the fact that a subjective maximum performance not only

---

1. This chapter has been adapted from Oliveri M: Arbeitsbezogene funktionelle Leistungsfähigkeit. In: Lendenwirbelsäule. Ursachen, Diagnostik und Therapie von Rückenschmerzen. Edited by J. Hildebrandt, G. Müller et M. Pfingsten. © 2005 Elsevier Gmblt, Urban & Fischer Verlag München.

depends on physical, but also on psychological factors such as willingness to perform and tolerance for strain or pain due to maximal effort. In a psychophysical test, the end point is determined by the moment when the test person breaks off the test, either as a result of tiredness or complaints or when the maximal test time per load level can no longer be maintained. Functional respectively ergonomic criteria for performance limits are not taken into account. This limits the significance of the maximum performance measured for the following reasons:

In the case of low load tolerance due to psychological reasons, test persons will break off a test prematurely by themselves, i.e. before an observable ergonomic performance limit has been reached. Particularly, the subjective physical stress tolerance of people with chronic pain usually is much lower than what could be expected from a somatic-functional point of view, due to symptom magnification and avoidance behaviour [8, 9].

In contrast, very performance-oriented subjects tends to overdo things and to tolerate a further load progression even when their ergonomic performance limit has already been exceeded or an ergonomic and safe test performance is no longer guaranteed. This can lead to longer lasting acute pain episodes, particularly if the subject already had back problems before [10].

Kinesiophysical performance tests

In the work process or in a work-oriented rehabilitation, not primarily maximum psychophysical performance, but daily safe and ergonomic performance of any work or exercise activities is required. A physical test procedure should thus provide information on ergonomic limits of performance. In addition, particularly when assessing clients with chronic pain and disability for a medico-legal purpose, self-limitation should be recognised using plausible criteria, in order to permit a fair judgement of work-related physical capacity (in comparison with disabled subjects showing a good effort), and to avoid unjustified pension payments.

These concerns were the starting point for the development of an alternative test procedure. In *kinesiophysical* performance tests [11, 12], it is not the test person who subjectively sets the performance limits, but the examiner observes the test person during the progressive load levels of a test and evaluates the load at each level on the basis of standardised ergonomic observation criteria (Table 2) as *light, medium, heavy or maximum*. The comprehensive observation in different test situations also allows well-founded statements on effort (willingness to perform) and consistency.

The observing method that focus on safe and ergonomic performance is also linked to an important psychological aspect of a work-oriented assessment: many clients are afraid of movements and physical activity because of pain or fear of increase in pain or even harm, which has a negative effect on their effort and test performance. To support their willingness to perform, test persons are therefore informed during the tests that the safety of test performance is being very carefully monitored and that the test will be stopped as soon as this can no longer be guaranteed. If necessary, an explanation is also given as to why a difference should be made between function and pain: "*Chronic pain is an unpleasant companion, but not a measure of the body's ability to function safely – a certain physical per-formance is possible despite pain and also beneficial in order to avoid permanent disability and restore function in daily life."* Thanks to such test management, the evaluation often has also a certain therapeutic effect in that initially self-limiting persons find out in the course of the tests that they can actually perform better than they had supposed.

Prerequisites for quality and reliability of kinesiophysical tests are good education and the experience of the examiner in terms of ergonomic observation criteria. It is also important for the examiner to have received medical education (physio- or ergothera-pist) to ensure that the functional observations can be correctly interpreted in connec-tion with the medical findings [6].

Extrapolation of the test results into the physical capacity during a working day

One important step when evaluating the test results is the extrapolation of the observa-tion during the relatively short time of a test into the client's physical capacity during a 8-hour working day. This extrapolation is based, firstly, on the principles of sports and occupational medicine and, secondly, on the DOT classification of work (Dictionary of Occupational Titles) [13]. This means for instance for lifting:

A load that is *light* for the test person can be lifted *very frequently* while a *very heavy* load can only be lifted *rarely*.

In psychophysical tests, the entire extrapolation is based only on the reached maxi-mum performance. In kinesiophysical tests, *light* means that no signs of effort are observed (Table 2), thus no particular fatigue is to be expected if the task should be per-formed frequently during a working day. In contrast, *maximum (very heavy)* means the observation that maximum effort was needed to perform the task (Table 2), thus rapid onset of fatigue is to be expected in the case of many repetitions. In the DOT classifica-tion (slightly modified), the following frequencies or duration of working tasks during a normal working day are defined: *rarely* = 5% (up to 1/2 hour), *occasionally* = 5-33% (1/2 to 3 hours), *frequently* = 34-66% (3 to 51/2 hours), *continuously (very frequently)* = 67-100% (5 1/2 to 8 hours). According to this classification, a very heavy load should not be handled more than 30 minutes during the day (altogether), a light load, however, can be handled more or less the whole day (in a usual work rhythm with usual breaks). Also the evaluations for the middle categories *occasionally* and *frequently* are derived from the observation protocol in most of the tests. In the extrapolation of other test results such as endurance for elevated work, normative reference data based on investigations of S. Isernhagen are taken into consideration [11, 14].

Working reality and standardised work-related tests

Of course, the evaluation of a real work performance in a company or in a vocational training centre would be the most reliable method. However, this would take a lengthy period of time and could also not be done in many companies. In addition, a specific work evaluation in a certain professional activity provides too little information on general work-related physical capacity and suitability for any work on the labour market. For these reasons, an assessment using work-simulation tests is beneficial. An assessment of this type should contain a *set of relevant, work-related key functions*, which are *as realistic as possible but standardised and not too specific*. This contradiction cannot be fully solved: the more realistically the tests are intended to represent specific job requirements, the more specific tests should be included in the set of tests, which would rapidly exceed the limit of what is feasible. However, if we work for practical reasons with a limited number of standardised "laboratory tests", we are moving a little away from reality. For example, there is more or less a major *difference between* the test *lifting a box with weights* and the real *material handling in the workplace* – possibly important additional factors such as large volume or bulkiness of the load, difficult to grip, uneven or slippery flooring are not shown in the test. Aggravating factors like these must be taken into consideration, based on the experience of the examiner or based on supplementary work-specific tests, when judgements are made regarding specific material handling in the work place. Of course, this restricts validity of judgement to a certain extent, but this problem is inherent to all standardised work-related assessment systems.

Also *Motivation*, which is a result of differently acting mental factors, can vary a lot between the test situation and working reality and thus may falsify the judgements based on the results of the test observation in terms of physical performance capacity at the workplace.

The *overall duration of the tests* is also relevant. The aspect of working endurance should be appropriately evaluated in any case even if the working reality can only be simulated to an approximate degree. Beside the quantitative test results, a lengthy test period also makes it possible to acquire many observations as well as verbal and non-verbal expressions by the client and thereby examine the consistency of the surveys.

In order to evaluate the *daily reproducibility of performance* required at work, the tests should take place on two successive days and, in particular, the lifting tests repeated on the second day. In the case of patients with non-specific back pain, it is true that Reneman [15] found a high correlation for the lifting and carrying tests with test repeats on two successive days. Experience shows, however, that in some cases the performance on the second day can no longer be reproduced due to longer-lasting irritation symptoms that appeared with latency after the first test day. In cases like these, it is not permissible to rely on the better test results of the first day for judgement of the physical capacity. In contrast, it occasionally happens that client's performance on the second day is better, because, after his or her test experience on the first day, he or she gains more trust in his or her body and thus partially overcome self-limitation.

Another blur comes from the above-mentioned *method of extrapolating the test results* into the physical capacity during an entire working day. It is not known with accuracy, which bandwidth for the assumptions of such extrapolation can be considered reliable.

Due to the restrictions mentioned, judgements in a standardised work-oriented assessment can only be considered as the best possible approximation of working reality (in the sense of the best possible probability).

Relevant characteristics of assessment systems for work-related physical performance capacity

The currently most important assessment methods established in Europe for work-related performance capacity are the *PILE lifting test* (Progressive Isoinertial Lifting Evaluation) [16] and, in particular, the comprehensive systems *Functional Capacity Evaluation according to Isernhagen* (FCE) [11] and the *ERGOS work simulator* [17]. The *BTE work simulator* and the more recent unit *E-Link* were primarily designed for the functions of the upper extremities. Other assessment systems such as ARCON, Blankenship, ErgoScience, EPIC, KEY, Lido, etc. are barely present in Europe and therefore only mentioned here. Further information on them can be obtained from Innes [3] and King [5]. The IMBA system (vocational integration of people with disabilities) is a superordinated profile comparison system, into which the data of different assessment systems can be integrated. Some important characteristics for the comprehensive assessment systems are discussed below using FCE and ERGOS[2] as typical examples.

Test methods
In the kinesiophysical test procedure (FCE), maximum physical performance capacity is evaluated using standardised observation criteria. This valuation procedure is more complex in comparison to psychophysical test methods but, as mentioned, provides more information on ergonomic load limits and their functional causes as well as on any non-organic barriers. Test monitoring that is based on careful observation by the examiner and the associated extensive communication with the client during the tests also promote their cooperation and willingness to perform. In the psychophysical test procedure, that is machine controlled in the case of ERGOS, the end point of the tests corresponds to the maximum achieved by the test person. A test observation by the examiner also takes place, but this does not have the same significance as with FCE.

Standardisation and flexibility
The compactly built and computerised workstation with the full installation of all test elements as well as machine-audiovisual test instructions (ERGOS) results in a high degree of standardisation and methodical reliability. The primary evaluation of the test data acquired is automatic. For the job match, i.e. the comparison between job (demands of work) profile and physical capacity profile, a large database containing thousands of job profiles is available. However, the following disadvantages must be stated: the data-

---

2. As some improvements have been introduced in Germany for the use of ERGOS compared with the description provided by the American company, the information is based on current practice in Germany.

base with the job profiles comes from the USA. A large number of these profiles are only applicable to a limited degree to European workplaces; this applies in particular to workplaces in small and medium-sized companies that are very common in European countries. In addition, these profiles are not continuously updated in line with the rapidly changing occupational world. Retrieved ERGOS profiles can be modified to a limited degree: some features such as weight or frequency of a working process can be adapted to a specifically obtained job profile of a single case. However, additional features cannot be entered. The consequence of this is that occupational features of relevance for the work concerned in connection to relevant functional deficits of a client may not be able to be taken into account in the ERGOS job match. The validity of the profile comparisons is thus in question. Also at legal level, a Swiss court, for example, would not accept a judgement of work ability that is based on a job match between the test person's physical capacity and a job profile from the USA (without proof that this corresponds to a comparable workplace in the client's region). It must also not be forgotten that a test machine with audiovisual on-screen instructions designed typically for industrial production is, from the design aspect, not necessarily suited to the evaluation of an immigrant employed in a gardening company with low linguistic and poor reading skills. In contrast, the more flexible test system FCE with somewhat less standardised devices and defaults offers better possibilities for addressing the specific properties of the test persons and of workplaces. The relevant job requirements are in each case specifically acquired and integrated into the profile comparison whereby standard job descriptions can be used as "raw material". If necessary, the standardised FCE tests are supplemented with work-specific tests. One disadvantage must, of course, be noted here in that the methodical reliability of FCE is largely linked to the education and experience of the examiners due to the evaluation being based on observation criteria and to the flexibility of the test application.

Transparency

A further important point is the possibility to comprehend the results and judgements. In the case of automated data analysis (ERGOS), the impression is gained of a "black box", as the programmed defaults and rules of the analysis are barely known to the users. The results thus do not appear to be transparent to the recipients of the report (insurance company administrators, rehabilitation professionals, lawyers, etc.). The plausibility of the assessment cannot be checked as with a simple and open test and evaluation system (FCE). ERGOS also appears to be less transparent and realistic to the clients than FCE, for example, with simulated lifting on a measuring machine in comparison with the realistic free lifting of boxes containing weights.

Expense

The equipment for FCE is simple and inexpensive. ERGOS is, however, a sophisticated work simulator with very high acquisition costs and considerable annual costs for updates and maintenance. In addition, the dependence on one single company must be considered a disadvantage.

Test duration and examination of reproducibility on the following day
FCE tests last a total of 5-6 hours, ERGOS tests take 4-5 hours (excluding the time for evaluations and reports). FCE is a two day procedure to evaluate reproducibility of performance, in particular of the lifting tests.

Effort rating
The significance of the test results regarding judgment of physical capacity is highly dependent on the effort of the test person. Therefore, the assessment of effort and consistency is a very important component of a work-related assessment *(cf. § [Evaluation of effort and consistency])*. An evaluation of this type is done both with FCE as well as with ERGOS.

Interdisciplinarity
Close cooperation between doctor and therapist for the assessment and reporting is vital since the reports often have the status of medical expertise. It is not only a question of combining knowledge and findings from different specialist fields: as a Swiss Federal Appeal Court judge recently stated at a conference, interdisciplinarity is also an important correction factor for the inevitable subjectivity of the individual examiner (influences exerted by personal values, sympathy/antipathy). Interdisciplinarity is considered highly important both with FCE as well as with ERGOS; the type of cooperation between doctor and therapist is, however, different in practice among users of both systems.

Role of clinical findings and diagnoses
While the diagnoses or clinical findings are not a criterion as such for physical capacity judgement, they provide – as background information – references concerning the plausibility of restrictions. They are sometimes also important for the judgement for prognosis regarding physical capacity, e.g. when a future deterioration is probably to be expected due to medical experience with a given diagnosis, or when the occupational stress should be reduced to prevent any further deterioration. The clinical findings in terms of mobility and strength also serve in the cross-comparison with observations made during the activity tests (evaluation of consistency). The clinical background of the examiners is guaranteed both with FCE as well as with ERGOS.

The kinesiophysical test procedure, in particular, permits an evaluation of the relevance of clinical findings for daily and work activities: the detailed observation of body functions during the tests clarifies to what extent different clinical diagnoses/findings (in cases of several disorders) really are limiting the activities. This is particularly important if assessment of functional limitations due to different disorders (e.g. sequels of different injuries) is required for medico-legal reasons. Furthermore, lifting, for example, as a stress for nearly all body parts (legs, trunk and neck area, arms, circulation) offers the doctor or therapist an excellent possibility of analysing in an easy way different body functions in action respectively under gradually increased stress and thus observing functional findings that supplement substantially the usual clinical investigation. From this, relevant functional goals for rehabilitation may be derived.

Quality assurance
Reliability of the assessment is only guaranteed by good praxis of well-trained and experienced examiners. A quality assurance system for the users has been established both for the FCE system as well as for ERGOS.

Areas of use
A study by the Federation of German Pension Insurance Institutes (VDR) and IQPR (Institute for Quality Assurance in Prevention and Rehabilitation, German Sport University, Cologne) of FCE or ERGOS using facilities in Germany revealed that FCE is primarily used for the clarification of functional performance in general as well as for the assessment of suitability for the previous job and secondarily for the judgements on generic physical capacity with regards to the labour market; ERGOS, however, is primarily used for the clarification of suitability for certain activities in general as well as in the field of vocational reorientation and secondarily for the clarification of suitability for the previous job. In Switzerland, FCE is still required mainly for judgement of generic physical capacity (for medico-legal purposes). This means that FCE is, with the exception of the FCE assessment integrated into a work-hardening program, (unfortunately) not used most often to support a return to work. FCE or part of it has proved to be of optimum value as assessment within a work-hardening program: Some tests such as lifting or carrying can be taken over directly as a training element. In addition, the kinesiophysical viewpoint is very helpful for monitoring the exercises in strength and work-simulation training.

PILE test (Progressive Isoinertial Lifting Evaluation)

The PILE test [16, 18, 19] can be called the classic psychophysical lifting test. A lower and upper lifting test (0-75 cm or 75-135 cm height) is carried out. With successive increase in loads at a fixed increment (men 5 kg, women 2.5 kg), clients lift the box with the weights four times per load level for a maximum of 20 seconds until they break off the test. Apart from a maximum weight limit of 55 to 60% of body weight and a heart-frequency limit of 85% of the maximum heart rate (appropriate for the patient's age), there are no criteria for breaking off the test. In the PILE test, people willing to perform often lift substantially more than would be permissible from an ergonomic viewpoint according to the criteria of the kinesiophysical observation. Within a pre-employment test for healthy candidates for a job as ambulance man, a comparative test evaluation of the lower psychophysical PILE test[3] and of the kinesiophysical FCE lifting test was carried out at the Bellikon rehabilitation clinic. 137 people (62% men and 38% women) were examined. The average of the maximum weights lifted was 28.9 kg in the FCE test and 43.3 kg in the PILE test. The correlation coefficient between the two tests was 0.58. In the PILE

---

3. Due to the high physical demands for ambulance officers regarding lifting, the test limit of maximum lifting weight and maximum heart rate not used for the young and healthy subjects (verified by a health check by questionnaire), and the increment of 5 kg was also set for women.

test, 50% more weight on average was thus lifted than in the FCE test. The result of the higher load values in the psychophysical PILE test in comparison to the kinesiophysical FCE lifting test is also corresponding to an unpublished study by I. Farag (1995) [4]. However, we assume that a load tolerance that is so much higher (50%) in comparison to the observable ergonomic load limit will only be found among healthy and highly motivated test persons (they all wanted the job). As no ergonomic observation criteria are set for breaking off the PILE test, various non-ergonomic techniques such as swinging the load in order to lift a weight that was already too heavy (from an ergonomic standpoint) were frequently observed. Nevertheless, the PILE test can be considered fairly safe, which is probably due to the gradual and slow progression of the load. In the project 26B of the Swiss National Foundation for Research [10], no acute or long-lasting increase in complaints in the PILE test was observed also with people with chronic back pain. A test is naturally only a single event, and the hypothesis from an ergonomic viewpoint would be as follows: in the case of daily exposure to loads corresponding to the psychophysically established maximum (much higher than the ergonomically evaluated one), impairments would occur more frequently in the long run.

Functional capacity evaluation (FCE) according Isernhagen

The FCE system developed in the USA by S. Isernhagen [www.isernhagen.com] [11, 14], was introduced in 1991 by M. Oliveri and M. L. Hallmark Itty in Switzerland [www.sar-rehab.ch → Who is who → Interessengemeinschaften → IG Ergonomie] and later from there also in Germany [www.efl-akademie.de], Austria, Lithuania. It is also in use in the Netherlands and in Ireland. The FCE system according to Isernhagen includes a test battery with 29 standardised functional performance tests (Table 1, figs. 1-3), supplemented by a survey in terms of physical job requirements, self-perception of abilities in the PACT Spinal Function Sort test (*cf. § [PACT Spinal Function Sort (self-perception of physical abilities)]*) and pain. Sometimes, additional work-specific tests are also required for certain work activities such as highly repetitive work cycles or working in long-lasting static postures. Besides the quantitative load values, effort, consistency and pain behaviour are also

Table 1 – Test elements in the FCE according to Isernhagen.

Handling loads/strength	*Posture/Flexibility*	*Ambulation*
Floor to waist lift	Elevated work	Walking
Waist to overhead lift	Forward bending sitting/standing	Stair climbing
Horizontal lift	Rotation sitting/standing	Step ladder climbing
Push/pull	Crawl/kneel/crouch-deep static	Balance
Right/left carry	Repeated squat	*Hand coordination*
Front carry	*Static work*	Right/left hand coordination
Right/left grip strength	Sitting/standing tolerance	

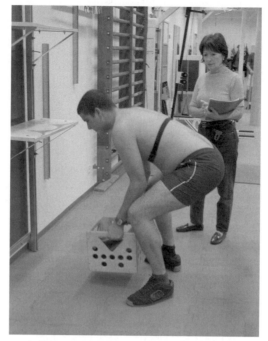

Fig. 1 – FCE: Floor to waist lift.

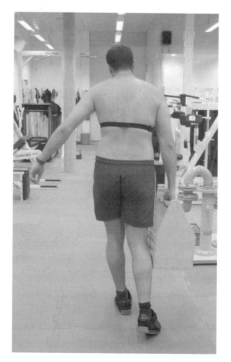

Fig. 2 – FCE: Right carry.

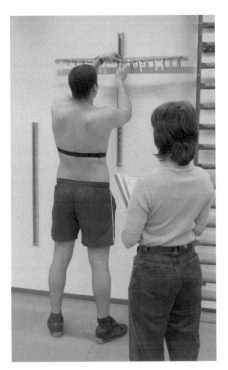

Fig. 3 – FCE: Elevated work.

evaluated *(cf. § [Evaluation of effort and consistency])*. The tests are carried out by trained physio- or ergotherapists.

Procedure using observation criteria with the lifting test as an example

The lifting and carrying tests are performed using a box filled with weighted bags of 2.5 kg or 5 kg. The individual load levels *light* to *maximum* are established with the observation criteria (Table 2) in about 5 to 6 tested progressive load levels (without fixed increment). In order to allow the observation of the muscle recruitment pattern and the stabilisation of the body parts under load, the clients are stripped to the waist (women with bras), and wear shorts during the test. When the point is reached at which the ergonomic and safe test performance turns into one that is no longer ergonomic or safe (e.g. unsafe handling, inability to stabilise properly, using swing techniques for lifting, avoiding certain movements or doing false movements, trembling of the muscles), the test is stopped by the examiner even if the test person would be ready to continue. Sometimes, a clearly recognisable deterioration of the clinical findings (e.g. increased pain radiation into the leg) must also be taken as a criterion for the maximum tolerated load. If, on the other hand, the test person breaks off one or several tests prematurely despite explanation and encouragement, this is recognised and noted down as a self-limitation.

Table 2 – Standardised ergonomic observation criteria for lifting and carrying.

	Light	Medium to heavy	Maximum
Muscles recruitment	Only prime movers (quadriceps, trunk stabilisers, biceps, hand grip)	Beginning to pronounce recruitment of accessory muscles (neck flexors, upper trapezius, deltoids, rhomboids)	Bulging of accessory muscles (neck flexors, upper trapezius, deltoids, rhomboids)
Base of support	Natural stance (hip wide)	Stable to wider base	Very solid base
Posture	Upright posture	Beginning to increased counter balancing	Marked counter balance
Control and safety	Easy movement patterns	Smooth movements to using a slight impetus	Still safe but unable to maintain control if any more weight is added
Pace	Fast movement possible	A little to clearly slower, cautious	Very slow, no longer controlled with faster movement
Circulation, breathing	Minimal increase in heart rate	Slight to greater increase in heart rate* and respiration	Substantial increase in heart rate and respiration

* An increase in pulse rate at loads that are still low should sometimes also be interpreted as a sign of an increased vegetative pain reaction

The evaluation of tests in respect of postures, flexibility and ambulation is based on comparable observation criteria, with the tolerated duration, number of repetitions or distance to be used as a measure.

Physical capacity profile and job match

The extrapolated values for physical abilities in relation to a normal working day are shown in a physical capacity profile. Table 3 contains the values of a 50-year-old sawmill worker, showing a good effort, with chronic back complaints after previous lumbar herniated disk operation, recurrent disk herniation for 1 1/2 years and beginning hip-joint osteoarthritis on both sides. For horizontal lift, for example, a weight up to 10 kg was evaluated as light, the weight of 40 kg as a maximum, this leads to the following extrapolation: 10 kg can be handled continuously (very frequently) 40 kg rarely.

Based on the physical capacity profile (Table 3), the generic significant abilities and deficits (without reference to a specific job) are summarised in the report. If a job is available, the job description and profile respectively, the critical job demands are explored (cf. § [Job

Table 3 – FCE form: Physical capacity profile (selection of tests)

Duration of load per 8 hrs	Never	Rarely	Occasionally	Frequently	Continuosly	Limit, comments, observations
Strength (kg, kp)						
Floor to waist lift		30	22.5	15	7.5	Strength limit of the back
Horizontal lift		40	30	20	10	Ditto
Pull		42	30	20	10	Ditto
Posture/flexibility						
Forward bending standing				X		Can only straighten up again with difficulty
Kneeling		X				Limited hip extension prevents an upright working posture, hip pain
Standing tolerance				X		Restless, constant weight shifting on the right/on the left. Hip pain and pain radiation into the left leg
Ambulation						
Walking				X		Not a problem on even floor, difficulties when walking uphill and downhill
Additional work specific test						
Standing, forward-bending with a weight of 10 kg		X				Obvious fatigue can be observed, pain radiation into the left leg

description (job profile) and sociodemographic data]). The job match (comparison of the job profile and the physical performance profile) for the sawmill worker is given in Table 4.

ERGOS

Developed in the USA, the ERGOS work simulator [Work recovery / www.simwork.com] was first introduced in Europe in the Netherlands and from there in Germany since 1995 [17]. For the machine-based tests, a compactly built work simulator of industrial-style design is available with 5 units:

  unit 1: Static and dynamic lifting, pushing and pulling (fig. 4);
  unit 2: Full-body flexibility;
  unit 3: Work endurance, carrying;
  unit 4: Standing and walking tolerance, forward bending;
  unit 5: Sitting tolerance.

Table 4 – Job match (FCE according to Isernhagen [11]).

Critical job demands	Physical capacities (according to tests)	Requirement fulfilled?
Putting boards (60 to 100 kg) on the saw table (lifting at least on one side to do this) – frequently on some days	Horizontal lift frequently up to 20 kg (rarely up to of 40 kg)	No
Loading beams (up to 25 kg) onto a truck – occasionally	Floor to waist lift occasionally up to 22.5 kg (rarely up to of 30 kg)	Yes
Long standing and frequent walking	Without problems	Yes
Operating a nailer with body leaning forward – frequently	Clear restriction for forward-bending posture, in particular, with additional holding of weight; only rarely	To some extent
Kneeling – rarely	Rarely possible	Yes
Pulling a loaded trolley (pull strength up to 60 kp) – rarely (one can put less load on the trolley but then more time is required)	Pulling rarely a maximum of 42 kg	To some extent

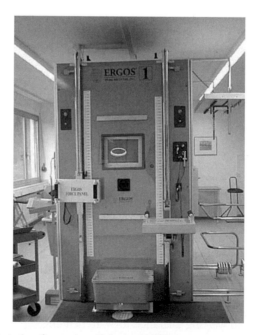

Fig. 4 – ERGOS: Test station for static and dynamic lifting.

The key functions such as lifting, carrying, elevated work, etc. correspond largely to those of the FCE. Some functions such as lifting are, however, structured in greater detail, and additional elements can also be found in the field of hand functions. Apart from the different testing principle, the extrapolation of the test results and description of abilities and deficits are basically comparable with the FCE system. In comparison to FCE, the quantification of the individual functions is more detailed with ERGOS, although the systematic observation of reactions to the test loads and the recognisable functional restrictions, of performance behaviour as well as consistency are less strongly weighted. Table 5 contains an extract from an ERGOS evaluation. ERGOS users in Germany emphasise that the assessment in the ERGOS report or expertise is not only based on the primary automatic evaluation by the system but also takes into account the observations during the tests and the medical assessment.

Table 5 – ERGOS evaluation (extract).

Type of workload	Occasionally		Frequently		Continuously	
	kg	hours	kg	hours	kg	hours
Static lift to ...						
height of metacarpus	38 (22)	8+ (8)	19 (12)	8+ (8)	7 (5)	8+ (8)
height of bench	22 (15)	8+ (8)	11 (8)	8+ (8)	5 (4)	8+ (8)
height of ankle	25 (17)	8+ (8)	13 (8)	8+ (8)	6 (4)	8+ (8)
height of shoulder	16 (17)	8+ (8)	8 (8)	8+ (8)	3 (4)	8+ (8)
Dynamic lifting to...						
height of bench, left-hand	*19 (23)*	8+ (8)	*10 (12)*	8+ (8)	5 (6)	8+ (8)
height of bench, front	*19 (23)*	8+ (8)	*10 (12)*	8+ (8)	5 (6)	8+ (8)
height of bench, right-hand	*19 (23)*	8+ (8)	*10 (12)*	8+ (8)	5 (6)	8+ (8)
height of shelf, left-hand	15 (11)	8+ (8)	6 (6)	8+ (8)	3 (3)	8+ (8)
height of shelf, front	15 (11)	8+ (8)	6 (5)	8+ (8)	3 (3)	8+ (8)
height of shelf, right-hand	15 (11)	8+ (8)	6 (5)	8+ (8)	3 (3)	8+ (8)
Reaching						
forward		8+ (8)		8 ( )		6 (8)
overhead		8+ (8)		8 ( )		5 (8)
bended repeatedly		8+ (8)		(8)		(8)
Grip strength ...						
on the right	34.2 kg (28 kg)					
on the left	8,2 kg (28 kg)		*very easy* work			

Italicised print = deficits; Figures in () = Job requirements

BTE and E-Link

For quite some time, the *BTE simulator* [Baltimore Therapeutic Equipment, USA / www.bteco.com] has been used in hand rehabilitation centres, in particular for the evaluation of upper extremity functions, whereby an examination of general work-related functions is also possible. The system consists of a computer and an exercise head onto which different tools such as a gripper, a steering wheel, differently sized levers or screw-driver handles or a cable system for the performance of a lifting test can be attached. The exercise head produces an adjustable resistance and measures performance. BTE has proved to be valuable both as a test unit as well as a training unit in the field of hand rehabilitation.

The *E-Link* unit [Biometrics, UK / www.biometricsltd.com] has recently come onto the market. Substantially smaller than the BTE unit, this device also permits the computerised measurement of hand and finger strength as well as the flexibility of all the hand joints. Various levers and handles as well as a small force plate can also be attached. The interesting thing about E-Link is that videogames can be operated by all the connectable tools - according to the goal of the test or the treatment, the control system works more with the strength used or with movement (such as, for example, pronation/supination). Further meaningful applications are also found for coordinative and cognitive disorders, or as entertaining training of sitting tolerance, for example for patients with back pain.

Surveys within the of work-oriented assessment

Job description (job profile) and sociodemographic data

If the assessment is to refer to the previous workplace, the job profile (physical job demands) must also be evaluated. A suitable basis for this is a structured survey of the client in the following fields:

 – job designation, tasks and working procedures;
 – lifting and carrying heavy loads, handling tools requiring physical effort;
 – repetitive activities;
 – postures, static loads;
 – locomotion;
 – special aspects (e.g. working clothes or protective equipment, special tools, particular exposures);
 – general information on the company and work organisation.

This evaluation should also record duration or frequency of certain jobs or work cycles. An alternative suitable grid for the job description is given by Laurig [20]. We are aware that the reliability of the client's information on his or her job requirements is not always satisfactory, particularly in the case of clients with questionable willingness to work and consistency. In the case of uncertain data, additional information is requested from the employer. Sometimes, a job description put together by a case manager of the insurance company is also available. If necessary, an on-site workplace evaluation in the company may be arranged in addition to the physical performance tests. As the method for workplace assessment, a Finnish system has proved valuable [21]. For a comprehensive work-oriented assessment, some sociodemographic data such as the current job situation and working ability, the duration of absence from work, the pension situation, school and vocational education as well as the family situation should also be collected.

PACT Spinal Function Sort (self-perception of physical abilities)

The client's self-perception of their own physical abilities controls their willingness to perform work and activities. In the case of symptom magnification, clients substantially underestimate their physical abilities and will thus limit their activity level to a substantial degree. However, overestimating their own abilities is also problematic with respect to the potential risk for (re)injuries. It is therefore very informative to compare the self-perception of abilities prior to physical tests with the test results, and to evaluate self-perception once again after the physical tests (learning effect using the experience of the performance testing?). The PACT Spinal Function Sort [22, 23] has proved to be a particularly suitable tool for measuring self-perception of the own abilities. This assessment system consists of a test book with 50 pictures of working or everyday activities (fig. 5). For each of the 50 pictures, the client marks on a separate evaluation sheet (Table 6) whether he or she feels *able* (=1) or *unable* (=5) to perform the task, or if performance is rated *slightly* (=2), *moderately* (=3) or *substantially* (=4) *restricted*.

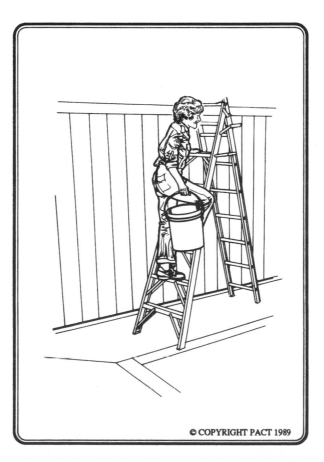

© COPYRIGHT PACT 1989

Fig. 5 – PACT Spinal Function Sort: Carrying a 10 kg bucket up a step-ladder.

Table 6 – Spinal function form (two sample items).

	Possible	Restricted	Impossible	?
18. Hammer nails	① 2 3 4		5	?
38. Carrying a 10 kg bucket up a step-ladder	1 2 ③ 4		5	?

One of the substantial advantages of the PACT assessment is its clear orientation towards physical abilities (the word "pain" is not to be found anywhere) as well as the information transfer using pictures, which makes it far easier to use with clients with lower levels of education and/or poor language ability. In the analysis, the PACT Spinal Function Sort score is calculated (0-200) and compared with the classification of physical demand level according to the DOT classification [13] (Table 7). The PACT test is used on a standard basis with FCE.

Table 7 – Interpretation of the PACT Spinal Function Sort index in terms of physical demand levels.

Physical demand level (DOT)	(Maximum) occasional load	PACT index
Mainly sedentary	Up to 5 kg	100-110
Light	5-10 kg*	125-135
Medium	10-25 kg	165-175
Heavy	25-45 kg	180-190
Very heavy	> 45 kg	> 195

* Supplementary criteria: or either with substantial share of walking or standing; or mainly sitting, but arm or foot control functions required

Pain survey

A pain drawing and pain measurement scale are meaningful on the 1st and 2nd test day before the start of the test. A careful pain survey at the start is also important to establish a good and confidential relationship with the client. After that, it makes it easier to explain to the client that the pain will be taken into account but, in the tests, it is the recognition of functional abilities and deficits that is important.

Survey of cardiovascular risk factors

As the tests represent a physical strain, risk screening is essential (with the aid of a health questionnaire for example). The doctor is responsible for a specific risk assessment and any test restrictions.

Symptom magnification and self-limitation

A work-oriented assessment often takes place when symptom magnification and self-limitation is presumed and the willingness of the client to perform work or activities is questionable – this also applies to a work-hardening program to a certain extent (cf. § .7). Therefore a short overview of these issues and the discussion of evaluation options within a work-related assessment is presented [24, 25, 26]. The term symptom magnification describes an excessive topographic spread of pain and pain intensity as well as excessive disability and losses in social participation in comparison to doctor's and therapist's normal expectations based on clinical findings and general experience. Thus symptom magnification describes an observed phenomenon, not a diagnosis. There are numerous publications on different concepts and models regarding abnormal illness behaviour, we have based our concept, in particular, on the work done by Matheson, Waddell and Main [9, 26, 27]. Important causes of symptom magnification and self-limitation include, in particular:

– Fear of increased pain or harm when performing physical activity, of a serious diagnosis that the doctor has not recognised or would not like to pass on, or of an uncertain future with pain and disability.

– Social reinforcement of symptom behaviour; this includes for example the medicalisation of the problem and excessive medical investigations, lengthy treatment with mainly passive modalities, and advice to avoid movements and activities (beyond the acute stage of pain), increased attention and support in the role of patient, high social benefits, lack of possibility to early return to work with restricted duties ("please come back to work only when you are able to do full work"), imminent loss of job.

Fear and avoidance behaviour often leads to the vicious circle of *pain → fear of movement and avoidance of activities → increasing deconditioning and reduced stress tolerance → more pain (even with low physical activity) → etc.* Occasionally, a symptom magnification is associated with a clinical relevant psychiatric disorder such as phobia or depression.

According to Matheson, a symptom magnification can be recognised on the three dimensions *symptom perception and dealing with symptoms, social role of the symptoms* as well as *effort (willingness to perform) and consistency* (Table 8).

The first two dimensions can be evaluated in an interview. In 1991, Matheson published a concept for a structured interview for the evaluation of symptom magnification [28] that contains 14 items, such as perception of the symptoms (localised and differentiated or diffuse and general), goal setting (functional goals or only freedom from pain and regaining one's health), social consequences of symptom behaviour (active social role despite pain or barely performing everyday tasks) or control of symptoms (differentiated description of the effect of different measures or "Nothing has helped in any way at all so far"). Important aspects of symptom magnification are also represented by the "Yellow Flags" [27, 29]. For the third dimension, the evaluation of effort and consistency, a work-related assessment is naturally predestined.

Table 8 – Three dimensions of symptom magnification according to Matheson.

I. Symptom perception and dealing with symptoms
Diffuse description of symptoms. Very high pain level (e.g. value 8 and more, measured on a 10-point scale); no knowledge of what increases or reduces the pain. No strategies to control symptoms: inability to "negotiate" with the symptoms (i.e. looking for the best possible adaptations in order to perform activities and control the pain, pacing, etc.). All treatments fail, no positive approach anywhere.

II. Social role of symptoms
Delegation of control of personal environment and future goals to the symptoms: everything in life revolves around the symptoms. Imprisonment in a world of symptoms (Statement: "The pain dominates all my life").

III. Effort and consistency
Implausible extent of demonstrated disability in comparison to clinical findings and general experience. Lack of willingness to tolerate (even low) loads and gradually increased activities in a test or in a training program (which could be reasonably expected based on clinical experience); no functional limit observable, when the client breaks off. Inconsistencies concerning clinical findings, performance behaviour and results in physical tests, client's information about his daily life. Inadequate adherence to rules, not very cooperative behaviour.

Evaluation of sincerity of effort and consistency

Concerning effort (willingness to perform), already general behaviour in the tests usually provides a spontaneous impression, that, however, can not be justified in a report. Using the kinesiophysical test procedure, it is possible to rate effort more precisely: if a client's effort is good, it is possible to subject the test person to loads up to an observable somatic-functional performance limit whereas, in contrast, the test person with sub-optimal effort breaks off the test much earlier. Sometimes, functionally plausible observations in terms of performance limits (e.g. load-dependent increasingly evasive movements or trembling muscles) must be distinguished from theatrical behaviour when symptom magnification is substantial (often seen at very low loads and often does not increase with a progression of loads).

The evaluation of consistency results from comparisons between performances in different tests, between tests and the PACT Spinal Function Sort or anamnestic information or between tests and clinical findings. The FCE system according to Isernhagen has a check list with a total of 15 consistency points, whereby further observed inconsistencies are also to be listed (e.g. when a client drives for at least 1 hour without a break to the clinic for the assessment, but claims in the survey part of the tests that he can only remain seated for a maximum of 10 minutes). The reliability of an effort evaluation based on the coefficient of variation of 3 repeat test performances (as provided for by the ERGOS original protocol) is put into question by different studies [24, 30]. In the ERGOS application in Germany, the effort evaluation is also supported by further criteria and observations. As certain inconsistencies are found very often and the positive predictive value of isolated single findings is usually low, Matheson recommends a scoring of several features for the effort valuation [24]. Waddell had also established a scoring of this type for the evaluation of "non-organic or behavioural signs"[26]. Some additional contributions offer an interesting overview of the evaluation options of effort and consistency [31, 32, 33, 34].

The establishment of self-limiting behaviour and inconsistencies may have far-reaching consequences for the client and must therefore be carefully recorded in the report with observed facts. The evaluation must not be limited exclusively to the initial situation - a positive change occasionally observed in the course of the tests must be taken into account. In the face of a clear lack of effort and self-limitation, the level of physical capacity that could reasonably be expected should be judged at least higher than the performance demonstrated by the client (after checking plausibility of such a statement based on somatic diagnoses and clinical findings). If there is a confirmed or presumed psychiatric diagnosis that can affect the client's willingness to perform, such a statement must, however, be put into perspective dependent on the case.

Client management within the framework of the tests

As an examiner, one should give the client the best opportunity to do a good test in the interest of the optimum rehabilitation and reintegration chances as well as to avoid any permanent disability. As mentioned, fear of movement and physical activity is a frequent cause of self-limitation. *Up to now, being careful and avoiding (painful) activities were what was required, the doctor gave injections and prescribed x-rays, massage or electrotherapy and possibly cautious movement therapy – and now one should lift a box with weights all of a sudden!* As was previously mentioned, the examiner can encourage the client more or less as follows to continue the tests: "*I understand that you are in pain. But I can see that your movements are still safe. It is important for you that we find out what your real performance limit is. We will break off the test immediately if I see that the test performance is not safe anymore.*" Such an approach, with conversation, understanding and interest on the part of the examiner seeking information from the client helps to build up confidence. In the case of self-limitation and inconsistency, the clients should also be confronted skilfully with this and given another chance to perform a particular test. In this way, "difficult" clients can often be encouraged to overcome their initial avoidance behaviour (which is often also iatrogenic in nature), at least to a certain extent.

Validity and reliability of the test procedures

Up to now, only few studies on the reliability of the test procedures are found. Undoubtedly, this is also related, to a certain extent, to the fact that good studies are methodically difficult in this complex field of physical, psychosocial and contextual factors influencing work ability and return to work. Smith [35], Isernhagen [12] and Gross [36] found good test-retest and inter-tester reliability for the evaluation of lifting tests using observation criteria. Reneman found good test-retest reliability for the FCE lifting test according to Isernhagen on 2 successive days [15]. He also found good test-retest reliability for the static tests "elevated work", "crouch-deep static" and "kneeling", also under the following different conditions: a) standard method, b) very fast manual activity with screws during the relevant static position tests, c) standard method in noisy surroundings [37]. Brouwer investigated the test-retest reliability of different tests of the FCE according to Isernhagen, when the test was repeated after an interval of 2 weeks. In most tests, an acceptable test-retest reliability was found: Cohen's kappa > 0.6, percentage accordance > 80%, intra class correlation >= 0.7 [38]. In a study by Matheson, FCE lifting tests proved to be predictive for return to work, whereas grip strength was not [39]. In an already older study, an evaluation of functional performance capacity according to Smith also proved to be predictive for a return to work [40]. Lechner found an average correlation between a prediction based on a similar assessment system with FCE according to Isernhagen and the physical demand level of the actually performed work activity, only at 14-18% work activity was much more demanding than the performance level identified in the assessment [41]. Reneman found in younger subjects (20-29 years old) a maximal endurance for static elevated work (over shoulder height) of 14.5 minutes and for work in forward bending position of 16.2 minutes. No predictors have been found, and the authors concluded that only the practical test performance allows a judgement on the endurance for these tasks [42]. Dusik examined the construct validity of ERGOS and found a significant accordance in the investigations being compared [43]. Construct validity of FCE (in comparison with the Pain Disability Index and the Pain Visual Analogue Scale) was confirmed in a study by Gross [44]. Reneman examined the relation ship between disability (measured with the questionnaires Roland, Oswestry and Quebec) and FCE tests according to Isernhagen in patients with chronic back pain: whereas the disability was considered to be moderate to substantial based on the questionnaires, a work-related physical strength level of moderate to heavy was found based on the FCE tests. The correlations between the surveys and FCE tests were only slight to moderate. The authors concluded from this that both the survey and the tests were required to gain a comprehensive picture of the disabilities of patients with chronic back pain [45]. Gross et al. [46, 47] investigated the prognostic value of FCE according Isernhagen and concluded that the validity of FCE is questionable. But due to serious flaws and shortcomings in the study design regarding predictor variable, outcome variable and concept of use and utility of FCE, the conclusion of this study can not be accepted as valid [48]. For the question of extrapolation, the study by Saunders is interesting [49]. He investigated a functional work-related assessment based on ergonomic observation criteria extended to 22 hours (over 6 days). The results were as follows: a) the reliability of the tests carried out was good; b) the extrapolation of the loads that could be handled in the DOT category *often* (based on the maximum according the test results noted for the category *sometimes*) proved to be reliable (declared variation of 73-84%). Further references to studies on work-related test systems can be found in the work by Innes [3, 4]. For the Spinal Function Sort, good reliability and construct validity were found [22, 50]. In future, not only further studies on methodology, but also studies on the outcome and, in particular, the economic effects of work-oriented assessments would be of major interest.

Acknowledgements

The author would like to thank Franziska Denier-Bont (Rehaklinik Bellikon), Marie Louise Hallmark Itty (Küsnacht), Verena Fischer (Rehaklinik Bellikon) and Peter Oesch

(Clinic Valens) for their contributions and Verena Küng (Rehaklinik Bellikon) for revising the manuscript.

References

1. Hadler NM (1995) The disabling backache. An international perspective. Spine 20: 640-9
2. WHO (2003) ICF [International Classification of Function]. Funktionsfähigkeit, Behinderung und Gesundheit (Bearbeitung: Deutsches Institut für Medizinische Dokumentation und Information). Verband Deutscher Rentenversicherungsträger (www.dimdi.de → Klassifikationen → ICF)
3. Innes E, Straker L (1999a) Reliability of work-related assessments. Work 13: 107-24
4. Innes E, Straker L (1999b) Validity of work-related assessments. Work 13: 125-52
5. King PM, Tuckwell N, Barrett TE (1998) A critical review of functional capacity evaluations. Physical Therapy 78: 852-66
6. Hart DL, Isernhagen SJ, Matheson LN (1993) Guidelines for functional capacity evaluation of people with medical conditions. J Orthop Sports Phys Ther 18: 682-6
7. Snook SH, Irvine CH (1969) Psychophysical studies of physiological fatigue criteria. Hum Factors 11: 291-300
8. Kopp HG, Oliveri M, Thali A (1997) Erfassung und Umgang mit Symptomausweitung. Medizinische Mitteilungen der Suva 70: 56-78
9. Matheson LN (1988) Symptom Magnification Syndrome. In: Work Injury: Management and Prevention. (Ed. Isernhagen SJ). Gaithersburg, Maryland, Aspen p 257-82
10. Oliveri M, Kopp HG, Läubli T (1993) Die Bedeutung von körperlicher Aktivität und physischer Leistungsfähigkeit für die Prävention und Behandlung chronischer Rückenbeschwerden. Forschungsprojekt des Schweizerischen Nationalfondsprogramms NFP/26B. Wissenschaftlicher Schlussbericht
11. Isernhagen SJ (1988) Functional Capacity Evaluation. In: Work injury: Management And Prevention. (Ed. Isernhagen SJ). Gaithersburg, Aspen p 139-91
12. Isernhagen SJ, Hart DL, Matheson LN (1999) Reliability of independent observer judgments of level of lift effort in a kinesiophysical Functional Capacity Evaluation. Work 12: 145-50
13. US Department of Labor (1986) Dictionary of Occupational Titles. 4th, revised. Washington DC, Employment and Training Administration
14. Isernhagen SJ (1995) Contemporary Issues in Functional Capacity Evaluation. In: The Comprehensive Guide To Work Injury Management. (Ed.Isernhagen SJ). Gaithersburg, Maryland, Aspen p 410-29
15. Reneman MF, Dijkstra PU, Westmaas M et al. (2002a) Test-retest reliability of lifting and carrying in a 2-day functional capacity evaluation. J Occup Rehabil 12: 269-75
16. Mayer TG, Barnes D, Kishino ND et al. (1988a) Progressive Isoinertial Lifting Evaluation I. A Standardized Protocol and Normative Database. Spine 13: 993-7
17. Kaiser H, Kersting M (2000) Der Stellenwert des Arbeitssimulationsgerätes ERGOS als Bestandteil der leistungsdiagnostischen Begutachtung. Rehabilitation 39: 175-84
18. Mayer TG, Barnes D, Nichols G et al. (1988b) Progressive Isoinertial Lifting Evaluation II. A Comparison with Isokinetic Lifting in a Disabled Chronic Low-Back Pain Industrial Population. Spine 13: 998-1002

19. Mayer TG, Gatchel R, Barnes D et al. (1990) Progressive Isoinertial Lifting Evaluation. Erratum Notice. Spine 15: 5
20. Laurig W (1992) Wie lassen sich Belastung und Beanspruchung ermitteln? In: Grundzüge der Ergonomie, Erkenntnisse und Prinzipien. (Ed.Laurig W). Berlin, Beuth p 104-106
21. Ahonen M, Launis M, Kuorinka T (1989) [Ergonomic Workplace Analysis] Ergonomische Arbeitsplatzabklärung (Kursmanual: Schweizer Bearbeitung durch Huwiler Hj; Hallmark Itty ML; Klipstein A). [[Finnish Institute of Occupational Health, Ergonomic Section] Schweizerische Arbeitsgemeinschaft für Rehabilitation SAR, Interessengemeinschaft Ergonomie, 2. Auflage 2000 (www.sar-rehab.ch → Who is who → Interessengemeinschaften → IG Ergonomie)]
22. Matheson LN, Matheson ML, Grant J (1993) Development of a Measure of Perceived Functional Ability. J Occup Rehabil 3: 15-29
23. Matheson LN, Matheson ML (1996) Spinal Function Sort (PACT-Test, edited in different languages). Swiss Association for Rehabilitation SAR, Working group Ergonomics (www.sar-rehab.ch → Who is who → Interessengemeinschaften → IG Ergonomie)
24. Matheson LN, Bohr PC, Hart D (1998) Use of maximum voluntary effort grip strength testing to identify symptom magnification syndrome in persons with low back pain. Journal of Back and Musculoskeletal Rehabilitation 10: 125-35
25. Mayer TG, Gatchel RJ (1988) Functional Restoration for Spinal Disorders: The Sports Medicine Approach. Philadelphia, Lea & Febiger, p 1-321
26. Waddell G (1998) The Back Pain Revolution. Churchill Livingstone, p 223-40
27. Main CJ, Spanswick CC (2000) Pain Management. An Interdisciplinary Approach. Churchill Livingstone
28. Matheson LN (1991) Symptom Magnification Syndrome Structured; Interview: Rationale and Procedure. J Occup Rehabil 1: 43-56
29. Kendall NAS., Linton SJ, Main CJ (2004) Guide to assessing psychsocial yellow flags in acute low back pain: risk factors for long term disability and work loss. Wellington (N Z), Accident rehabilitation and Compensation Insurance Corporation of New Zealand and the National Health Committee [www.nzgg.org.nz → guidelines → musculoskeletal disease]
30. Hazard RG, Reeves V, Fenwick JW (1992) Lifting capacity. Indices of subject effort. Spine 17: 1065-70
31. Colledge AL, Holmes AB, Soo Hoo ER et al. (2001) Motivation Determination (Sincerity of Effort): The Performance APGAR Model. Disability Medicine (American Board of Indepent Medical Examiners) 1: 5-18
32. Fishbain DA, Cutler R, Rosomoff HL et al. (1999) Chronic pain disability exaggeration/malingering and submaximal effort research. Clin J Pain 15: 244-74
33. Hopf HC, Deuschl G (2000) Psychogene Störungen der Motorik, Sensibilität und Sensorik aus der Sicht des Neurologen – "bed-side" – Befunde bei somatoformen Störungen. Akt Neurol 27: 145-56
34. Kool J, Oesch P, de Bie RA (2002) Predictive tests for non-return to work in patients with chronic low back pain. Euro Spine J 11: 258-66
35. Smith RL (1994) Therapists' ability to identify safe maximum lifting in low back pain patients during functional capacity evaluation. J Orthop Sports Phys Ther 19: 277-81
36. Gross DP, Battie MC (2002) Reliability of safe maximum lifting determinations of a functional capacity evaluation. Phys Ther 82: 364-71

37. Reneman MF, Joling CI, Soer EL *et al.* (2001b) Functional capacity evaluation: Ecological validity of three static endurance tests. Work 16: 227-34

38. Brouwer S, Reneman M F, Dijkstra PU *et al.* (2000) Test-retest reliability of the Isernhagen Work Systems Functional Capacity Evaluation in patients with chronic low back pain. J Occup Rehabil 13: 207-18

39. Matheson LN, Isernhagen SJ, Hart DL (2002) Relationships among lifting ability, grip force, and return to work. Phys Ther 82: 249-56

40. Smith SL, Cunningham S, Weinberg R (1986) The predictive validity of the functional capacities evaluation. Am J Occup Ther 40: 564-7

41. Lechner DE, Jackson JR, Roth DL *et al.* (1994) Reliability and Validity of a Newly Developed Test of Physical Work Performance. JOM 36: 997-1004

42. Reneman MF, Bults MM, Engbers LH *et al.* (2001a) Measuring maximum holding times and perception of static elevated work and forward bending in healthy young adults. J Occup Rehabil 11: 87-97

43. Dusik LA, Menard MR, Cooke C *et al.* (1993) Concurrent validity of the ERGOS work simulator versus conventional functional capacity evaluation techniques in a worker's compensation population. J Occup Med 35: 759-67

44. Gross DP, Michele C (2003) Construct Validity of a Kinesiophysical Functional Capacity Evaluation Administered Within a Worker's Compensation Environment. J Occup Rehabil 13: 287-95

45. Reneman MF, Jorritsma W, Schellekens JM *et al.* (2002b) Concurrent validity of questionnaire and performance-based disability measurements in patients with chronic nonspecific low back pain. J Occup Rehabil 12: 119-29

46. Gross DP, Battié MC, Cassidy D (2004) The prognostic value for functional capacity evaluation in patients with chronic low back pain: Part 1: Timely return to work. Spine 29: 914-9

47. Gross DP, Battié MC (2004) The prognostic value for functional capacity evaluation in patients with chronic low back pain: Part 2: Sustained recovery. Spine 29: 920-4

48. Oliveri M, Oesch P, Kool J *et al.* (2005) Letter to the editor (Re: Gross *et al.* The prognostic value for functional capacity evaluation…). Spine 30: 1232-33

49. Saunders RL, Beissner KL, McManis BG (1997) Estimates of weight that subjects can lift frequently in functional capacity evaluations. Phys Ther 77: 1717-28

50. Gibson L, Strong J (1996) The Reliability and Validity of a Measure of Perceived Functional Capacity for Work in Chronic Back Pain. J Occup Rehabil 6: 159-75

Work rehabilitation programs: work hardening and work conditioning[1]

F. Franchignoni[2], M. Oliveri[3] and G. Bazzini[4]

Introduction

According to the American Commission for Accreditation of Rehabilitation Facilities (CARF), work hardening (WH) is "a highly structured, goal-oriented, individualised treatment program designed to maximise the ability to return to work, addressing the issues of productivity, safety, physical tolerances, and work behaviours" [1]. WH attempts to bridge the gap between the patient's residual functional performance capacity and the job requirements, focusing on physical (biomechanical, neuromuscular, cardiovascular/metabolic), functional, behavioural and vocational needs. WH involves a coordinated interdisciplinary team (including physiatrist, physical and/or occupational therapist, and – as needed – psychologist, vocational counsellor or other rehabilitation professionals) and consists of the following components: physical conditioning, simulated work activities, education, and psychosocial interventions. The duration of WH sessions is usually several hours (max. 8) daily, 5 days per week. In order to meet the need for a less comprehensive program, the American Physical Therapy Association (APTA) also defined a work conditioning program (WC). WC is a "work-related, goal-oriented treatment program for subjects with less complex conditions", provided by a single discipline, of up to 4 hours per day [2]. WC is limited to function and work related physical conditioning interventions and does not include behavioural and psychological components. WH or WC should be provided only to clients that are unlikely to return to work with less intensive and expensive treatments.

1. Some parts of this chapter have been adapted from Oliveri M: Work Conditioning and Work Hardening. In: Lendenwirbelsäule. Ursachen, Diagnostik und Therapie von Rückenschmerzen. Edited by J. Hildebrandt, G. Müller et M. Pfingsten, Urban & Fischer, 2005 (with permission of Urban & Fischer).
2. Unit of Occupational Rehabilitation and Ergonomics, Rehabilitation Institute of Veruno (NO), "Salvatore Maugeri" Foundation, Clinica del Lavoro e della Riabilitazione, IRCCS, Italy.
3. Unit of Occupational Rehabilitation and Ergonomics, Rehaklinik Bellikon, Bellikon, Switzerland.
4. Unit of Occupational Rehabilitation and Ergonomics, Rehabilitation Institute of Montescano (PV), "Salvatore Maugeri" Foundation, Clinica del Lavoro e della Riabilitazione, IRCCS, Italy.

The first WH program was established in 1977 by the American psychologist Matheson [3]. In 1988, Mayer and Gatchel described the functional restoration program they had developed for spinal disorders [4]. WH and WC programs were subsequently described by many authors in the nineties [5, 6, 7, 9, 10], and their components have been extensively commented in occupational therapy books [11, 12, 13] and supplements of rehabilitation journals devoted to industrial rehabilitation medicine [14, 15, 16].

Clients

The APTA guidelines state that WH should start after resolution of the initial or principal injury/illness [2], when subjects are medically stable and without serious diagnosis as documented by a recent medical examination prior to program entry. As time off work is inversely correlated to the rate of return to work, early intervention is strongly recommended. When time of inactivity is kept short and use of passive modalities (physical agents, manual therapy, massage, etc.) is limited, individuals are less likely to develop symptom magnification and to assume a "sick role". Most of the studies in this field involve industrial "blue-collar" workers (mean age ranging from the mid-30s to the mid-40s) suffering from activity-related spinal disorders, particularly low back pain. For low back pain, admission to a WH program is recommended 6 to 12 weeks after the onset of acute symptoms [4, 17, 18, 19, 20]. Clients enrolled in WH programs are usually physically deconditioned, and their physical abilities do not meet the physical demands of a targeted job. A psychosocial dysfunction such as abnormal illness behaviour, fear and depression is often present, but important mental disorders should be excluded. There should be a reasonable expectation that the client can be reintegrated in a specified occupation. Motivation, of course, is crucial for the success of a WH or WC program. However, before starting the program it is often impossible to separate true motivation from a convincingly expressed pseudo-motivation like *"Of course, I will do anything that is good for my back"*. For this reason, it is advisable in doubt to enrol the client on a trial basis.

Program

Programs include flexibility, strength and endurance exercises (specific treatments can be added whenever necessary), and a highly individualised job-specific training (if return to previous job is possible, otherwise the goal is to get the person fit for any suitable work). The program follows an active therapy approach, requiring the "temporarily disabled" individuals to participate in a daily structured routine that mimics their job (in its physical, temporal and procedural structure) and minimises incentives for illness behaviour. The tasks are structured and graded to progressively improve physical and psychosocial work functions: functional performance capacity, psychomotor skills, work habits and rules (such as punctuality, attendance, compliance to safety instructions), work procedures and work-related skills (such as task completion, quality standards, productivity), interpersonal and communicative skills (with supervisors and peers). The training is based on the worker's specific job demands and functional deficits, as defined by a WH assessment. The ultimate goal of WH is to help the client to achieve, in a safe and quick way, a level of acceptable productivity for the competitive labour market, increasing confidence for the resumption of productive work [21]. The duration of daily participation should begin at a comfortable level (based on baseline assessment), gradually increasing – as work tolerance improves – to the full-work level. Return-to-work rate is a common measure of success. Some clients may return to a modified light-work schedule and/or part-time work.

Equipment and space

WC and WH needs equipment for gym and work simulation activities. In order to simulate physical work demands, the latter should approximate as closely as possible to the actual work environment in terms of noise, light, humidity, etc. Rooms for counselling and additional treatments should be available, access to a gym hall for group exercise (e.g. aerobics, low impact, games) is recommended. In European countries, WH is usually located in a rehabilitation centre. For out-patients, return to part-time work may be implemented already during the program, and on-site work evaluation and/or rehabilitation can be added, if appropriate. In general, there is no need for expensive high-tech equipment. A set of devices for resistance training and simple work-simulation systems (such as bolt box, brick wall, assembly etc.) is usually sufficient; job-specific work stations are added for individuals with special work demands.

Assessment

A work-related baseline assessment should consider the physical and psychosocial factors affecting the person's ability to participate in the program and later return to work. Assessment should take account of neuromusculo-skeletal and cardiovascular status, work-related functional capacity, vocational status (including work demands) and incentives for return to work, behavioural issues (including strategies to cope with the actual disability and motivation to improve function, symptom magnification tendencies, abnormal pain behaviours, and work motivation), and other psychosocial or financial factors.

Structured interview and questionnaires on medical and psychosocial issues

The evaluation starts with a review of the worker's medical history and condition. The client should carefully report pain and other symptoms and how he copes with them, perceived functional limits and work tolerance, and use of medication or other treatments prior to the program. The key questions are: is the client's description of symptoms and limitations clear and specific, or is it vague, generalised and leaning to catas-trophising *(cf. § [Recognition of symptom magnification and self-limitation])*? Is this des-cription consistent with medical findings or not? Does the client use active strategies to cope with symptoms or to overcome limits? Did he/she have mainly passive modalities and medications or also active training as previous treatment, and what was the reaction to the treatments? Evaluation proceeds with a job description *(cf. § [Job evaluation])*, the person's work-related abilities and interests, the social environment and its interaction with the disability, and non-vocational activities involving employment-related beha-viours (hobbies, sport, social groups, etc.) [7, 12]. A useful questionnaire for assessing clients' beliefs about their work-related abilities and deficits (which can differ from results of functional capacity evaluation) is the *Spinal Function Sort* [22]. A systematic and very helpful checklist of possible barriers for rehabilitation and return to work are the *yellow, blue and black flags* [23, 24]. Parts of this intake evaluation can be re-admi-nistered at discharge, for outcome evaluation.

Physical assessment

The clinical examination includes generalised testing of range of motion, manual muscle testing, sensory screening and tests for motor coordination and manual dexterity.

The main part of physical assessment is a work-related *Functional Capacity Evaluation* (FCE) *as described in chapter 6*. In addition to the FCE battery, an assessment of cardiovascular endurance (e.g. ergometer test or a walking test) is recommended, because a deficit in this field is common in clients with chronic disorders. For a minimal functional evaluation, at least the following tests of FCE should be performed at the beginning and end of the program: *lifting floor to waist, horizontal (waist to waist) and waist to overhead, unilateral carrying, standing and sitting for longer time, walking*. Other FCE tests can be done as part of a standard test battery or according to the work demands of the client: *pushing and pulling, grip strength, elevated work (overhead), forward bending (stooping), crawling, kneeling, crouching, squatting, stair and step ladder climbing, balancing, hand coordination*. In some cases, work-specific activities should be assessed as well (e.g. building a wall with bricks). The main criteria for these evaluations are: safety of adminis-tration, reliability, job relatedness, practicality, and predictiveness [12]. The FCE measure-ments should be compared with the physical demands of the job to which the client is expected to return (job match grid), to ensure a properly designed rehabilitation plan and reasonable return to work decision making. As discussed in the chapter of this book on FCE *(cf. § [Functional Capacity Evaluation])*, assessment of work-related functional capacity is complex and therefore a methodical challenge for studies. Only few studies on FCE have been carried out, and there is no universally accepted operational definition for FCE batteries [25, 26]. Nevertheless, many tests have reasonable content validity and good reliability, particularly those consisting of simulation of critical demands or func-tional tasks performed with standardised procedures [27]. For this reason, at present FCE is the best available option for assessment in work-related rehabilitation (widely reco-gnised by rehabilitation professionals, by insurance companies and also in court). In addition, FCE helps in identifying symptom magnification and self-limitation (*cf. §* *[Recognition of symptom magnification and self-limitation]*). In this case of observed self-limitation, the "maximum" performance does not represent the true functional capacity; the observations referring to this and the consequent drawbacks in the results' interpretation should be documented in the report on the assessment.

Recognition of symptom magnification and self-limitation

Recognition of any symptom magnification and self-limitation is crucial, not only for judging the validity of the FCE results, but also for optimising program management and, in particular, training dosage. The rehabilitation team should therefore be able to assess whether clients are really working at their physical boundary or are limited by psychological factors. Self-limitation is mostly due to fear of movement (threat of tissue damage or pain aggravation). However lack of understanding of the program principles, unwillingness to return to work (e.g. due to problems at the workplace) and/or secondary financial sickness gain can also play a role. Symptom magnification and self-limitation are discussed in detail in the chapter of this book on FCE by Oliveri. For their evaluation, the following issues – based on the interview or questionnaires and physical examination – are most important:

– description of symptoms and limitations: specific or vague and global with catastrophising?

– social role of the symptoms: does the client have some control over the symptoms and does he/she still participate in various social activities, or do the symptoms dominate all aspects of life (the client as prisoner of the pain)?

– does the client estimate his/her own functional abilities as very low, e.g. resulting in a very low index of the Spinal Function Sort?

– does he/she clearly underestimate the level of function compared to results of functional test?

– is the client willing to perform the physical tests and continue until observed functional limits in spite of some pain increase or discomfort, or does he/she stop very early, before the therapist identifies any functional problem?

– are there important discrepancies between clinical examinations (e.g. Waddell signs), answers in the interview or questionnaires, and FCE-tests, or between different physical tests with comparable physical demands? [23, 24, 28, 29];

– is the client willing to perform a minimum of training tasks at a reasonable performance level and to gradually increase the performance level within the first week of the program (provided that any severe and strongly restricting clinical condition has been excluded)?

Clients focusing on pain should learn to accept that a quick resolution of their pain problem is not realistic, and that the primary goal of WH is restoration of function. In order to change the focus from pain towards function, weekly assessment of functional evolution (FCE tests or training performance level) and a formal feedback of the results for the client is critical. The clients should learn to really appreciate their functional improvements in spite of the fact that some pain is persisting.

Job evaluation

A job description from the client and/or company is the first preliminary method for obtaining a report of the worker's job tasks, including duration, the physical, functional, and psychological demands of the job, and the use of specific equipment, tools and materials [7]. Work-related sensory components and environmental conditions are also important.

An early visit to the workplace (usually by the therapist together with the client and possibly with an outside case manager) can play a significant role in the rehabilitation program. Such a visit can be part of both assessment and intervention:

– it shows the client the central value of his/her return to work within the WH program;

– it engages the employer and those in charge at the company in the WH concept and process, in order to find the best solutions for client's re-entry and maintenance at work, and remove prejudices towards the "handicapped" member of staff;

– it helps understanding of the exposures of a specific job and problems the client must overcome to return to the job, and it is essential for planning ergonomic modifications at the work site if needed (cf. § [Ergonomic interventions at the work site]);

– it makes it possible to design an accurate environment to simulate the job-specific tasks and establish the job performance criteria on which program goals are based. It also offers an opportunity for borrowing actual tools and materials that are appropriate for work-simulation training (if needed).

Sometimes, telephone contact with the company is sufficient or the only realistic option for geographical reasons.

In other cases an extended job analysis is compulsory [30, 31]. Furthermore, it is important to be aware that there are notable differences in workers' physical performance depending on gender (women have on average 65% of the strength of men), age (people at 55 years have lost on average 15% of the strength they had at 25 years of age) and inter-individual differences (both due to constitutional factors and specific skills acquired during work experience).

Intervention

General considerations regarding intervention

Relationship between psychologically-oriented interventions and physical training

As mentioned, many clients with (a tendency to) chronic musculo-skeletal disorders present not only severe deconditioning but also important psychological and behavioural problems. The latter include fear of movement, symptom magnification, disorganisation of daily activities, stress, depression, loss of hope and life perspectives, problems related to financial uncertainty, etc. Psychological or behaviour-oriented interventions (such as the goal setting process, information and education on coping with pain, and symptom-negotiation training (*cf. § [Goaling process/Structured information and education on coping with pain/Enhancing self-efficacy beliefs]*) pave the way for the physical training as they build up knowledge of the WH concept and willingness to tolerate intense physical training (in spite of pain and discomfort that often accompanies it, especially in the first period). These psychologically-oriented interventions may require a considerable amount of time: from 2 hours/day [32] to around half the daily duration of the program [33].

The client's role: personal responsibility and self-treatment

Patients' healing expectations – in particular the belief that passive modalities such as manual therapy or massage or extended medical investigations will heal their pain – often result in a dependence on doctor and therapist (that is sometimes also promoted by the two professionals). Waddell associated this medicalisation and extensive medical investigation of unspecific back pain and lack of self-activity and responsibility with the epidemic-like increase in disability due to back pain [29]. Matheson called the therapeutic approach to chronic pain that primarily aims at pain reduction "the feel good trap" [34]. Patient and therapist may be satisfied by the temporary effect of such modalities, but in the long term this approach is counterproductive. In contrast, clients in WH must take responsibility for their treatment, supported by the therapist and the whole rehabilitation team. They are learning to perform the training by themselves and to "negotiate" with their symptoms (*cf. § [Symptom negotiation training]*).

Role of the rehabilitation team: uniform treatment planning and patient management

The rehabilitation team (which comprises the doctor and therapist involved, as a minimum) is responsible for assessment, treatment planning – including the global and weekly goals – and therapy. The team approach must also guarantee the "unité de doctrine" [uniform doctrine] regarding method and program structure as well as the information that is given to the client.

Role of the therapist as a coach

In WH, the therapist is not a helper or a healer, but mainly a coach. The coach must be aware of the psychological implications of his/her therapeutic conduct, and behave as an enabler, not as a manipulator or someone who gives orders. He/she should not just confront his/her concepts and decisions, but merely holds up a mirror to the clients, i.e. presents them with the consequences their own ideas and behaviour. Coaching is thus an aid towards self-help, whereby other ways of thinking and action patterns should be stimulated. The coach should ask the correct questions, leaving the client to find the correct answer.

The greatest challenge in the art of coaching is the ability to negotiate and determine weekly goals at the crossing point between the requirements imposed by the primary goals of the program and the clients' capacity for achievement based on his/her current physical and mental state.

Goaling process

Primary goals

The selection of primary goals is one of the first steps in the WH program. It assists the client in communicating their concerns, preferences and attitudes and acquiring a sense of responsibility for their own behaviour, it also helps to develop a rational basis for planning and monitoring the interventions. The goals are both personal and job-related and must be negotiated with the client (taking also into account the targets of the employer and insurance company that pays for the program). Goals can be determined on an activity level (e.g. climbing stairs, carrying a shopping bag, putting goods on overhead shelves, or driving a car) and on a more global participation level (e.g. return to previous work, or pursuing a certain sport again). The goal setting process can include the following steps [34]:

– listing of occupationally-significant and personal goals by a structured interview;

– ranking of goals in ascending priority of importance (discussing first what is considered least important and ending with the most important item – this direction is easier for the client). Then the list is rewritten in the order of descending priority. The client is now asked to go through this list with at least one confidant and make meaningful corrections;

– formalization and distribution of the goal document: the client must hand copies of the definitive list to some confidants to inform them of his/her goals.

Many clients initially mention freedom from pain as their most important goal. After further discussions, most acknowledge that this goal is unlikely to be achieved in a few weeks after long-lasting pain. They then usually accept the formulation of more realistic and functional goals and give them higher priority than pain relief. Therefore, discussions about the goaling process also help to shift the client's focus from pain towards function and activities.

A useful tool for activity goal setting, the SMART form (Specific-Measurable-Acceptable-Realistic-Time), has been developed by the Pain Management and Research Centre of the University of Maastricht. It has proven its value at different pain clinics in Holland. Clients are asked to note down 5 activities in which they feel limited. They should then note how important each activity is for them (rating of 1 to 5) and how well they would assess their current ability to do that activity (1 to 5). Based on these answers, goals and time limit to achieve them are negotiated between the therapist and client and noted on the lower part of the sheet.

Role of weekly goals and visits in the goaling process

Measurable weekly goals can be derived from the primary goals. The art of setting weekly goals lies in "neither raising the bar too high nor leaving it too low". If goals are too ambitious they will remain unachieved, which demotivates the clients and undermines their self-efficacy *(cf. § [Enhancing self-efficacy beliefs])*. Conversely, if goals are too easy, the primary goals will not be achieved within the requisite time. Moreover, inadequate challenges do little to develop enthusiasm and self-confidence.

In weekly visits or conferences, goal achievement of the previous week is examined and the goals for the next week set. At least the doctor (senior physician or resident), the therapist in charge for treatment and the client should take part. A psychiatrist or psychologist, vocational counsellor or social worker may also be present if necessary. The visit should take place directly in the training premises, so allowing to look together at relevant or problematic exercises and make observations and proposals on the spot. Doctors can thus evaluate clients directly "at work" in the program, and – with their "authority" – praise or encourage them or admonish them for inadequate effort. The aim of combined on site observations is also to cross-validate the observations and assessments made by individual members of the team during the week. A central working instrument is the goal and progress form, in which the primary goals, problems, relevant weekly goals and goal achievement as well as the tasks of team members are continually updated. As already mentioned, most of the weekly goals should be measurable (e.g. weight or walking distance, number or duration of repetitions, number of series or laps per day) in order to monitor the performance and give objective feedback to the client (also in graphic form). Prior to the visit, the therapist's job is to enter the goal achievement of the past week with comments as well as proposals for next goals and proper pacing of the level of progressive challenges.

Structured information and education on coping with pain

The information and messages to the clients on coping with pain as well as behavioural therapy should be closely linked to clients' experience in practical training and possibly include additional measures for stress management, relaxation or pain treatment.

Contents

The pain concept of many clients is related to experience of acute pain: these clients associate pain with threat and fear of tissue damage, thus pain-producing activities are avoided and disability increases. This belief is also supported by damage-associated information from some doctors or therapists, for example, about "arthritis" or "slipped disks", and recommendations (beyond the acute phase) such as "*You shouldn't put any strain on your back, don't bend and don't pick up anything heavy*" [35]. Fear and stress lead in turn – via an increase in muscle tension and a lowering of pain threshold – to increasing pain. Explaining the difference between acute and chronic musculo-skeletal pain can help clients to reduce fear and stress and improve their willingness to participate in a WH program. Information and training should be behaviourally oriented (cf. below in this § and also [Symptom negotiation training]) and not largely consist of medical explanations based on anatomy and pain physiology [20].

Important core messages to give the back pain client are:

– chronic pain does not mean harm! It is not dangerous to move and stress your body when you are in pain! In fact, this is necessary in order to escape from the vicious circle of avoiding physical activity, loss of fitness and pain;

– chronic pain usually cannot be reduced in a short time. However, it is possible to increase performance capacity with intensive training despite pain. In many cases, a reduction in pain will then occur in the long term;

– some pain increase usually occurs at the start of the program as under-used muscles and joints are now trained, and the body has to readapt to higher activity level. This is normal!

– in this program, the primary goal is not pain reduction but *increasing your performance capacity*. This will be measured weekly as the main criterion for your success. An intensive training program creates the prerequisites for successful return to work.

It is well-known that psychological factors play an important role in chronic pain. To explain the interdependent functioning of physical and mental factors, information may begin with the message: "*Psyche and body are not independent of each other. A physical change has an effect on the psyche and vice versa. For example, experiencing fear or stress leads to an increase of muscle tension, heart beat or sweating. The response from the emotions and the behavioural reactions can influence personal experience of pain. This is good news, because this offers possibilities to gain a certain control over back pain*" (*cf. § [Techniques of relaxation, awareness and diversion]*).

One important goal of psychologically-oriented intervention is to overcome fear-avoidance behaviour [24, 29, 36]. Fear cannot be "talked away": overcoming fear is a cognitive-behavioural therapeutic task. The goal is to create challenging situations in which clients can learn from their own experience to reduce their exaggerated fear about tissue damage during painful activities and thereby approximate their expectations to reality (*cf. § [Symptom negotiation training]*). In addition, the connection between fear and chronic pain can be illustrated using the Vlaeyen model "Fear of movement/(re)injury" [36, 37], that postulates two opposed reactions to fear of movement or tissue damage: *confrontation* and *avoidance*. If there is no serious back pathology, the confrontation with everyday challenges and more or less normal daily activity despite back pain probably leads – as an adaptive response – to a fear reduction and promotes functional recovery. In contrast, avoidance leads to the maintenance or exacerbation of fear and possibly to a phobia-like condition. Avoidance maintains the vicious circle of *feeling pain → catastrophic ideas of pain → fear of pain → avoidance of activities → reduction in tolerance to strain → (even more) pain.* Clients should be aware that back pain mostly is a harmless everyday problem that they can check themselves and not a serious illness that requires particular caution and care. This applies also to back pain after resolution of the primary damage in case of an injury.

If necessary, behavioural training regarding communication about back pain is also meaningful. It can help to get rid of the habit of talking incessantly about pain and frequently showing that one is in pain (e.g. limping, supporting one's back with the hand or even using a stick when walking). Clients should understand that this behaviour promotes focusing on pain, and also leads to their complaints being taken less and less seriously. In contrast, communication on other topics helps to keep pain at a distance. Within the framework of the WH program, "rules of the game" can be agreed upon, e.g. *"In the morning, we discuss your pain because we take your pain seriously and would like to be informed about it. After that, however, you should not talk about it any more if possible until the next day and also show your pain as little as possible. Instead, try to find some diversion from pain. Think of all the other things in your everyday life, which are important to you and which you can talk about with others".* In order to train this communication excluding pain issues, the therapist and doctor should show interest in other areas of the client's life (e.g. hobbies, things that happened at work or with the children, politics, etc.), and try to draw the patient out on these themes.

Methods for structured information

An individual explanation by a doctor, therapist and/or psychologist has many advantages: the information and advice can be tailored to intellectual levels and individual problems, the client is addressed directly, discretion is guaranteed, and the best language for communication can be selected (language is a problem for rehabilitation clinics with many immigrants). In comparison to group discussions, however, individual talks preclude any exchange of information and interaction between clients. From the clients' viewpoint, statements made by fellow patients often appear more credible than those made by seeming healthy doctors, psychologists or therapists who do not know what it means to suffer pain every day. Therefore, it is often worthwhile introducing information using the following approach: *"Just the other day, a patient told me that…"* *"Other patients have found that…".* This is better accepted than a theoretical approach. In the case of people from other cultures, it can be useful to have a mediator. A written booklet on how to learn to cope with pain can be very helpful in supporting education. The client is asked to read it and prepare questions for the next consultation with the psychologist, therapist or doctor. Stimulated by the patient pamphlet "The Back Book" [38], which gives advice on coping with acute or subacute back pain, the WH team of the Rehabilitation Clinic Bellikon has issued a learning program on coping with chronic pain [info@rehabellikon.ch]. The inclusion of such an assisted self-study task within the information process emphasises the principle of self-responsibility and provides a tool for evaluating the client's willingness to learn about coping with pain.

A closed education group can also be meaningful if the usually referred clients are linguistically and culturally fairly homogeneous. A combination of preliminary individual information and education and then participation in an open education group with exchange of experience may be a valid compromise.

Enhancing self-efficacy beliefs

In his important work *"Getting a handle on motivation: self-efficacy in rehabilitation"*, Matheson set out the basic principles of self-efficacy, goaling process and motivation referring also to works by Bandura and White [34]. Self-efficacy is based on the perception of personal competence and skills. It influences people's behaviour, motivation, ways of thinking as well as emotional reactions to challenging circumstances. According to Bandura, self-efficacy beliefs is an important component of motivation, it encourage one to carry out new activities. White postulated an urge towards competence (i.e., sense of the ability to influence and control one's surroundings) and self-assertion, and he positioned this urge at the same level as the urges for satisfaction of hunger, sex and safety. Specific goals in the occupational and private field can be understood as an expression of this urge. Normally, temporarily disabled people are motivated to discover every day what they can still do or do again in order to regain their skills as fast and completely as possible. In some people, however, this urge towards competence appears to be blocked, and they develop avoidance behaviour, mostly because they feel threat of damage or pain when performing movements. This results in lack of control over symptoms, increasing disability, hopelessness and poor motivation. Sometimes a more or less conscious sickness gain also plays a role. The result is not only persisting disability and lack of participation in social life but also, in particular, the feeling of being an invalid, i.e., an overall lack of self-efficacy.

How can this destructive process be stopped and reversed? There are two main means: the goaling process, and symptom negotiation training.

Goaling process as a means to enhance self-efficacy

The feeling of competence and/or trust in one's own strength is based on success. According to Harding, *"Increased self-efficacy is closely linked to successful rehabilitation... To increase confidence, patients need to attempt something previously feared, achieve it, and recognise it as their own achievement. Thus, persistent goal attainment will reinforce self-efficacy and lead to a perception of mastery over the problem and the task.... Goals must be personally relevant, interesting, measurable and achievable. Goal setting should be a matter of negotiation between the patient and the therapist"* [39]. The goaling process as a whole, the consistent, realistic and measurable weekly objectives, the relevant achievement of these weekly goals and the associated feeling of success are thus the cognitive-behavioural therapeutic alpha and omega of the rehabilitation process. In this way, clients learn to recognise and appreciate an improvement in their functions as a result of rehabilitation instead of clinging to a "pain barometer" as they had largely been doing before.

Symptom negotiation training

Many clients with chronic back pain cannot "negotiate" effectively with their symptoms or cope with their pain. They experience their symptoms as being more or less beyond their control. As they cannot predict the pain behaviour, they feel unable to exert control over their pain, themselves and their environment. This, in turn, increases the lack of self-efficacy. Symptom negotiation training is therefore an important training element for these clients in a WH program [34]. It is based on the following principle: when symptoms can be predicted, they can be better controlled. To achieve this, the therapist must create situations in which the symptoms appear in a predictable way and for which prediction and control by the client are facilitated.

The most important strategies for symptom negotiation training are:

Graded activity

This approach is based on a tasks presenting a gradually increased activity level. The starting point and the increment are set by the therapist in such a way that a clear relationship between activity and symptoms can easily be felt by the client. For example, in a progressive lifting test, load, lifting height, speed or rate can be increased. The purpose of this exercise is not, however, to evaluate lifting performance, but to clarify the connections between stress level of the task and symptoms. Some clients have initially to learn to differentiate pain levels as shades of grey rather than as black-or-white (i.e., either no pain or catastrophic pain).

Graded exposure to feared movements

This method [36, 37, 40] resembles the "graded activity", but clients are exposed as realistically as possible to the specific physical stress that they are afraid of: "*For example, if the patient fears the spinal compression produced by riding a bicycle on a bumpy road, then the graded exposure should include an activity that mimics that specific activity, and not just a stationary bicycle. Such an approach gives the individual an opportunity to correct the inaccurate predictions about the relationship between activities and harm*" [36].

Pacing

Clients with painful disabilities often function according to an "on/off" principle ("Yes, I can" or "No, I can't"). They should experience that by adjusting their working pace there are intermediate options: e.g., doing things slower, making short breaks, doing some stretching, loosening up or relaxing exercises in between, alternating work activities, etc.

Modification of working techniques, tools or workplace

Many clients with pain-related disabilities have not yet learnt to appreciate the value of working smart rather than working hard. They keep on working as uneconomically as they did before the accident/disease or even worse. Ways of modifying working techniques and requirements as well as tools and workplace (*cf. § [Tool modification]/ § [Job site modification]*) should be evaluated [41].

Coping with exacerbated pain

An exacerbation of pain during rehabilitation is a challenge for a client's self-management and should be used for education of proper pain behaviour [39]. Clients should learn to avoid panic and assess the pain situation realistically, and to avoid, for instance, alarmed consultations at emergency wards. They should apply the learned self-treatments for pain relief (e.g. cool packs, relaxation technics, the meaningful use of medicaments) and analyse the likely causes of the acute pain attack.

Physical conditioning and functional restoration

The avoidance of pain-producing activity generates physical deconditioning that should be treated through an exercise program aimed to increase muscle strength and endurance, flexibility, motor coordination, and cardiovascular fitness. The terminology for describing such programs includes "functional restoration", "physical reconditioning", "dynamic strength exercises" and so on [42].

Increasing strength

The prescription parameters for optimal strength training are as follows [43]:

Mode and intensity

The training stimulus to produce resistance can come from the weight of the body or any of its segments, from free weights, elastic bands or tubing, or weight machines. The exercise can be isotonic (alternating concentric and eccentric muscle activation that moves a body part through a range of motion against resistance), isokinetic (involving specialised equipment that provides "accommodating" resistance so that the joint moves at a constant angular velocity), isometric (muscle action that is performed against resistance at any point in a joint's range of motion, for periods of 5-10 seconds, and that produces no joint movement), or plyometric (requiring eccentric activation of muscles against a resistance, followed by a brief amortisation period, and after by "explosive" concentric activation).

When isotonic exercises are performed, the concept of a "Repetition Maximum" (RM) should be used to prescribe the weight or load that one lifts: "n" RM represents the maximal load a person can move for n repetitions before fatigue in conditions of good technique, for example a 1 RM is the maximal load for one (and only one) repetition. To elicit improvements in both muscular strength and endurance, the American College of Sports Medicine recommends performing 8-12 repetitions (i.e., 8-12 RM, corresponding or 60-70% of 1RM). Some other programs suggest 15-20 repetitions (corresponding 50-60% of 1 RM) for patients with musculo-skeletal disorders or older persons in order to avoid tissue strain, but there is no evidence to justify this precaution, with the exception of evident lack of tissue tolerance to strain (in such case, a starting dosage of 20 RM is usually adequate). A training for local muscular endurance (e.g., > 20 RM) is recommended when more repetitive activity is needed at work. Furthermore, also power development programs (using light to moderate loading for 6-10 repetitions with high repetition velocity) may help to optimise functional abilities.

Conversely, in some specific working activities the loads and repetitions established in the FCE tests can be transferred directly to training, e.g., the 5 repetitions used in the FCE lifting tests have proved appropriate also for lifting training.

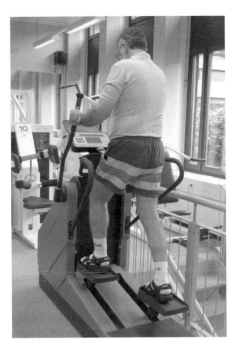

Fig. 1 – Training of cardiovascular endurance and back stabilisation.

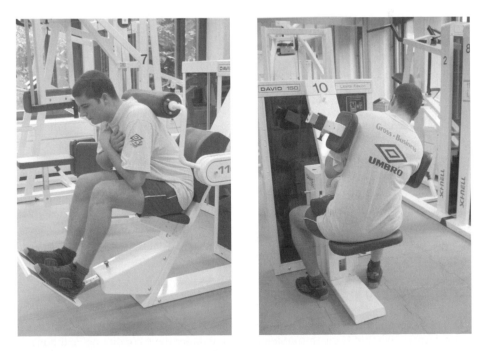

Figs. 2a and 2b – Training of back strength and flexibility.

Number of sets

One set of 8-10 exercises that conditions the major muscle groups might be enough for strength training in healthy subjects, but a 2-3 set regimen may provide greater benefits in the case of important deconditioning and pain, or when strength endurance is required at work.

Frequency per week

Two to five times a week (5 times applies more for rehabilitation of important deconditioning and/or self-limitation due to symptom magnification).

All three parameters (intensity, duration, frequency) contribute to the training volume. The volume should exceed that which the muscles normally encounter. This "overload" induces muscles to adapt and progressively increase their ability to generate force. Dynamic muscular strength improvement is greater when eccentric actions are included in the repetition movement. The training program should emphasise multiple-joint exercises and functional closed kinetic chain movements. Also free weights (e.g., dumbbells or exercise ball) are important because they produce patterns of intra- and intermuscular coordination that mimic the movement requirements of specific tasks. Coordination is also improved when doing work simulation training (cf. § [Work simulation training]).

The responses to strength training are both functional and structural [44]. Functional changes include more motor units recruited during a task, more synchronised recruitment of motor units, and less activation of antagonist muscles. Structural changes are increased activity in muscle metabolic enzymes, hypertrophy of muscle fibres, increased size and activity in mitochondria, and splitting of fibres (without true hyperplasia). Strength gains that occur in the first two to three weeks of an exercise program are due to functional changes. Structural changes take longer. The exercise prescriptions produce changes that are specific to: 1) muscle group; 2) joint angle or range of motion; 3) type of muscle action; 4) speed of muscle action; 5) muscle fiber type; 6) metabolic energy system. For these reasons, general motor performance and coordination improve more when the training exercise components also address the specific tasks or activities of the individual worker (cf. § [Work simulation training]).

Particular exercises can sometimes reduce muscle pain, especially when a more intense muscle training (at 10 RM) is performed. Possibly, a high recruitment demand has greater impact on muscle areas respectively fibres that are tense and painful (which do no longer react normally to a low level of neuromuscular recruitment). As a consequence, these areas get (better) activated, local blood circulation and metabolism will improve, and their increased contraction is then followed by (better) relaxation.

Strength training in painful conditions

Many clients with persistent or chronic pain feel pain or even more pain when doing resistance exercises. Should strength training take place under these conditions? Is it possible to gain strength and endurance when exercise performance is limited by pain? In general, persisting or chronic pain is not a reason for avoiding resistance exercises, nor is it an absolute limit for dosage (dosage should be monitored by criteria of safety and fatigue) but appropriate consideration should be given to the pain behaviour. When clients are reliable and willing to join in, less "pushing" is necessary and you have to check that they do not overtrain. Conversely, self-limiting clients should be pushed as far as they tolerate the loads: it is essential to negotiate a compromise that permits both progress in training as well as client's cooperation. Under this condition, the "strength training" will be initially more akin to a pain tolerance training until the client tolerates weights that really produce a physical training effect. Given a linear ratio of pain and load, it is always possible to ask for a "more courageous" level without risk of delayed long-lasting pain or soreness, but particular caution is needed concerning initial performance levels if delayed and/or long-lasting pain due to exercises are known or expected by the patient. In selected cases, electromyostimulation can be added, especially when pain significantly inhibits active muscle recruitment. Strength training should not be applied in case of substantial painful muscle irritation, and people suffering from inflammatory musculo-skeletal disorders and fibromyalgia are not eligible for training in painful conditions.

Strength training through full range of motion?

As already mentioned, strength, coordination and stabilisation ability are specific for range of motion (ROM). If part of ROM is not loaded or trained for a long time (e.g. pronounced lumbar flexion), a local deficit of stabilisation ability will develop and persist. However, loading for instance in lumbar flexion occurs from time to time in daily activity or during work, and damage can easily occur. Therefore it is important perform strength training over the whole ROM. If tolerance to resistance is considerably diminished in the more painful part of ROM, temporarily splitting the movement into two arcs and training the more painful part at a lower resistance than the rest. A similar choice is recommended for a middle painful arc, where training should focus on both sides of ROM leaving out the painful area and aiming to progressively bring closer the two training sections. Appropriate maximal loading throughout the entire ROM can be obtained also with the accommodating resistance of a isokinetic device.

For certain disorders (e.g. osteoarthritis, disc herniation, spinal stenosis or spondylolisthesis) where repeated movements produce important pain increase, stabilisation training with only minimal movement in the middle part of ROM should be prescribed, as the "lesser of two evils". A good option therefore is the training concept "neutral spine" [45, 46], which is based on old well-known back exercises, but forms a unique concept because of its consequent instruction and implementation of the stabilisation principle. First of all, clients learn how to find and maintain their best individual (lumbar) "neutral spine" position (when pain is minimal). In the course of further training, they practise keeping this position stable at all times while increasing movements and exercises of the arms or legs. Corresponding training on weight machines can be done in such a way that the weight is only lifted and moved little in the "neutral spine" position.

Increasing flexibility

Flexibility exercises should be incorporated into the overall fitness program to improve and maintain range of motion (ROM) [43]. Daily exercises should stretch the major muscle groups. A greater flexibility improves joint function, enhances muscle performance, prevents muscle injury (especially during eccentric exercise) and other soft-tissue injury, and decreases post-exercise soreness. Furthermore, more flexible muscles permit greater storage of elastic strain energy and greater force production during plyometric activities. Relevant parameters for stretching protocols include intensity of stretching force, and duration and frequency of stretch. The most widely used protocols consist of static elongation for 10 to 30 sec at a range that causes mild discomfort. The majority of stress relaxation takes place during the initial 12-18 seconds. Slow rates of elongation permit greater stress relaxation than faster rates and generate lower tissue forces. For restriction of lumbar flexibility, repetitive self-mobilisation exercises according to McKenzie appear valuable [47]. A high number of repetitions (e.g., 10 x every hour) and effective stretch at the end of the movement is decisive in order to stretch also structures such as shortened ligaments or joint capsules. For flexibility training, strength training machines are also suitable: a low weight is chosen and full range of movement during the concentric and eccentric phase is emphasised.

Increasing cardiovascular endurance

Many clients with long-lasting musculo-skeletal disorders have poor cardiovascular endurance. The endurance training is thus an important component in a work conditioning or hardening program. The prescription parameters for optimal endurance training are as follows [43]:

Mode and intensity

Exercise should train large muscle groups (at least 1/6 of the global muscle mass), be continuous, and involve aerobic, rhythmic activities (e.g., walking or hiking, running or jogging, cycling, cross-country skiing, aerobic dance or group exercise, rope skipping, rowing, stair climbing or step trainer, swimming, skating). The most effective exercise prescription begins with an aerobic activity that the client enjoys. A prescribed schedule of stepwise increments in intensity, duration and frequency should gradually lead to a maintenance level of fitness. Exercise intensity is calibrated by establishing a training heart rate at 65%-90% of maximum heart rate (MHR, equal to 220-age in years) or 50-85% of HRR reserve (HRR = MHR − resting heart rate). Other widely used formulas for the training heart rate are 190-age or 170-[age/2]. Lower intensity exercise (55-64% of MHR or 40-49% of HRR) is appropriate for unfit individuals. While the equation based on MHR is easy to teach to clients, applying it to older people can be problematic, because it may calculate a training value that is too close to the resting heart rate (so forcing the person to exercise at only the most trivial intensities). In these cases, the intensity should be based on a HRR percentage or the "rating of perceived exertion", which rates the individual feeling of the exercise intensity by an ordinal scale from 6 ("very, very light) to 20 ("very, very hard") (Borg scale). The latter also may be a relevant measure with clients using beta-blocker medication, where heart rate recommendations based on MHR do not apply.

Duration

It depends on intensity, and activity can be continuous or intermittent. Lower-intensity exercise should be performed for at least 30 to 60 min, whereas more intense exercise should last at least 20 min. The first type of exercise is safer and often associated with better adherence than the latter. Less fit individuals can start "building up" exercise bouts throughout the day as long as each bout lasts at least 10-15 minutes (including 3 minutes to achieve the steady state).

Frequency per week

Three to five times a week.

The main benefits of endurance training are:

1) it maintains and improves cardiovascular function; 2) it reduces risk factors associated with many common chronic diseases (coronary artery disease, diabetes mellitus, hypertension, obesity, etc.); 3) it improves bone health and reduces risk for osteoporosis (especially in postmenopausal women); 4) it improves postural stability and reduces risk of falling; 5) it improves general health status, and particularly mood and concepts of personal control and self-efficacy. Some of these features, of course, also apply to resistance training. Matheson demonstrated that both strength of back muscles as well as cardiovascular endurance contribute, independently of each other, to lifting performance capacity [48].

Circuit weight training

Circuit weight training (sequence training) is a useful compromise that allows to train strength, muscular endurance and cardiovascular endurance fairly efficiently in one training session [49]. Individuals proceed immediately from one weight machine (10 repetitions) to the other without any rest interval in-between. The sequence of the equipment is arranged so that the body region trained varies when the weight machine is changed. This prevents muscular fatigue from becoming a limiting factor in producing a cardiovascular effect. The choice of exercises includes about 8 to 12 machines that cover a wide spectrum of functions. Typical equipment includes a back extension and trunk bending, pull-down, shoulder press and leg press. For back training, the inclusion of trunk rotation, lateral flexion as well as hip abduction is important to train also stabilisation in the frontal plane and during rotation. This is important in asymmetric pain patterns (single-sided pain, radiating in the direction of the buttock or leg and/or with single-sided loads). Circuit training is a well-standardised form of basic training and can be quickly developed with clients as a basic module. Depending on the disorder, some of these exercises also address specific problems. In addition to sequence training, other more specific training exercises can be implemented if needed, for stabilisation of spine or peripheral joints, for example.

Work simulation training

Work simulation is the crucial part in the functional training of a WH program. It mimics many job situations, functional postures and tasks, so offering clients the opportunity of practising work activities and procedures in a "therapeutic" framework, in order to train job-specific deficits step by step. Moreover, this training allows one to monitor the client's safety practices, productivity, work behaviours, use of tools and equipment, and complex functions. In this way, clients can progressively regain confidence in their work-related abilities, e.g. when coping with loads and handling tools, in terms of endurance over several hours, and thus eliminate their fears of strain and demands in the workplace before they return to work. Work simulation training also emphasis the clear focus on return to work. As work-simulation training is related to real everyday and work activity, there are also some elements of "play": sometimes clients partially "forget" their pain and restrictions and work in this setting better than in other therapeutic surroundings. Observation of the client during work simulation activities will yield information also regarding cooperativeness, ability to follow instructions, reliability in following schedules or keeping appointments, and ability to get along with others.

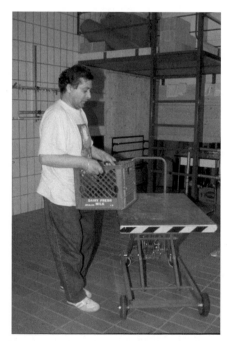

Fig. 3 – Lifting and carrying.

The basis for work simulation is a work-oriented functional assessment: on the basis of the client's work-related deficits, the most suitable work samples (work stations) are selected for training. A work sample may address a single work trait (e.g. manual dexterity), a collection of tasks common to various jobs (e.g. a mix of strength, endurance,

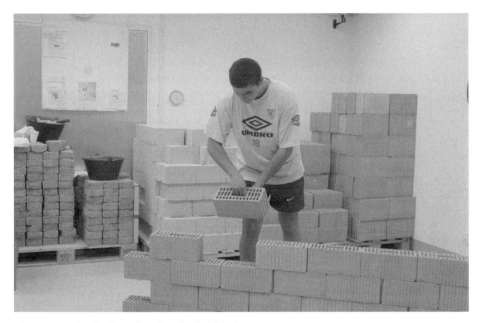

Fig. 4 – Standardised workstation for bricklaying.

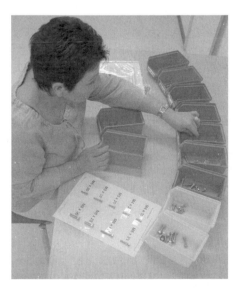

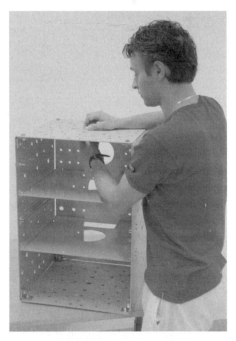

Fig. 5 – Standardised workstation for sorting and assembly (screws and nuts).

Fig. 6 – Bolt box – assembly in various body positions.

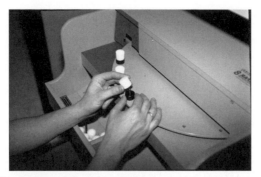

Fig. 7 – Standardised assembly work station (3 components) – performance standing or sitting.

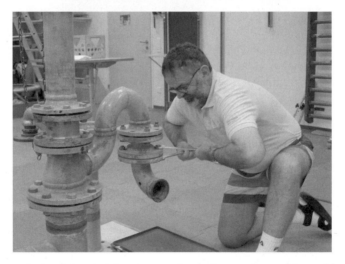

Fig. 8 – For work simulation training, inexpensive devices can be used (assembly system of old tubes).

range of motion, etc.), the common critical factors of a job (but not all factors affecting it, e.g. not including the environmental stress), or all the key tasks of an actual job (e.g. in pipe fitting or electronic assembly) [11, 50, 51]. There are two main kinds of work station used in work-simulation training: standard or job-specific work stations, and computer-controlled work simulators.

Standard and job-specific work stations

Standard work stations are designed to ensure that important work-related skills can be simulated in a simple way. Typical examples are: *lifting, carrying, sorting, brick wall building, tool use (bolt box), electrical installation, installation of a sanitary pipe system*. With this kind of workstations (many are polyvalent with regard to the functions being trained), a wide range of work-related functions can be covered.

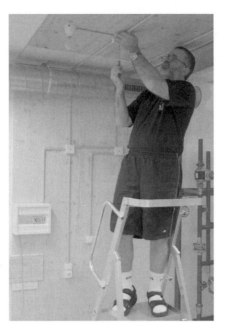

Fig. 9 – Work station for electro-installation.

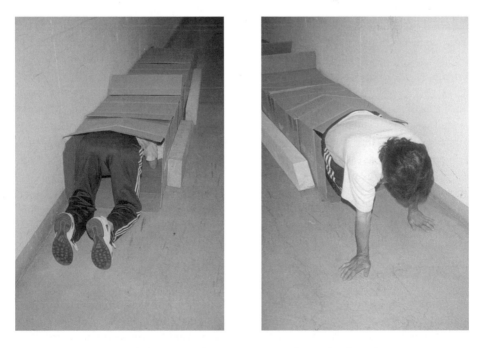

Figs. 10a and 10b – Simple work-specific device conceived with the client for training to move in narrow tunnels (after hip injury).

Important features of standard workstations are:

– standardised working procedure, with clear instructions to the clients. Time to complete the task may be 20-30 minutes or more per station;

– the work done on a standard work station must be measurable in terms of completion time or number of parts per set time or error quota, etc. This allows reasonable goal setting;

– work-simulation training should be competitive for two reasons. Firstly, to provide an incentive for a successive increase in the work load (for example, clients should not simply set up and dismantle any brick wall several times a day, but should measure the time for a defined wall with "n" bricks, try to progressively improve their performance, and compare their current performance with that of a reference population). Secondly, the competitive work input required later in the workplace should be prepared for;

– availability of reference data (e.g., from groups of healthy people or groups such as low back pain patients) to allow comparison with the client's current performance, and help the rehabilitation team to better interpret the client's performance.

Most work stations can be set up by rehabilitation centres themselves with simple means. Some specially designed workstations are offered by companies, e.g. multifunctional work station or work bench (sets for screwing bolts) from Rolyan' [www.smith-nephew.com], or the Valpar Component Work Samples, such as "*Simulated assembly*" or "*Whole-body range of motion*" [www.valparint.com, under "product line/work samples"]. Basic sets of work material (e.g., bricks, shuttering planks, sandbags, ladders for construction workers) should be available. For those occupational requirements less covered by standard workstations, specific working procedures can be simulated providing actual working materials and tools.

Computer-controlled work simulators

Such machines can be used for the computer-controlled testing and training of work-related sets of movements for strength and endurance. The results can be printed out as a report and also in the form of charts. BTE Work Simulator [Baltimore Therapeutic Equipment, USA/www.bteco.com] and E-Link [Biometrics, UK/www.biometricsltd.com] are particularly well-suited to the evaluation of the upper extremities; E-Link also offers computer-animated training, firstly for movement and strength exercises for arms and hands and, secondly, for attention and concentration. Consideration must, however, be given to the relatively high cost of such devices.

Education of ergonomics

At common back schools, the usual choice of activities for training working techniques, and duration and frequency of such training are often too limited to consistently modify the worker's behaviour [20]. Evidence that these ergonomic recommendations are effective (in chronic low back pain) has only been shown when they are carried out at the workplace [19]. But education of ergonomic working techniques may be just as effective during work simulation training as in the workplace. The information must be carefully adapted to the individual's understanding [52] and should be given consistently and repetitively by the members of the rehabilitation team [53]. An educational program may cover body mechanics and proper posture (and eventually a simple review of the anatomic and physiologic background), means for prevention of strain or pain at work, clarification of the role of exercise, and – most important – practical training in safe and economic work performance. In education, direct therapist/client interaction is required. Also videotapes of the client performing simulated work tasks can provide an opportunity for group discussion and be an effective instructional aid.

Education of a worker who manually handles materials should include training to: 1) estimate one's own capacities and limits; 2) always keep the weight to be moved as close to the body as possible; 3) lift the weight slowly and gradually and avoiding brisk movements; 4) divide the weight and distributing it evenly on the upper limbs; 5) distribute very heavy weights into more than one container or between people; 6) use the free hand as a support or rest the foot on a small box/step when flexing the trunk. Conversely, subjects working mostly sitting or standing during the work shift should be aware of how to correctly adjust office furniture and to create conditions of postural changes. The significance of pacing, in particular the structuring of breaks during training or prolonged work activity breaks (e.g., getting up and moving about for a while) and/or monitoring working speed, has already been explained (cf. § [Symptom negotiation training]). Work pacing is a very important ergonomic tool for enhancing work performance and limiting activity-related pain.

Ergonomic interventions at the work site

Depending on the clients' work, an in-depth analysis of the working tools and workplace, and possible adaptations, may be appropriate. A work conditioning or work hardening program that regularly treats clients of a particular company may establish a closer relationship between the centre for rehabilitation ergonomics (that provides the program) and the company, leading to collaboration regarding ergonomic interventions at the work site in order to prevent work-related disorders and long-term disability.

Tool modification

In order to reduce the risk of developing work-related musculo-skeletal disorders, tools should: 1) allow work to be done with the wrist in a neutral position, avoiding excessive flexion, extension, ulnar and radial deviations; 2) be of a congruous and balanced weight (the centre of gravity must correspond to the centre of the hand grip, in order to avoid the tool sliding or rotating); 3) include functionally advantageous levers, particularly if the task requires great strength; 4) have a large area of contact with the hand in order to avoid excessive localised pressure; 5) be usable by both hands so that the hands can be alternated during the task [54]. Biomechanical analysis is basic for identifying stress points [55]. For example, conventional pliers produce a significant pressure on the palm of the hand, thus compressing vessels and nerves, while pliers with asymmetrical handles shaped according to the hand form, with a wider diameter and covered with soft plastic, reduce the pressure on palm and interphalangeal joints. Scissors and pliers should also have automatic opening to avoid local trauma to the dorsal surface of the fingers. The high and low frequency vibrations of electrical instruments can be isolated or reduced by using special covers over the areas in contact with the worker. Gloves incorporating vibration-absorbing materials are commercially available.

Job site modification

There are well-established ergonomic rules and criteria which apply to designing/modifying a workplace [30, 41, 56]. The systematic approach should consider spatial arrangements, the nature and variety of work tasks to be carried out, and the anthropometric characteristics of the employee. The analysis should include the following:

– movements carried out during the work and awkward postures associated with fixed or constrained body positions. For instance, for the upper limbs: raised elbows and arms, manoeuvres involving rotational movements, lack of alignment of the axis object/hand-wrist; for the back: abrupt straightening and bending movements especially if associated with rotation;

– frequency and duration of the work cycles. For instance highly repetitive movements, with cycles lasting less than 30 seconds; frequency and length of breaks;

– strength needed in different tasks. For Instance knobs to rotate and equipment with short levers that require excessive force to move; the frequent need to use a hand strength greater than 20% of the maximum isometric force; use of inappropriate gloves (worn to protect against abrasions, cuts and blisters, but which reduce the coefficient of friction between the hand and the instrument: consequently a stronger grip must be produced during the task); excessive weight of the material being moved (acute dynamic overload).

Characteristics of the workplace, which can cause exposure to mechanical trauma. For instance a table with sharp edges; slippery surfaces; lack of mechanical aids; vibration stress (electrical equipment); thermal stress.

The importance of a properly structured workplace (together with correct positions and work manoeuvres) should not be overlooked, remembering that during heavy tasks: 1) bending forward to lift a weight can increase the load on the back by up to 2.5 times that of the same weight lifted with a straight back and the knees bent; 2) lifting a weight above shoulder height decreases the tolerable weight by 25-30% of that which can be lifted to lower heights; 3) a load held at arms' length produces five times more stress on the spine than does the same weight held close to the body; d) the maximum load that can be lifted highly varies according to lifting frequency, and so on. Such considerations highlight the importance of structuring the workplace where manual material handling is performed, in order to: 1) arrange the materials to move at a height between the hands and the shoulders, and minimise all distances with respect to hand positions; 2) use appropriate work surfaces; 3) minimise the length of transports; 4) optimise the grip of the weight and accessibility (and robustness) of storeroom shelves; 5) minimise the weight of containers and study their best shape; 6) use mechanical systems for lifting (elevators) and transport (trolleys) for heavy or cumbersome loads.

Similarly, when manual work is carried out in the sitting position, the workplace must be planned in such a way that: 1) the height, distance and any slope of the work bench are appropriate; 2) the parts on which the forearms and elbows rest are padded; 3) no postures or movements are necessary that involve joint excursions to the maximum limits, but rather the task can be performed while maintaining the joints in a neutral position for as much time as possible; 4) containers for objects are at bench height, slightly tilted towards the worker and have low sides. In VDT workstations, the choice of a work chair should be based not only on anthropometric criteria but also on ergonomic principles such as the presence of: 1) adjustable seat height; 2) adjustable, tilting, body-contoured back support; 3) prong base with no-slip swivel casters; 4) armrests. As for computer screens, there must be at least 50-70 cm between the screen and the person looking at it and the screen must not be placed in front of light sources, such as windows. Moreover, the desk should have a sufficient width and depth and its height should assure leg room (the usual range is 65-85 cm.). The use of a footstool could be also considered if height of the desk is not freely adjustable.

Likewise, the main ergonomic parameters for a driver's seat are: 1) that the back rest is inclined at about 30° with respect to vertical, encompassing the thoraco-lumbar tract, and has a lumbar support cushion about 5 cm thick; 2) that there is a reasonably firm seat, slightly inclined with respect to the horizontal plane; 3) possibly, an automatic gear box, for those who drive for many hours in city traffic.

Further measures regarding stress and pain management, specific counselling

Stressors lead to increased mental as well as muscular tension. Examples of stressors are troubles at the workplace, family problems and vocational or financial insecurity, disturbed sleep. In addition, pain of course is a stressor itself, often connected with fear of no improvement (or even further deterioration) or fear of a severe disease. Stress-related muscular tension, in turn, is a very important pain factor, probably due to a worsening of local blood circulation and metabolic processes with the distribution of pain mediators into the tissue. Stress probably also lowers the pain threshold via direct psychosomatic mechanisms. The relationship between pain and stress is a vicious circle. An important means of stress management is information and education on coping with pain (cf. § [Structured information and education on coping with pain]). Further measures are explained below.

Techniques of relaxation, awareness and diversion

Interesting "mind/body techniques" such as progressive muscle relaxation (first described by Jacobson) or other relaxation concepts [57, 58], meditation [59], "creative visualisation" [60], autogenous training, yoga or other methods have proved to be valuable components of psychological intervention. Sometimes, individual psychological advice on how to cope with stressors is needed.

Therapeutic modalities and medication

Therapeutic modalities can support training by helping to reduce pain and tension, improve mobility and promote the healing soft-tissue disorders. Primarily, self-treatment measures should be taught wherever possible. Sometimes clients can also benefit from massage, physical agents or other modalities and thus train better, but there is the previously mentioned risk of the "feel good trap" *(cf. § [The client's role: personal responsibility and self-treatment])* and of therapeutic dependence. For this reason, the benefits and chances of success must be carefully balanced against any possible disadvantages regarding the individual client. The following modalities might be used: self-application of cold or heat; manual soft-tissue treatments like trigger-point or fascia massage techniques, classical massage techniques; manual therapy; electromyostimulation (inducing repetitive muscle contraction), TENS, targeted pain-point electrotherapy; complementary medicine interventions, etc.

Many clients that are sent for WH take a lot of pain medicaments, including also opioids. Often this medication is not even helping much, but the clients feel dependent on such daily medication. In most of these cases (there might be a few exceptions), it is mandatory to cut the medication down to zero or an absolute minimum (preferably only paracetamol and only when needed, e.g. if pain prevents sleep) prior to the program, in order to allow a realistic and optimal training dosage. Pain management by reasonably adapted activity, pacing, diversion and relaxation techniques and self-application of modalities such as cold packs is much more help in building up self-efficacy than taking a lot of chemicals.

Psychological/psychiatric evaluation and counselling

If needed, specific psychiatric/psychological evaluation and counselling can help to reduce stress and tension and support the training program, especially if the therapist or doctor has communication problems with the client, or when special psychological advice/care is required by the team (e.g. in significant psychiatric disorders such as anxiety and depression, neurosis, post-traumatic stress disorder) or by the client. However, not all clients with problems or signs of symptom magnification are a "case for the psychiatrist". The "small psychological counselling and support" is also one of the tasks of doctor or therapist in their position as coach. The function of a psychologist or psychiatrist is also to supervise the therapists and doctors when dealing with challenging clients.

Occasionally, in connection with stress management, advice should be focused on the way clients run their life. Aspects such as disadvantageous sleeping habits (fatigue because clients do not sleep enough), overweight, excessive coffee drinking (sleeplessness, nervousness, stomach problems), excessive consumption of medicaments, alcohol or drugs, smoking and a lack of meaningful daytime activity (boredom also promotes a focusing on pain) are stress factors. However, it must taken into consideration that these problems not only may cause stress but can themselves also be a consequence of stress.

Vocational evaluation and counselling, social advice

Quite a number of clients have problems regarding their vocational prospects, in particular when they are without secure employment or do not have the possibility to return to their company. In these cases, vocational evaluation or counselling may be required. Additionally, other non-clarified or unsolved socio-economic questions can have a substantial effect on the client's motivation; in such cases, social advice or advice regarding insurance issues may be important.

Discharge from a WH or WC program

Recommendations at discharge

To recommend discharge with return to a specific job, the team has to demonstrate, based on results of FCE tests, that the worker has reached the goals stated in the plan or a plateau in his/her functional levels. For those clients with a specific job to return to, the care providers must document the worker's ability in relation to the job requirements, and the discharge recommendations may consist of the following options: return to work with full duty, modified duty, or reasonable accommodations [7]. If, after training, the worker's residual physical and behavioural functions do not meet the requirements of the job, a further vocational planning, possibly including vocational training, is necessary. Occasionally, additional medical investigation and therapeutic measures may be recommended. In cases of lack of cooperation and willingness to perform the training program and to accept weekly increases of activity level (which should be tolerated based on the functional test or training observation according to the FCE-criteria), the program should be terminated prematurely, and the relevant observations regarding behavioural issues should be documented in the discharge report.

Case management as a means to support return to work

In order to support a successful return to work in some difficult cases, case management in terms of communication with all the important "players" is recommended. The first step is an analysis of the client's environment, which may include protagonists such as partner or other important family members, family doctor, employer, insurance company, lawyer, etc. It is important to gain a picture of this environment and, in particular, to identify possible "brake blocks". It may be useful to contact the negative protagonists, to explain the program and the goals agreed with the client and enlist their support of the client on the way to achieving the goals. Naturally, the inclusion of positive protagonists can also support clients. Sometimes, an external case manager works in close cooperation with the rehabilitation team. There is a moderate evidence for case management that promotes communication, cooperation and the joint goal setting between clients, the rehabilitation team and other medical specialists involved, and employers or supervisors at work [20].

As the work-hardening programs are particularly focused on work, contact with employers is essential. If the client's workplace is in the neighbourhood and reintegration at the regular workplace appears realistic, a visit to the workplace, usually by the therapist together with the client and, possibly, with an external case manager, is highly recommended (*cf. § [Job evaluation]*). External contacts must be carefully planned: the people to be contacted and the right moment have to been determined, and the team member in charge for organising the visit has to be selected.

Quality assurance

A system of quality assurance and certification for the cost-intensive work conditioning or work hardening programs is needed and also required by the insurance companies. This includes guidelines for quality standards or minimum criteria for the program structure, process and outcome evaluation [8], as well as a control system that certifies providers and then checks for quality at regular intervals. One important prerequisite for quality is a structured training for the therapists and physicians for WH. The only WH training of this type so far on offer in Europe is from the Swiss Association for Rehabilitation [www.sar-rehab.ch → Who is who → Interessengemeinschaften → IG Ergonomie].

The main focus for quality assurance is outcome. A continuous review of the results by means of a simple cohort study (including soziodemographic data, some of the questionnaire and functional test results, the judgement of readiness for work at discharge and if possible a follow up regarding return to work) is crucial to reflect on the rehabilitation team's results and compare them with benchmarks provided by published studies. However, such comparisons are complicated by the great differences in outcomes in terms of return to work after WH or functional restoration programs. For example, the following return to work rates in a follow-up of 1 to 2 years have been reported: 87% [61], 77% [62], 63% [32], 32% [63]. These differences may be partially due to differences in quality and intensity of the programs, but many other factors play an important role in the substantial differences in outcome [10]. Some of these factors are:

– differences in patient groups – in terms of medical problems, vocational and social features (e.g. work status, level of physical demands of work), proportion of immigrants (and degree of their integration), proportion of clients in litigation, general motivation. These features are highly relevant but sometimes difficult to measure;

– different environmental factors relating to the social security and public health systems (e.g. legislation and rules regarding working ability, work-related benefits, or pensions), pre-evaluation and expectations of the referring institution (e.g. insurance company) as well as the family relationships, doctors providing primary care for a WH program, more or less restrictive medical assessment of ability to working (before and after the program), workplace security for clients with limited abilities, and labour market situation. With these factors it is a question of the degree of support and the incentive to resume work;

– different determination of relevant outcome parameters.

Such wide dissimilarities make it difficult to compare studies and benchmark a team's own results. At least, it is important to analyse and recognise the factors that may be responsible for important differences in outcome.

Discussion

WC and particularly WH programs are critical when return to work after injury or illness is expected (from a medical point of view), but the usual care and physical therapy have not attained this goal. There are many possible reasons for this failure:

– important client's deconditioning: there is a big gap between actual functional capacity and the physical demands of the specific job;

– lack of work-oriented goals in usual care and physical therapy (these treatments often are pain oriented and do not focus on prompt increase of work related functional capacity, nor do they include work simulation tasks, and they are usually not intensive);

– relevant psychosocial barriers, many of them are listed in the yellow and black flags [23, 24]. They include high levels of pain perception, stress, and depression; catastrophising; hysteric symptoms and hypochondria; low self-esteem; dissatisfaction with the program, poor cooperation and willingness to perform; low job satisfaction; low expectation/intention of return to work, conviction that pain is work-related or that one will no longer be able to restart working; alcohol abuse and other chemical dependence; resentment, anger and frustration; sickness gains – such as avoidance of responsibility, and attention received from others); pending litigation; other financial opportunities – such as unemployment benefits, welfare benefits, worker's compensation, etc. [11, 20, 36, 42, 64, 65, 66].

In order to overcome the multiple barriers to recovery as far as possible, work hardening is not only based on intense and function – and work-oriented physical training (gym and work simulation), it also emphasises education and extensive psychosocial interventions. Important issues are goal setting, self-efficacy, self-responsibility and self-management of pain.

Optimisation of working techniques, tools, equipment and work organisation should be emphasised as well. This approach focuses on adapting the methods of carrying out a task to best suit the individual worker. For example, employee rotation between different tasks would be very useful, alternating the main job with a lighter one, training the subject to early recognise development of health problems and thus call quickly for advice and help. It has been clearly demonstrated that intermittent work with brief pauses (1-2 minutes) alternated with intense efforts is more efficient and healthier than prolonged work with pauses of 20-30 minutes. The ideal option would be to identify the best pace to carry out repetitive tasks (at any rate) and teach it to workers, starting from a lower grade.

A recent Cochrane review concluded that work-related physical conditioning programs including a cognitive-behavioural approach plus intensive physical training seem to be effective in reducing the number of sick days for workers with chronic low back pain when compared with usual care [42]. Similarly, two systematic reviews concluded that there is moderate evidence showing that multidisciplinary biopsychosocial rehabilitation offers some benefit for adults with chronic/subacute low back pain [67, 68]. Nachemson came to the following conclusions in a comprehensive review: 1) concerning prevention of back pain, there is strong evidence for strengthening back muscles, general body building and fitness training; 2) with regard to conservative treatment for chronic back pain, there is strong evidence for training therapy and in the short term for a multidisciplinary treatment program [19]. According to a review by Waddell [20], there is moderate evidence for a comprehensive rehabilitation program, particularly in a work-related setting, and when associated with an organisational intervention (case management) to support the return to work. Haldorsen found in an Norwegian study that multidisciplinary treatment is effective concerning return to work when given to patients who are most likely to benefit from that treatment [69]. A recent meta-analysis on randomised controlled studies regarding non-acute and non-specific back pain came to the following conclusions: treatment sessions with training therapy alone or as part of a multidisciplinary program reduce the number of days off work. The effects are stronger in patients with longer duration of back pain and diminish over time [70].

Because many of the analysed studies have some methodical shortcomings and multidisciplinary return-to-work programs are expensive and need to demonstrate their cost-effectiveness also in the long term (to demonstrate their benefit and justify reimbursement), there is still the need for high-quality trials in this field to address issues such as patient selection, the optimal intensity and duration of programs, and the most effective treatment components.

References

1. Commission for Accreditation of Rehabilitation Facilities (CARF) (1988) Work Hardening Guidelines. Tuscon
2. American Physical Therapy Association (APTA) (1992) Guidelines for programs in industrial rehabilitation. Magazine of Physical Therapy 1: 69-72
3. Matheson LN, Ogden LD, Violette K et al. (1985) Work hardening: occupational therapy in industrial rehabilitation. Am J Occup Ther 39: 314-21
4. Mayer TG, Gatchel RJ (1988) Functional Restoration for Spinal Disorders: The Sports Medicine Approach. Philadelphia, Lea & Febiger, p 1-321
5. Campello M, Weiser S, Van Doorn JW et al. (1998) Approaches to improve the outcome of patients with delayed recovery. Baillieres Clin Rheumatol 12: 93-113
6. Darphin LE (1995) Work-Hardening and Work-Conditioning Perspectives. In: The Comprehensive Guide to Work Injury Management. (Ed. Susan J, Isernhagen P). Gaithersburg, Maryland, Aspen Publishers, p 443-62
7. Demers LM (1992) Work hardening. A practical guide. Boston, Andover Medical Publishers

8. Hart DL, Berlin S, Brager PE *et al.* (1994) Development of clinical standards in industrial rehabilitation. J Orthop Sports Phys Ther 19: 232-41

9. Isernhagen SJ (1991) Functional Capacity Evaluation and Work Hardening Perspectives. In: Contemporary Conservative Care for Painful Spinal Disorders. (Eds. Mayer TG, Mooney V, Gatchel R). Philadelphia/London, Lea & Febiger, p 328-345

10. Lechner DE (1994) Work Hardening and Work Conditioning: Do they affect disability? Physical Therapy, p 74

11. Burt CM (2001) Work evaluation and work hardening. In: Occupational therapy. (Eds.Pedretti LW, Early MB). St. Louis, Mosby 5: 226-36

12. Fenton S, Gagnon P (1998a) Evaluation of work and productive activities: work performance assessment measures. In: Willard & Spackman's Occupational Therapy. (Eds.Neistadt ME, Crepeau EB). Philadelphia, Lippincott William & Wilkins 9: 208-13

13. Fenton S, Gagnon P (1998b) Treatment of work and productive activities: functional restoration, an industrial rehabilitation approach. In: Willard & Spackman's Occupational Therapy. (Eds.Neistadt ME, Crepeau EB). Philadelphia, Lippincott William & Wilkins 9: 377-82

14. Industrial rehabilitation medicine (1992) Arch Phys Med Rehabil 73[5-S]: 3-28

15. Industrial rehabilitation medicine (1997) Arch Phys Med Rehabil 78[3 Suppl]

16. Industrial medicine and acute musculoskeletal rehabilitation (2002) Arch Phys Med Rehabil 83[3 Suppl 1]: 1-39

17. Andersson GBJ, Frymoyer JW (1991) Treatment of the Acutely Injured Worker. In: Occupational Low Back Pain. (Eds.Pope MH, Andersson GBJ, Frymoyer JW, Chaffin DB). Mosby Year Book, p 183-93

18. Krause N, Ragland D R (1994) Occupational disability due to low back pain: a new interdisciplinary classification based on a phase model of disability. Spine 19: 1011-20

19. Nachemson AL, Jonsson E (2000) Neck and Back Pain. Lippincott Williams & Wilkins. Philadelphia USA, p 1-473

20. Waddell G, Burton A K (2001) Occupational health guidelines for the management of low back pain at work: evidence review. [www.facoccmed.ac.uk → Publications]. Occup Med (Lond) 51: 124-35

21. Foye PM, Stitik TP, Marquardt CA *et al.* (2002) Industrial medicine and acute musculoskeletal rehabilitation. 5. Effective medical management of industrial injuries: from causality to case closure. Arch Phys Med Rehabil 83: 19

22. Matheson LN, Matheson ML (1996) Spinal Function Sort (PACT-Test, edited in different languages). Swiss Association for Rehabilitation SAR, Working group Ergonomics [www.sar-rehab.ch → Who is who → Interessengemeinschaften → IG Ergonomie]

23. Kendall NAS, Linton SJ, Main CJ (2004) Guide to assessing psychosocial yellow flags in acute low back pain: risk factors for long term disability and work loss. Wellington (NZ), Accident rehabilitation and Compensation Insurance Corporation of New Zealand and the National Health Committee [www.nzgg.org.nz → guidelines → musculoskeletal disease]

24. Main CJ, Spanswick CC (2000) Pain Management. An Interdisciplinary Approach. Churchill Livingstone

25. Fishbain DA (2000) Functional capacity evaluation. Phys Ther 80: 110-2

26. King PM, Tuckwell N, Barrett TE (1998) A critical review of functional capacity evaluations. Physical Therapy 78: 852-66

27. Jones T, Kumar S (2003) Functional capacity evaluation of manual materials handlers: a review. Disabil Rehabil 25: 179-91

28. Waddell G, McCullock JA, Kummel E *et al.* (1980) Nonorganic Physical Signs in Low-back pain. Spine 5: 117-25

29. Waddell G (1998) The Back Pain Revolution. Churchill Livingstone, p 223-40

30. Grandjean E (1991) Fitting the Task to the Man. A textbook of Occupational Ergonomics. London, Taylor & Francis

31. Rajan JA, Wilson JR (1997) Introduction to task analysis. In: Musculoskeletal Disorders in the Workplace: Principles and Practice. (Eds. Nordin M, Andersson GBJ, Pope MH). St. Louis, Mosby, p 167-90

32. Pfingsten M, Hildebrandt J, Leibing E *et al.* (1997) Effectiveness of a multimodal treatment program for chronic low-back pain. Pain 73: 77-85

33. Gatchel RJ, Mayer TG, Hazard RG *et al.* (2002) Editorial: Functional Restoration. Pitfalls in Evaluating Efficacy. Spine 17: 988-95

34. Matheson LN (1995) Getting a Handle on Motivation: Self-Efficacy in Rehabilitation. In: The Comprehensive Guide to Work Injury Management. (Ed.Susan J.Isernhagen). Gaithersburg, Maryland, Aspen, p 514-42

35. Kopp HG, Oliveri M, Thali A (1997) Erfassung und Umgang mit Symptomausweitung. Medizinische Mitteilungen der Suva 70: 56-78

36. Vlaeyen JW, Linton SJ (2000) Fear-avoidance and its consequences in chronic musculoskeletal pain: a state of the art. Pain 85: 317-32

37. Vlaeyen JW, De Jong J, Geilen M *et al.* (2001) Graded exposure in vivo in the treatment of pain-related fear: a replicated single-case experimental design in four patients with chronic low back pain. Behav Res Ther 39: 151-66

38. Burton AK, Waddell G, Tillotson KM *et al.* (1999) Information and advice to patients with back pain can have a positive effect. A randomized controlled trial of a novel educational booklet in primary care. [www.coventrypainclinic.org.uk → Spinal Pain → The Back Book]. Spine 24: 2484-91

39. Harding VR, Simmonds MJ, Watson PJ (1998) Physical Therapy for Chronic Pain. Pain Clinical Updates VI

40. Vlaeyen JW, De Jong J, Geilen M *et al.* (2002) The treatment of fear of movement/(re)injury in chronic low back pain: further evidence on the effectiveness of exposure in vivo. Clin J Pain 18: 251-61

41. Kroemer KHE, Kroemer HB, Kroemer-Elbert KE (1994) Ergonomics: How to design for ease and efficiency. Englewoods Cliffs, Prentice Hall

42. Schonstein E, Kenny DT, Keating J *et al.* (2003) Work Conditioning, Work Hardening and Functional Restoration for Workers with Back and Neck Pain (Cochrane Review). The Cochrane Library [4]. Chichester, John Wiley ans Sons, Ltd

43. Kraemer WJ, Adams K, Cafarelli E *et al.* (2002) American College of Sports Medicine position stand. Progression models in resistance training for healthy adults. Med Sci Sports Exerc 34: 364-80

44. Deschenes MR, Kraemer WJ (2002) Performance and physiologic adaptations to resistance training. Am J Phys Med Rehabil 81: 3-16

45. Saal JA (1991) The New Back School Prescription: Stabilization Training Part II. In: SPINE: State of the Art Reviews. (Ed.White LA). Philadelphia, Hanley & Belfus, Inc. p 357-66

46. Saal JA, Saal JS (1991) Postoperative Rehabilitation and Training. In: Contemporary Conservative Care for Painful Spinal Disorders. (Eds.Mayer TG, Mooney V, Gatchel RJ). Philadelphia, Lea & Febiger 1: 318-27

47. McKenzie RA, May S (2003) The Lumbar Spine. Mechanical Diagnosis and Therapy. 2[1 & 2]. Waikanae, New Zealand, Spinal Publications

48. Matheson LN, Leggett S, Mooney V *et al.* (2002) The contribution of aerobic fitness and back strength to lift capacity. Spine 27, 1208-12

49. Gunnari H, Evjenth O, Brady M (1984) Sequence exercise. The sensible approach to all-round fitness. Oslo, Dreyers Forlag, 1:1-151

50. Bernard BP (1997) Musculoskeletal Disorders and Workplace Factors. Cincinnati, NIOSH

51. Pruitt WA (1986) Vocational evaluation. In: Menomonie, W. Pruitt Associates, p 105-35

52. Cedraschi C, Nordin M, Nachemson AL *et al.* (1998) Health care providers should use a common language in relation to low back pain patients. Baillieres Clin Rheumatol 12: 1-15

53. Nordin M, Cedraschi C, Balague F *et al.* (1992) Back schools in prevention of chronicity. Baillieres Clin Rheumatol 6: 685-703

54. Putz-Anderson V (1988) Cumulative trauma disorders: A manual for musculoskeletal diseases of the upper limbs. London, Taylor & Francis

55. Amstrong TJ (2000) Analysis and design of jobs for control of work related musculoskeletal disorders. In: Occupational Ergonomics: Work Related Musculoskcletal disorders of the Upper Limb and Back. (Eds.Violante F, Amstrong T, Kilbom A). London, Taylor & Francis, p 51-81

56. Chaffin DB, Andersson GBJ (1991) Occupational Biomechanics. New York, John Wiley & Sons

57. Benson H (2000) The Relaxation Response. New York, HarperTorch/HarperCollins Publishers, p 1-227

58. Bernstein DA, Borkovec TD, Hazlett-Stevens H (2000) Progressive Relaxation Training: A Guidebook for Helping Professionals. Praeger Publishers. München, Verlag J. Pfeiffer, p 1-176

59. Kabath-Zinn J (1991) Full Catastrophe Living. Using the Wisdom of Your Body and Mind to Face Stress, Pain, and Illness. New York, Delta; Dell Publishing, 1:1-467

60. Gawain S (2002) Creative Visualization. Use the Power of Your Imagination to Create What You Want in Your Life. Novato (California), Nataraj Publishing/New World Library, 1:1-175

61. Mayer TG, Gatchel RJ, Mayer H *et al.* (1987) A Prospective Two-Year Study of Functional Restoration in Industrial Low-Back Injury. An Objective Assessment Procedure. Jama 258: 1763-7

62. Lanes TC, Gauron EF, Spratt KF *et al.* (1995) Long-term follow-up of patients with chronic back pain treated in a multidisciplinary rehabilitation program. Spine 20: 801-6

63. Corey DT, Koepfler LE, Etlin, Day HI (1996) A Limited Funcitional Restoration Program for Injured Workers: A Randomized Trial. Journal of Occupational Rehabilitation 6

64. Beissner KL, Saunders RL, McManis BG (1996) Factors related to successful work hardening outcomes. Phys Ther 76: 1188-201

65. Niemeyer LO, Jacobs K, Reynolds-Lynch K *et al.* (1994) Work hardening: past, present, and future – the work programs special interest section national work-hardening outcome study. Am J Occup Ther 48: 327-39

66. Petersen M (1995) Nonphysical factors that affect work hardening success: a retrospective study. J Orthop Sports Phys Ther 22: 238-46

67. Guzman J, Esmail R, Karjalainen K *et al.* (2001) Multidisciplinary rehabilitation for chronic low back pain: systematic review. Bmj 322: 1511-6

68. Karjalainen K, Malmivaara A, Van Tulder M *et al.* (2003) Multidisciplinary biopsychosocial rehabilitation for subacute low back pain among working age adults. Cochrane Database Syst Rev CD002193

69. Haldorsen EH, Grasdal AL, Skouen JS *et al.* (2002) Is there a right treatment for a particular patient group? Comparison of ordinary treatment, light multidisciplinary treatment, and extensive multidisciplinary treatment for long-term sick-listed employees with musculoskeletal pain. Pain 95: 49-63

70. Kool J, De Bie R, Oesch P *et al.* (2004) Exercise reduces sick leave in patients with non-acute non-specific low back pain: a meta-analysis. J Rehab Med 36: 49-62

Vocational rehabilitation and low back pain

V. Fialka-Moser, M. Herceg and E. Hartter

Low back pain – a leading work-related musculo-skeletal disorder

Low back pain (LBP) is one of the major problems among work-related musculo-skeletal disorders. Its lifetime prevalence among workers and the general population is 60% to 80%, with a yearly incidence of 6% to 20%. Most episodes are mild and self-limited. Approximately 90% recover spontaneously and return to activity within one month, 20% seek health care, and only about 10% of the affected workers seek compensation [1]. Epidemiologic studies have investigated the recovery time of workers with low back pain: 40% to 50% of them are back at work by 2 weeks, 70% to 80% return by 4 weeks. Those workers who are still absent from work at 6 months are at progressively higher risk for becoming chronically disabled [2]. The small number of cases that become chronic account for a large part of the compensation expenses [3]. Webster *et al.* stated that low-back injuries constitute 16% of all workers' compensation claims, but consume 33% of all claim costs [4].

Work-related and personal risk factors

Work-related risk factors for back injuries have been identified, such as heavy physical work, repetitive work tasks, exposure to vibration, frequent bending and twisting, static work postures, and lifting or forceful movements [5]. Wanek *et al.* [6] stated that psychosocial stressors such as time pressure, conflicts with co-workers and superiors are also important. The frequency of chronic back pain, working conditions and requests for workplace modifications were investigated among 974 employers of a metal company. Prolonged exposure to physical stressors was associated with a strongly elevated risk for chronic back pain. In addition, research has linked work-related musculo-skeletal disorders to stressful aspects of work organization, such as machine-paced work, inadequate work-rest cycles, wage incentives, time pressure, overload, low job control, low social support, and repetitive work, and lack of task variability [7].

Garg *et al.* [8] identified personal risk factors such as age, gender, anthropometry, physical fitness and training, lumbar mobility, strength, medical history, years of employment, smoking, psychosocial factors and structural abnormalities.

Factors affecting outcome of vocational rehabilitation and return to work time

For the physician in charge, a thorough medical history taking is very important for a proper diagnosis. It is also important for prognosticating and managing the individual's return to work. A history of previous injuries on the job and recovery periods can be very helpful. An exact description of the incident is essential; the same is true for the work tasks and the frequency of performing these tasks. The nature of pain, the postures that induce difficulties, and the effects of medication should be inquired. The worker's perception of his functional ability or rather disability is also important, because sometimes a return to light duty is possible and this would mean less absent workers on compensation. The individual's attitude towards the job may affect his/her speed of return to work; the attitude towards the boss or work culture may be useful in making a prognosis. Finally, work environment, job requirements, and the patient's perception of the employer's flexibility are important, since the worker is often expected to perform the original job to its full extent [2].

Selander *et al.* [9] reviewed publications from 1980 through to 2000 to overview factors which are associated with return to work following vocational rehabilitation for problems in the neck, back, and shoulders. A variety of (risk-)factors are associated with return to work in numerous ways.

Demographic factors are age, gender, nationality, income, level of education, marital status, living situation, legal claim working status and earlier sick leave.

Possible psychological and social factors would be self-confidence, life satisfaction, and level of experienced health, depression, health locus of control, cooperativeness, hypochondria, motivation and belief in return to work as well as social situation.

Medical factors are medical history, level of disease/injury severity, pain, and neurological symptoms during treatment as well as activities of daily living.

Furthermore factors can also be either rehabilitation related (type of rehabilitation measure, timing of vocational rehabilitation, understanding of work place, programme completion, patient influence, satisfaction with rehabilitation programme), or workplace related (changing jobs, working environment, modified work, early return to workplace, unscheduled breaks, vocational sector, job seniority, work history, size of workplace, public sector vs. private) but also benefit-system-related (disability benefit status, level of compensation, unemployment rates).

An important point is to carefully match workers and jobs. To achieve this end, a job analysis should describe the physical requirements for the tasks involved. Standardised tests of the essential functions of the specific job should exist. Work stations and tasks should be ergonomically designed, taking into account variations in physical size and capacity.

Gender differences, i.e., gender-specific vulnerabilities and advantages should also be considered. Headapohl [10] stated that there are differences not only between sexes but also among individuals of the same sex. An increasing number of women are now engaged in traditionally male occupations. Gender, pregnancy and individual differences have to be taken into account in job placement, worker protection and the ergonomics of accommodation.

Prevention and intervention

To maximize safety and efficiency at the workplace, Scheer et al. [11] recommended ergonomic assessment which included job analysis from the biomechanical, physiological and physical viewpoint. This review identified workers' training (fitness and stretching exercise, back support belts, postural instruction and back goniometric warning alarms), selection of workers (matching of workers' capacity and job requirements) and job/workplace redesign (to eliminate or lessen unfavourable mechanical stresses) as the three most commonly described categories of ergonomic intervention. Workplace redesign, using both engineering (directly affecting the job) and administrative methods (affecting the worker), is likely to be the most effective intervention.

A review of 14 randomized controlled trials made by Staal et al. [12] showed the need for effective treatment interventions for low back pain. The aim was to prevent chronic disability and achieve return to work. The results revealed different approaches using various physical exercises (muscle strengthening, coordination exercises, ROM exercises for the spine, cardiovascular fitness programs and reduction of muscle tension), education (to increase the patients' understanding of their disorder and treatment), and behavioural treatments (based on the gate control theory and/or the operant conditioning hypothesis). No concepts for ergonomic measures were presented [12].

Investigations by Schmidt et al. [13] demonstrated a significant impact of vocational rehabilitation (provided at the rehabilitation centre) and working on a trial basis (real work environment) on employment after rehabilitation. The likelihood of return to work was two-fold higher for people who participated in vocational rehabilitation than for those who did not, and three-fold higher for those who were involved in both vocational rehabilitation and work on trial than for those who were only involved in a vocational rehabilitation program. Thus, the study suggests that programs specifically aimed at promoting employment for persons with disabilities are effective, especially when they take place both in a laboratory and a natural setting.

Torstensen et al. [14] demonstrated that medical exercise therapy and conventional physical therapy reduce the costs of low back pain, even in chronic cases. Håland Haldorsen et al. demonstrated that multidisciplinary treatment (cognitive behavioural modification, education, exercise and occasional workplace interventions) was effective

in regard of returning to work, when provided for patients who were most likely to benefit from the treatment [15]. Butterfield *et al.* found out that injured workers who stopped exercising after a back injury had longer periods of disability than those who remained more active [16].

Gatchel was able to show the treatment and cost effectiveness of an early intervention
program for acute LBP patients. Seven-hundred patients with acute low back pain were
screened for their high risk or low risk status for developing chronicity. An early screening and intervention program (psychology, physical therapy, occupational therapy and
case management) among patients with acute low back pain could help to prevent high-
risk patients from becoming chronic and also save costs [17].

The role of the occupational or company physician

Obviously the key problems of occupationally acquired or occupation-associated LBP
are an ergonomic and satisfactory work place on the one side (primary prevention), and
early intervention on the other (secondary prevention). Ideally both should be provided
in close association to the work place. Recent literature indicates that the company physician or occupational physician might substantially contribute to the management of
both these problems [18, 19]. He/she is familiar with the work-place situation and the
resulting physical as well as psychomental stress and strain on the employees and usually
has knowledge about their health complaints at an early stage. Ideally he/she will make
suggestions on ergonomic workplace (re)design, on establishment of workplace safety
and healthy conditions of work, risk-management, instruct employees about safe work
techniques, as well as health hazards, and provide consulting about measures of general
as well as personal primary and secondary prevention. Occupational physicians should
recognize health complaints associated with or with relevance for the work-place at the
very early stage and provide or initiate adequate intervention (workplace-oriented, medical treatment). Integration of the occupational physician or company physician into the
process of vocational rehabilitation might substantially reduce the time until its onset,
the return to work time and the success rate [19].

Conclusions

This overview clearly indicates the need for a broad approach to the subject of vocational
rehabilitation. The need for improvement has been emphasised in many studies. Greater
efficiency, cost containment (less compensation and sick leave) as well as effective strategies for prevention, intervention and treatment methods are important topics [12, 17, 20].

Patients still have to accept prolonged waiting periods and processing times until
occupational rehabilitation can start. To improve communication between rehabilitation
centres and vocational training centres, cooperative approaches between these institutions were initiated in Germany. This resulted in a considerable acceleration of proce-

dures. Occupational reintegration of insured patients was improved to a high degree. The key term here is "occupationally orientated medical rehabilitation" [21].

Many different factors have to be taken into account. Communication between workers, business enterprises, occupational physicians, insurance companies, health care providers and the rehabilitation team is of great importance. From the rehabilitation point of view, it takes a team effort between doctors, therapists (physiotherapy and occupational therapy) as well as psychologists and social workers to provide the best possible care.

References

1. Hales TR, Bernard BP (1996) Epidemiology of work-related musculo-skeletal disorders. Orthop Clin North Am 27: 679-709
2. Scheer SJ, Robinson JP, Rondinelli RD et al. (1997) Industrial rehabilitation medicine. 2. Case studies in occupational low back pain. Arch Phys Med Rehabil 78: 10-5
3. Spengler DM, Bigos SJ, Martin NA et al. (1986) Back injuries in industry: a retrospective study. I. Overview and cost analysis. Spine 11: 241-5
4. Webster BS, Snook SH (1994) The cost of 1989 workers' compensation low back pain claims. Spine 19: 1111-5; discussion 1116
5. Andersson GB (1981) Epidemiologic aspects on low-back pain in industry Spine 6: 53-60
6. Wanek V, Brenner H, Novak P et al. (1998) Back pain in industry: prevalence, correlation with work conditions and requests for reassignment by employees. Gesundheitswesen 60: 513-2
7. Landsbergis PA (2003) The changing organization of work and the safety and health of working people: a commentary. J Occup Environ Med 45: 61-72
8. Garg A, Moore JS (1992) Epidemiology of low-back pain in industry. Occup Med 7: 593-608
9. Selander J, Marnetoft SU, Bergroth A et al. (2002) Return to work following vocational rehabilitation for neck, back and shoulder problems: risk factors reviewed. Disabil Rehabil 24: 704-12
10. Headapohl D (1993) Sex, gender, biology, and work. Occup Med 8: 685-707
11. Scheer SJ, Mital A (1997) Ergonomics. Arch Phys Med Rehabil 78: S36-45
12. Staal JB, Hlobil H, Van Tulder MW et al. (2002) Return-to-work interventions for low back pain: a descriptive review of contents and concepts of working mechanisms. Sports Med 32: 251-67
13. Schmidt SH, Oort-Marburger D, Meijman TF (1995) Employment after rehabilitation for musculoskeletal impairments: the impact of vocational rehabilitation and working on a trial basis. Arch Phys Med Rehabil 76: 950-4
14. Torstensen TA, Ljunggren AE, Meen HD et al. (1998) Efficiency and costs of medical exercise therapy, conventional physiotherapy, and self-exercise in patients with chronic low back pain. A pragmatic, randomized, single-blinded, controlled trial with 1-year follow-up. Spine 23: 2616-24
15. Haldorsen EM, Grasdal AL, Skouen JS et al. (2002) Is there a right treatment for a particular patient group? Comparison of ordinary treatment, light multidisciplinary treatment, and extensive multidisciplinary treatment for long-term sick-listed employees with musculoskeletal pain. Pain 95: 49-63

16. Butterfield PG, Spencer PS, Redmond N *et al.* (1998) Low back pain: predictors of absenteeism, residual symptoms, functional impairment, and medical costs in Oregon workers' compensation recipients. Am J Ind Med 34: 559-67
17. Gatchel RJ, Polatin PB, Noe C *et al.* (2003) Treatment – and cost-effectiveness of early intervention for acute low-back pain patients: a one-year prospective study. J Occup Rehabil 13: 1-9
18. Hartmann B. (2003) Rückenschmerzen am Arbeitsplatz – Ursachen und Konsequenzen für den Betriebsarzt. Arbeitsmed Sozialmed Umweltsmed 38: 566-75
19. Haase I, Riedl G, Birkholz LB *et al.* (2002) Verzahnung von medizinischer Rehabilitation und beruflicher Reintegration. Arbeitsmed Sozialmed Umweltsmed 37: 331-35
20. Rondinelli RD, Robinson JP, Scheer SJ *et al.* (1997) Industrial rehabilitation medicine. 4. Strategies for disability management. Arch Phys Med Rehabil 78: 21-8
21. Winkelhake U, Schutzeichel F, Niemann O *et al.* (2003) Occupationally Orientated Medical Rehabilitation (BOR) for disabilities caused by orthopedic diseases. Rehabilitation (Stuttg) 42: 30-5

Vocational rehabilitation in musculo-skeletal disorders – with examples mainly from the neck and shoulder region

J. Ekholm and K. Schüldt Ekholm

Particular principles of vocational rehabilitation of musculo-skeletal disorders

The literature on medical rehabilitation of patients with musculo-skeletal disorders is extensive [1, 2, 3], but the literature about vocational rehabilitation of those patients is considerably less [4, 5, 6]. What then, are the characteristics of vocational rehabilitation? One particular feature is that a job is involved in the process. The present chapter is focused on job-related factors of rehabilitation and will not describe general principles of medical rehabilitation of patients with diseases, disorders or injuries of the locomotor system.

If musculo-skeletal disorders, in this context, are divided into two main categories, one part can be musculo-skeletal painful conditions where the specific origin of the pathogenesis is not proven to be loading events of the work place, but for the patient still involve easily elicited pain in situations of load during working, e.g. arthrosis of cervical spinal joints, coxarthrosis, gonarthrosis.

The second part of the musculo-skeletal disorders can be the work related musculo-skeletal disorders (WMSDs) where loading situations of the patients' work tasks are associated with the etiology of the painful disorder [7], e.g. rotator cuff tendonitis, trapezius pars descendens myalgia, levator scapulae tendalgia, cervical spine extensor myalgia/tendonitis (or "tension neck syndrome"), lateral epicondylitis, hand-wrist tendonitis.

For both above mentioned categories the vocational rehabilitation measures must include improvement of the patient's work situations. In the second category with WMSDs it is crucial to eliminate the pathogenetic factors that have caused the patient's disease or disorder. Without changes in the working conditions the patient will get a recurrence after resuming work with the same tasks unchanged. This means that a thorough investigation of the patient's work history and work tasks must be performed, as well as inspection of the work place. In many countries the employer has an extensive responsibility to participate in vocational rehabilitation of this kind of patients. The preventive aspect is important [8]. If the patient is merely put on another task and his/her previous work station is unchanged some other employee will be at risk of getting the same WMSD.

For patients in the first mentioned category with disease or disorders not directly generated by the work load, the situation is somewhat different. In principle even modest loading can generate troublesome pain because the disease may generate easily elicited pain even if the load is light [9]. For these patients, too, the analysis of the work task is of great importance, since it might be possible to improve the situation by means of ergonomic measures. In addition, it may be important to inform the patient that the underlying disease is not produced by the work load itself. However, even for these patients the risk of recurrence exists, without changes in the working conditions.

Rough categorization of muscular and tendinous pain affected by external load

A rough grouping of common muscular pain conditions with tendon disorders included, related to vocational rehabilitation needs is *(i) regional pain which has a load-related pathogenesis including work-related musculo-skeletal disorders (WMSDs) containing neck and/or shoulder pain, with or without pain of upper limb, and tendon disorders of hand and forearm, certain forms of hip and knee arthrosis; (ii) regional pain with no proven load related pathogenesis as, for example, arthritis and spondylosis, myofascial pain syndromes and (iii) widespead pain conditions e.g., fibromyalgia syndrome.*

Occurrence of musculo-skeletal disorders in the context of vocational rehabilitation

The prevalence pattern of acute or subacute diseases or injuries and short-time sick leave is different from persistent (chronic) conditions common in long-term illness absence. The selection of patients influences the prevalence pattern. Often patients who have been assessed as having vocational rehabilitation needs have been sick-listed for a long time.

In many of those on long-term sick leave, musculo-skeletal disorders are the dominating factor.

About half of those on long-term sick-leave, awaiting decisions about a disability pension or vocational rehabilitation, will have musculo-skeletal diagnoses, of which low back pain and neck-shoulder pain represent a substantial portion [10, 11].

Vocational rehabilitation of patients with neck and shoulder pain conditions, with or without arm pain

Medical investigation

A medical examination must be undertaken to establish the diagnosis and pathophysiology underlying the symptoms. In principle, three different categories of load-related conditions can be identified. If the neck extensors are overused due to uninterrupted contraction of the dorsal neck muscles in situations where the head and neck are kept in a markedly bent position persistent pain may be generated in the dorsal neck muscles, their origins or insertions. This result in dorsal neck myalgia/tendonitis.

Overuse of shoulder girdle elevators may give persistent pain in one or more of the shoulder girdle elevating muscles – trapezius pars descendens, levator scapulae or the rhomboids with tendons.

Overuse of muscles and tendons involved in coordination of movements between the scapula and humeral bone may result in persistent painful conditions, such as rotator cuff tendonitis, biceps brachii proximal tendonitis.

It is important to analysis the type of pain involved; nocioceptive, neurogenic, psychogenic, or pain of unknown origin [12, 13]. Some patients have more than one type of pain, e.g. nocioceptive pain in cervical spine structures in combination with neurogenic pain in the form of radiculopathy. Different types of pain require different treatment strategies. A common combination of pain types is focal nocioceptive musculo-skeletal pain with referred pain in shoulders or upper extremity. In a selected group of women who were working in spite of pain, referred pain was present in about one third with focal pain in neck and/or shoulder [14]. Referred pain in combination with neck and/or shoulder pain as source of brachialgia is more common than neurogenic pain. An important step in the medical investigation is to map functional impairments, activity limitations and participation restrictions according to the ICF structure [15]. In vocational rehabilitation the analysis of environmental physical, social, and attitudinal factors is particularly important.

Vocational rehabilitation measures

Vocational rehabilitation measures must include efforts to improve the patient's working conditions. This requires ergonomic analyses which determine the actions taken. Individual ergonomic measures for patients with a cervical spine extensor myalgia or tendonitis should aim at producing working positions with less forward bend of the head and neck. For sitting postures, changes might consist of raising the computer screen, tilting the table surface for an work object, and similar changes aiming at a more vertical posture of the neck and head [16]. In addition to the loading moment of the head and neck, the level of muscle activity in the cervical spine extensors is influenced by the sitting angle of the trunk. If the trunk is slightly inclined backwards and supported by a backrest, the level of activity of the cervical spine extensors and the trapezius pars descendens is decreased [17, 18].

The shoulder girdle elevators are continuously active when the upper limbs are in abducted or forward flexed positions, common in a great number of working situations. It is therefore unsurprising that shoulder girdle myalgia/tendinitis is prevalent [7]. Ergonomic measures for this kind of patients aim at reducing the load on the elevators of the shoulder girdle. This can be achieved in different ways, e.g. arm support, arm suspension [7, 19], wrist support, the work object positioned closer to the trunk [16], and also suspension of the work tool. Some patients tend to elevate the shoulder girdle unconsciously even in less strenuous situations e.g. during work with computer stations. These patients may benefit from exercises related to writing on computer and can be trained in relaxation with EMG-biofeedback technique [20].

It has been shown that the duration of a muscle contraction is a major factor in creating muscular discomfort and pain [16], irrespective of whether the contraction is static or dynamic. This means that work tasks that imply contractions with few interruptions with low activity levels tend to be more risky than those in which there are frequent interruptions [16]. This can be utilized in vocational rehabilitation. Patients with myalgia can alter their work technique aiming to perform the task with more frequent short pauses in muscle contractions ("micro pauses").

Rotator cuff tendonitis (sometimes combined with subacromial bursitis), is related to the muscular moment of force needed to move the arm or keep the arm in a particular position in relation to the scapula. The rotator cuff muscles are active in almost all movements of the shoulder joints [21] to generate forces keeping the caput in the glenoid cavity. Individual ergonomic measures for patients with rotator cuff tendonitis should aim at reducing the load on the arm either by means of improved positioning with shorter lever arms or by means of suspension or support of the arm plus burden/tool. The maximum muscular torque in abduction is for women about 40% of that for men [22] which – for a given level of load – leads to a proportionally higher utilization of muscular capacity in women than in men (e.g. when women use work stations designed for men). Epidemiological studies [7] have shown that work with the upper extremities above the level of shoulder joints is a risk factor for "shoulder tendonitis", e.g. ship yard welders, women car fitters and other. Patients with rotator cuff tendonitis should therefore select work tasks where they don't need to work with hands above shoulder level.

Extreme-joint-position pain and its measures

Another variant of nocioception is the pain perceived when joints are kept in a sustained extreme joint position, i.e. at the limit of the range of motion [9, 23, 24]. This condition may occur, for example, when the cervical spine is kept rotated, forward flexed, and backward extended due to the content of work tasks. Examples of situations at the work place where there is a risk of extreme-joint-position pain are side-positioned drivers of trucks in a stock-in-trade, reversing a car or other vehicles, standing work at a low table, painting a ceiling and the like. The risk of extreme-joint-position pain is increased if the range of motion in the cervical spine is reduced and/or the patients have easily elicited pain due to e.g. spondylosis, arthritis, or the sequelae of traumatic cervical spine distortion. Vocational rehabilitation in these cases must entail an investigation of the patient's work with the aim of mapping the possible events where the extreme-joint-position may occur, for instance by means of video film. The next step is to make the patient aware of the situations where this occurs, e.g. by watching a video with the patient. With the goal of changing their work technique patients may begin to train in a program of body awareness to perform their tasks without extreme-joint-positions. The final step may be to train the patient in new work techniques.

Conditions with widespread pain, e.g. the fibromyalgia syndrome

The aetiology of the fibromyalgia syndrome (FMS) is unknown. However, some of the pathophysiology has been described. One theory is based on the concept of general impaired pain modulation [25]. The aetiology of the syndrome is not associated with physical work load, but pain intensity is usually increased by external load and FMS patients do not have the normal increase of pressure pain threshold during muscle contractions [26]. FMS patients often report increased pain intensity during muscular efforts either in the form of work or exercise [12]. The content of vocational rehabilitation of FMS should include body awareness training to avoid unnecessarily eliciting or increasing pain due to external load [27]. The likelihood of successful vocational rehabilitation increases if the patient can resume employment with low physical load and little stress.

References

1. Braddom R (1996) (ed) Physical medicine & Rehabilitation. Saunders Co, Philadelphia
2. DeLisa J & Gans B (1998) (eds) Rehabilitation Medicine. Lippincott Raven, Philadelphia
3. Grabois M, Garrison S, Hart KA et al. (2000) (eds) Physical Medicine and Rehabilitation: the complete approach. Blackell Science, Malden (MA)
4. Johnson KL & Haselcorn J (1997) (eds) Vocational Rehabilitation. In: Physical Medicine and Rehabilitation Clinics of North America. W.B.Saunders Company, Philadelphia
5. Hutson MA (1999) Work-related Upper limb disorders. Butterworth & Heinemann, Oxford
6. Gobelet C & Franchignoni (2005) (eds) Vocational Rehabilitation. Springer, Paris
7. Kourinka I & Forcier L (1995) (eds) Work related musculoskeletal disorders (WMSDs) – a reference book for prevention. Taylor & Francis. London. UK
8. Landstad Bodil (2001) At work in spite of pain. Prevention and rehabilitation in two predominantly female workplaces, their effects and further development of analysis methods of work place based rehabilitation and prevention. PhD thesis, Karolinska Institutet, Dept Public Health Sciences, Section Rehabilitation medicine, Stockholm

9. Harms-Ringdahl K & Schüldt K (1990) Neck and shoulder load and load elicited pain in sitting work postures. In: International perspectives in physical therapy (IPPT). Volume on ergonomics. (ed M.I. Bullock), Churchill- Livingstone, Edinburgh, 6: 133-47

10. John Selander (1999) Unemployed sick-leavers and vocational rehabilitation – a person-level study based on a national social insurance material. PhD thesis, Karolinska Institutet, Dept Public Health Sciences, Section Rehabilitation medicine, Stockholm

11. Marnetoft Sven-Uno (2000) Vocational rehabilitation of unemployed sick-listed people in a Swedish rural area. An individual-level study based on social insurance data. PhD thesis, Karolinska Institutet, Dept Public Health Sciences, Section Rehabilitation medicine, Stockholm

12. Mense S, Simons D, Russell J (2001) Muscle pain. Understanding its nature, diagnosis and treatment. Lippincott, Williams & Wilkins, Baltimore

13. Lundeberg T, Ekholm J (2002) Pain-from periphery to brain. Disabil Rehabil 24: 402-6

14. Landstad B, Schüldt K, Ekholm J et al. (2001) Women at work despite ill-health: diagnoses and pain before and after personnel support. A prospective study of hospital cleaners/home-help personnel with comparison groups. J Rehabil Med 33(5): 216-24

15. WHO (2001) International Classification of Functioning, Disability and Health, WHO library, Geneva

16. Chaffin D, Andersson G, Martin B (1999) (eds): Occupational biomechanics. Third Edition. John Wiley & Sons, New York

17. Schüldt K (1988) On neck muscle activity and load reduction in sitting postures. Revised version of PhD thesis. Scand J Rehabil Med Suppl No 19: 1-49

18. Boisset S, Maton B (1995) (eds): Muscles, posture et mouvement. Bases et applications de la méthode électromyographique. Hermanns Éditeurs des Sciences et des Arts, Paris

19. Schüldt K, Ekholm J, Harms-Ringdahl K et al. (1987) Effects of arm support or suspension on neck and shoulder muscle activity during sedentary work. Scand J Rehabil Med 19: 77-84

20. Basmajian J (1998) Biofeedback in physical medicine and rehabilitation. In: DeLisa J & Gans B (eds) Rehabilitation Medicine, Lippincott Raven, Philadelphia, p 505-20

21. Schüldt K, Harms-Ringdahl K (1988) Activity levels during isometric test contractions of neck and shoulder muscles. Scand J Rehabil Med 20: 117-27

22. Lannersten L, Harms-Ringdahl K, Schüldt K et al. (1993) Isometric strength in the flexors, abductors and external rotators of the shoulder. Clin Biomech 8: 235-42

23. Harms-Ringdahl K, Ekholm J (1986) Intensity and character of pain and muscular activity levels elicited by maintained extreme flexion position of the lower-cervical-upper-thoracic spine. Scand J Rehab Med 18: 117-26

24. Dalenbring S, Schüldt K, Ekholm J et al. (1999) Location and intensity of focal and referred pain provoked by maintained extreme rotation of the cervical spine in healthy females. Eur J Physi Med and Rehabil 8: 170-7

25. Henriksson KG, Mense S (1994) Pain and nociception in fibromyalgia: clinical and neurobiological considerations on aetiology and pathogenesis. Pain Rev 1: 245-60

26. Kosek E, Ekholm J, Hansson P (1996) Modulation of pressure pain thresholds during and following isometric contraction in patients with fibromyalgia and in healthy controls. Pain 64: 415-23

27. Gustavsson M, Ekholm J, Broman L (2002) Effects of a multiprofessional rehabilitation program for patients with fibromyalgia syndrome. J Rehabil Med 34: 119-27

Return to work after a traumatic brain injury: a difficult challenge

P. Vuadens, P. Arnold and A. Bellmann

Introduction

In spite of improvements in the prevention of car and work accidents, traumatic brain injury (TBI) is still devastating for the patients and their families and still constitutes a public health problem. In the USA, every year 1.5 million people sustain a TBI. Fifty-thousand persons will die from the consequences of brain injury, 230,000 will be hospitalised and 70,000 to 90,000 will experience a long term loss of functioning [1]. The precise financial costs of TBI are not well known and are probably underestimated. According to the data of the National Institutes of Health (NIH), the total annual cost for acute medical and rehabilitation services for new TBI patients in the USA is between $9 and $10 billion, with the average lifetime cost of care for a severe TBI patient ranging from $600,000 to $1,875,000 [2].

The benefit of work for the quality of life with TBI is well established and *job loss can be a frequent consequence of severe TBI* [3, 4, 5]. Many studies have demonstrated that TBI patients have significant difficulties returning to work after their injury [6, 7, 8]. Usually 20 to 30% of individuals with TBI return to work 1 year after injury [6, 8, 9]. Those with more severe injuries have much less chance of returning to work than those with mild injuries [10-15]. The rates range from 12.5% to 71% for severe TBI to 100% for mild TBI. This variability is, to some extent, a function of a large number of factors. The most important one is certainly the persistence of cognitive deficits after a severe TBI, and especially behaviour changes. Many brain injury patients are seen as inefficient at work, thus resulting in their termination, transfer or placement in a new assignment. In a survey, 70% of all previously employed TBI patients left their jobs, 10% were fired or laid off [16]. Only 2% continued their job.

Among the factors which determine the success of returning to work after a TBI, the bio psychosocial ones are also very important: level of education and vocational training, culture, familial support, psychiatric history, type of job [17]. These factors impinge at all stages of vocational rehabilitation. Vocational rehabilitation usually takes place at the end of neurological rehabilitation and is a project for the patient's future. It must take into account the past and the present of each individual who sustained a TBI. The process may fail otherwise. Moreover, the expectations of patients and their family must also be taken into consideration.

Epidemiological data of the silent epidemic

Vocational rehabilitation is necessary because the great majority of accidents injure young people of working age. Moreover, with the progressive improvement of intensive care and emergencies, more and more individuals survive severe TBI, but often with physical and cognitive difficulties [2, 18].

In Switzerland, in 2001, there was a car crash with one victim every 22 minutes and with a severely injured person every 29 minutes [19]. This means a total of 23,896 casualties with 30,704 victims and 5,458 severely injured persons. Sixty-eight percent of drivers were men and 60% of badly injured victims too. The great majority of wounded individuals were aged 15 to 50, the primary working population. In 1997, the same country spent 243,096,526 sfr. for acute medical treatment, rehabilitation, wages and pensions of TBI victims. More than 150 sfr. million were devoted to the pensions. In the USA, Johnstone et al. evaluated the financial and vocational outcomes of 35 TBI patients one year after trauma [20].

At least 5.3 million Americans (2% of the U.S population) live with disabilities due to a TBI [1]. Car crashes seem to be the primary cause of all TBI and about 40 to 50% of people do not use personal protective equipment (seat belts or helmets) [21]. In the USA, in 1995, the direct and indirect costs of TBI totalled approximately $56.3 billion of which 22 billion dollars were for lost productivity, wages, long-term care [22]. About 63% of TBI affect people aged 15-64, mainly the age group 15-19 years [1, 21, 23].

According to the data from 14 states that participated in an ongoing TBI surveillance system, the overall age-adjusted TBI-related live hospital discharge rate is 69.7/100,000 heads of population [21]. The rate for males is about twice as high as for females (91.9 versus 47.7/100,000 respectively). At discharge, the disability measured by the Glasgow Outcome Scale (GOS) was moderate in 9.6% of people, severe in 6.3%. In 73.9% of cases the recovery was good but 0.6% of patients were still in persistent coma. The GOS score was unknown in 9.6% of TBI patients.

In Argentina, TBI is also the primary cause of morbidity and mortality in young people, with an incidence of approximately 200 TBI per month in Rosario city [24]. This number is similar to the international figures suggesting a TBI incidence rate of 132 to 430 per 100,000 heads of population.

With the ongoing advances in medical technology, the number of TBI survivors is continuously increasing with its social and financial consequences of people with disabilities [25, 26]. Even if the handicaps of each individual may differ, the impact on the socioprofessional life is always devastating and many studies reveal that a great number of individuals with TBI do not return to work post-injury. From 248 brain injury patients of whom 94% were employed pre-injury, only 50% were competitively employed post-injury after two years and 6 months of rehabilitation; 11% had a non competitive work; and 39% did not work [27]. The results of another study seem more optimistic with 75% of 142 patients who successfully obtained employment [28]. In fact, one-half of those employed worked full-time and the average wage per hour was $8.50. At the last follow-up analysis, only 55% were still employed.

In reality, a significant proportion of persons disabled after TBI work less over a life-time and, on average, earn less compared with nondisabled people. JR Spoonsters, a vocational economic analyst, reports that in 1988, the mean earnings of all disabled workers was $12,253 and $18,951 for the healthy workers, a reduction of 35% due to the presence of a work disability [29]. According to him, the working-life expectancy of disabled people is also less than that of abled peers. This difference varies as a function of disability status.

From these data it is clear that neurological rehabilitation of TBI patients must be optimal and the vocational rehabilitation as appropriate as possible: return to work has positive effects on quality of life, social integration, and financial status [30, 31].

Factors influencing return to work and predictors

Unemployment rate is usually high in TBI patients. Estimates of return to work are often below 30%, depending on the study. The range of post injury employment is from 10% to 70% meanwhile it was from 61% to 75% pre injury. This relatively low rate of return to work is consistent with many studies [33-35]. According to the data of the National Institute on Disability and Rehabilitation Research (NIDRR) Traumatic Brain Injury Model Systems (TBIMS), only 22% of TBI patients have returned to work at 1 year after injury [36]. From the data of 15 different research studies, unemployment at admission to post acute brain injury rehabilitation was 80 to 90%. This rate decreased to 29% after rehabilitation, compared with 47% for patients who received no intervention [37]. In addition, people with more severe injuries have a lower probability of returning to work than those with mild injuries [8, 10, 11, 12, 13]. Limited employment opportunities in rural areas may also be a disadvantage for certain TBI patients [38].

In childhood, the incidence of severe traumatic brain injuries is also high (24%) [39]. The long-term outcome of TBI children is also related with the severity of the injury and the outcome in adulthood is worse than what their school performance predicted [40, 41, 42]. At 6 months post injury, the proportion of people who returned to school is 62% for former students. This rate increases up to 66% at one year [43].

This discrepancy between the studies is probably explained by the different predictors that may influence return to work after a traumatic brain injury. Many specific variables have been identified as either contributing to or inhibiting return to work after TBI, such as type of previous job, level of social support, the educational level and the number of psycho-social problems [14, 41, 44]. The combination of these variables will increase the predictability of return to work [3].

Brain injury severity

Follow-up studies have shown that severity of brain injury (time unconscious, length of hospitalisation) and severity of impairment (mobility and cognitive performances) are inversely related to employment [45-48]. In general, the more severe the brain trauma is, as measured by the Glasgow Coma Scale (GCS), the more dependent and less productive the patient is at follow-up [45]. The duration of coma is more important for patients who are severely injured, especially for long-term outcomes [40, 50]. In a multivariate correlational study to predict community integration and vocational outcomes 2-5 years after TBI, injury severity measured as GCS and length of post traumatic amnesia (PTA) is a predictor to discriminate the patients who will return to work [51]. In a German population of TBI with an initial GCS of 6.2 +/- 3.2, a duration of coma of 15.4 +/- 14.4 days, 42% of all patients have returned to their former work about 5.8 years after the accident, 32% were retrained to other professions, 5% were still in training or at college, 10% were unemployed, and 5% were retired. These outcomes were significantly correlated with age, injury severity, GCS, and duration of coma [52]. In another study the vocational status was lower in TBI patients with lower GCS and longer lengths of PTA. Among 131 males who worked full-time prior to the accident, only 55% were able to return to work full-time [47]. For other authors, only the length of APT determines the post-injury employment status. The duration of coma, the initial GCS do not seem to influence the outcomes of TBI patients [53]. Concerning the prediction of employment status 2 years after TBI, Ponsford *et al.* have shown by a stepwise discriminant function analysis that the total score on the Disability Rating Scale, the Glasgow Coma Scale Score, and the age allows to classify correctly 74% of grouped cases [54]. In 3 studies, the duration of PTS was not correlated with the possibility to return to work [6, 47, 55].

In childhood, the severity of head injury is also one of the major contributors in the prediction of long-term outcomes [40]. Children 7 years or younger at the time of the accident who sustained a severe brain injury, have more severe disability than the older children. Usually, they have worse social and vocational outcome and they are often incapable of independent employment [31].

Whatever the scale used for measuring the severity of traumatic brain injury (GCS, PTA, length of hospitalisation, Glasgow Outcome scale), they are weak predictors of returning to work. For example, in the study of Vogenthaler *et al.*, the results revealed that the lower the best GCS during the first 24 hours was, the more dependent and less productive the subject was at follow-up. However, several mildly injured subjects had poor outcomes, while several severely injured subjects had relatively good outcomes at follow-up [46]. We must keep in mind that all these studies and data show only tendencies within groups of people. None can predict what will happen to any individual of that group. The results of these scales must not be used to reject a candidate for vocational rehabilitation as having no possibility of returning to work.

Several authors propose combining different predictive factors to better assess the possibilities to return to work [32, 48, 56, 57]. It seems that the sequelae of the accident and the incapacities due to them are more important than the severity of brain injury.

Many studies report that physical impairment and above all the cognitive deficits interfere with vocational rehabilitation negatively [6, 9, 58-62].

Demographic, personal, and socio-professional factors

Much attention has been paid to factors independent of brain injury that may influence RTW after TBI [67]. Several demographic, personal, familial, social and professional factors have been cited although there is some inconsistency between reports probably to be explained by variations in population selection, method of RTW process, inconsistency of employment status, length of follow-up. For example, several studies only included hospitalized patients, either in acute care units, or in rehabilitation centres; in these studies patients were almost exclusively those with moderate to severe TBI [6, 5, 44, 64]. Traumatic injuries were not always separated from other non traumatic brain lesions [64, 65]. The patients studied might be all those with TBI identified in a centre, or only those working before injury [3, 5, 6, 44, 46, 64, 65]. Many selected sheltered, subsidized or unpaid (volunteer, homemaker) work in the RTW process [65, 66]. Difference between full- and part-time activities is not always considered. Stambrooks paid attention to the distinction between mild, moderate and severe TBI, but this separation is rarely specified in the literature, the nature of the evaluated TBIs being mostly dependant on the population selection [47]. We will here first consider the demographic, personal and socio-professional parameters most often evidenced in these studies. Patients with mild TBI (MTBI) have a much better prognosis, and factors influencing their RTW strongly differ from those of severe TBI patients, with sharper influence of pre-injury co-morbidity [47, 67, 63]. MTBI will so be treated separately.

For severe to moderate TBI, the demographic factor most often evidenced is age, with worse prognosis when the patient is > 40 years old [3, 5, 6, 44, 44, 46, 47, 54, 64, 65, 69]. This is especially significant when the economic context is unfavorable with important unemployment, and is associated to unwillingness of the employer to allow the patient back with limited working life ahead [6]. Worse prognosis is thus not solely a consequence of reduced adaptability of older patients. Females tend to have a better prognosis than males [66, 70]. This may be a consequence of bias due to mechanism of injury, with increased severity in males as a result of their risk-taking behaviours [70]; several authors however proposed an influence of hormonal status (protection through estrogens) and less lateralized brain in females [69, 70]. It is worth noting that some of the differences found may be attributed to the fact that some authors included homemakers when measuring RTW [69]. Being of an ethnic minority, particularly a black minority, has also been revealed to unfavourably affect outcome, but this is probably a consequence of other associated social and professional factors [5, 3, 71].

Some premorbid personality disorders have been associated with a poorer outcome. Anxiety and depression for example may unfavourably influence the person's progress after TBI, although this has been evidenced only by a few authors [47, 72]. Depressive mood after injury, however, negatively influences outcome, and since premorbid depressive mood is a risk factor for developing frank depression after trauma, it should then negatively affect evolution in TBI patients [73]. Except for drug and alcohol abuse, comorbid medical conditions have rarely been studied, and no conclusion can be drawn. Drug and alcohol abuse before injury so have been found to be factors associated with a bad prognosis, and their impact is probably underestimated, because these subjects were more likely to be lost of follow-up or even excluded from studies [44, 65, 71, 72, 74]. Surprisingly, other abnormal social behaviour such as violent or criminal behaviour had little or no influence on outcome [43]. It is further interesting to observe that pre-injury evaluation by close relatives of a patient as being energetic represented a favourable prognosis factor, as was patient's working alliance to vocational rehabilitation programs [6, 65]. The last statement also applied to family and social support [64, 65]. Nevertheless, patients seeking compensation showed less eagerness to work and achieved less productivity [65]. Social support to TBI patient is an important prognostic factor for outcome, materializing in better social integration after injury [64, 65, 72]. One would expect that marital status would have an influence on RTW, with married TBI patients doing better, but Ip showed that unmarried subjects had a better outcome [3, 5, 44]. This paradoxical finding might relate to the potential financial support afforded by the spouse, whereas unmarried TBI subjects were more motivated to return to gainful employment. Car driving aptitude is an important marker of independency, and in fact clearly favourably influences RTW ability when present [3].

Pre-injury professional status plays an important role on the RTW process. Subject who had an unstable professional situation, or those having not any work at time of injury, had a poorer vocational outcome [46, 69]. Individuals with higher level of education and skilled profession use to do better, as those who earn more money [3, 5, 46, 47, 64, 65, 70, 72]. Subjects working in a structural occupation are nonetheless more likely to return to their former occupation when compared to those who were professionals, managerial or service workers [10]. This can be explained by the fact that cognitive defects and behavioural abnormalities can be more tolerated in the former, which necessitate less speed, attention, concentration and organization abilities. It first appears to be in contradiction to the previous statement that individuals with more education and technical skills have a greater likelihood to RTW. It might be (at least partly) explained by the discrepancy between pre-injury and post-injury employment level of TBI patients, skilled patients having indeed more capability reserves [63]. Though sociodemographic factors clearly influence vocational outcome of moderate to severe TBI patients, neuropsychological deficits remain the most important feature in determining their ability to RTW [54, 75, 76] (see below).

Whereas seriousness of trauma strongly affects prognosis of severe TBI, either assessed in the acute phase or at time of rehabilitation, socio-economic background acts as a dominant parameter modulating evolution of mild TBI [67, 54]. A recent review of Van der Naalt treating mild and moderate TBI draws attention to the difficulty of analyzing the results of different studies, essentially because of the lack of a consistency of definition of the injury's severity, small samples' size and short length of follow-up, often not exceeding 3 months [67]. At that time, though the majority of patients still complained about persistent symptoms such as headache and memory impairment, most were nevertheless back to their work. Predisposing factors leading to failure of RTW after

MTBI have been addressed in 2003 by Reynolds and Vanderploeg [68, 77]. It is worth noting that strong demographic prognosis factors for severe TBI, such as age and gender, were here non-significant, whereas social and economic predisposing issues had the greatest influence. Profession-related parameters were low pre-injury vocational status, low level of motivation to work, and individuals whose occupation requires frequent personal interactions and necessitates managing many projects simultaneously [67, 78]. Financial compensation seeking, which is often present early after MTBI, strongly delays time of RTW, especially when through litigation [77]. The study did not indicate whether injury, patient, lawyer, insurance system or other variables accounted for these findings, but it is important to assess these at the beginning of the rehabilitation program, and prompt further studies in order to attempt explaining how financial compensation moderates outcome after MTBI [77]. Subjects at risk for failure to RTW tend to have lower general intellectual abilities, to have a past history of psychiatric disease such as anxiety, depression or psychosis, but often also medical co-morbidity [68]. Finally, chronic alcohol abuse and poor social support further unfavourably affect evolution of MTBI when considering RTW [67].

Neuropsychological factors

Cognitive impairment and employment after TBI

Studies having addressed the issue of employment status in relation with neuropsychological factors unanimously recognize the impact of cognitive and behavioural impairment on vocational outcome [46, 48, 55, 54, 79-82]). These variables interact with other measures such as traumatism severity and motor deficit [5].

Among cognitive deficits, the *dysexecutive syndrome* is certainly the most disabling in impeding return to work. It results from lesions of the frontal lobes, particularly vulnerable to closed head injury, and therefore is very frequently found among brain-damaged persons. Many authors have documented the negative impact of executive and attentional deficits on the vocational outcome [49, 83-87]. Executive functions are required for the genesis of any willed action which cannot be hold by routine operations, for instance coping with novelty, problem resolution, decision making, initiative taking, overcoming temptation, dealing with danger... When impaired, these abilities, which are required in most professions, may compromise different dimensions of work efficiency. Autonomy at work may be severely compromised by the patient's lack of initiative, his difficulty initiating something if not prompted to, organizing his actions, establishing priorities, adapting to new situations. Carrying responsibilities requires, among others, the ability to solve problems; it involves the ability to identify problems (potential dangers, for example), select a strategy, execute the operations, and evaluate the outcome [88]. All these steps or some of them may be impaired in patients with executive deficit. Quality and speed of performance may be compromised by the difficulties sustaining attention during long periods, ignoring distraction and performing dual tasks, as well as by mental fatigability and ideo-motor slowing which are currently found in brain-damaged people. Moreover, patients with executive deficits experience difficulties in projecting towards the future and elaborating realistic professional objectives taking their weaknesses into account; they are often tempted to follow immediately rewarding options rather than reasonable but more demanding ones.

Unawareness of deficit (anosognosia) and behavioural problems, commonly found in association with dysexecutive syndrome, are frequent sequels of brain damage. Many studies have found that acceptance of disability was significantly associated with work status in TBI patients [89, 90]. Impaired awareness of deficit decreases motivation for treatment and leads to inappropriate selection of long-term goals. Confronting the patients with their difficulties in a real setting may increase awareness, although their poor monitoring abilities often prevent accurate self-evaluation.

Neurobehavioural disability is very frequent in TBI patients and may have disastrous consequences on professional integration [91]. It ranges from simple impulsivity or lack of tact in interpersonal relationships, to rudeness, violent behaviour or sexual desinhibition. Authors have in particular documented the negative impact of agressivity, and aspontaneity [84, 91]. Brooks *et al.* have shown that behavioural disturbance and psychosocial maladjustment (as reported by relatives) intensify during the year and persist for at least seven years [6]. They have drawn the attention on their negative impact on social and professional integration.

Memory impairments rank also among the cognitive deficits having an impact on the return to work after TBI [81, 84, 85, 86]. Patients' anterograde memory problems may notably compromise their ability to remember instructions (especially after interference) or to learn new facts. It is important to address this point when a professional re-orientation is envisaged.

Role of neuropsychological assessment in the context of professional evaluation

Neuropsychological examination is concerned with the evaluation of the *nature* and the *extent* of cognitive and behavioural impairment. On the cognitive side, particular emphasis is placed on memory (in particular anterograde, prospective and working memory aspects), attentional functions (information processing speed, sustained, selective and divided components of attention) and executive functions (planning, flexibility, drive). Behaviour and awareness of deficit must be carefully investigated too, by means of validates questionnaires filled in by the patient himself or a relative.

Neuropsychologists must be particularly cautious in the extrapolation from psychometric scores to performance in everyday life. As stressed by Sbordone, no individual neuropsychological test was ever designed to predict how the patients are likely to live independently, return to work, or maintain competitive employment following brain injury [92]. Psychotechnic testing does bear only few relation to real-world settings: evaluations are conducted in a quite room with few distractions, the session is structured, with the patient having to execute tasks one after the other when told by the examiner;

the intellectual effort must be sustained during a limited period (rarely more than 2 hours) and a break may even be proposed by the neuropsychologist to make sure that the cognitive potential is not masked by the patient's fatigue. As a result, a standard neuropsychological assessment may fail to capture the patients dysexecutive symptoms and lead to an overestimation of their real functioning. On the other hand, patients performing complex but familiar or partially familiar activities in real life benefit from procedural skills and previous knowledge, and from the multiplicity of cues available in complex settings. Consequently, the patients may be more effective than predicted by the formal neuropsychological assessment in complex everyday activities such as driving or performing usual work, especially if there is no time constraint and no unpredictable event. For the reasons listed above, current methods of standardized psychometric assessment may not yield adequate estimates of functional capacity unless they are combined with more naturalistic methods. Assessment procedures that attempt to capture this more functional perspective utilize standardized tasks that more closely approximate activities in natural contexts, such as the "Multiple errand test" or "The six elements task" of Shallice and Burgess, where the patient is faced with a set of tasks and must organize himself respecting given rules [93]. Other options are questionnaires or situational observations [94]. However, usual neuropsychological tests assessing isolated cognitive functions are still very valuable, and must not be neglected [81]. They benefit from a better standardization. Compared to more global assessments where many variables are interlinked, they have also the advantage to focus more selectively on a given function or sub-function, and therefore allow a more subtle description of the deficit's nature. This specification is important for the elaboration of individualized rehabilitation objectives and for the proposition of adapted adjustments on the work place. For example, inefficiency to summarize the content of work meetings might result from deficits in memory, information processing speed, sustained attention, divided attention, working memory, abstraction, planning, etc... Providing a tape recorder to record the meetings will be useful if the problem concerns memory or information processing speed, but not if it arises from abstract thinking or planning difficulties

In our opinion, a neuropsychological examination carried out within the context of professional evaluation, should go beyond a list of deficits. It should also outline the preserved abilities (very important in the perspective of a professional re-orientation) and specify the circumstances in which problems arise (for example, a patient might be able to concentrate during 3 hours, but only in the morning, or only if there is no noise and distraction). On this basis, neuropsychologists can give an opinion about the patient's ability to go back to the anterior activity, provide concrete tracks regarding re-orientation and propose adjustments in the work place. Such adjustments range from simple environmental modifications (e.g. reducing the light intensity or closing the door, respectively against headaches and selective attention deficits) to compensatory external aids or strategies [63, 80, 95, 96]. For example, provision of a diary may help compensating anterograde memory problems; a programmed alarm may supply prospective memory deficits; giving instructions one after the other may help patients with organization deficits. In some cases, intensive neuropsychological rehabilitation centred on difficulties encountered on the working place can be proposed, as illustrated by Glisky and

Schacter's study [97]. They have used the preserved procedural memory competency of a severely amnesic patient to teach her with success the knowledge and skills needed to perform a complex computer data-entry job.

Employment stability

The employment stability is an important factor which determines the success of vocational rehabilitation programs. In fact, the data of different studies suggest that a substantial number of patients continue working for a number of years, whereas a larger proportion is entirely unsuccessful [3, 4, 5, 6, 16, 44]. In the study of Johnson, 42% of 64 patients sustained their work 10 years after severe TBI [3]. This percent is similar to findings reported by other investigators and confirms that only one-third of patients are able to maintain their job for a large number of years.

It seems that different variables including age, length of unconsciousness, and Disability Rating Score at 1 year after injury may predict employment stability [3]. Ethnicity, marital status, and education are also significantly related to employment stability [5, 98]. Non minority group members and married people are more than twice as likely to be stably employed [3]. On the other hand, lower education levels predict higher unemployment rates [5, 6, 44].

Conditions to facilitate return to work

A large variety of brain injury vocational rehabilitation services or programs are available, such as vocational assessment, social services, job training, vocational counselling, placement services, on-site support services, case management. Before starting to look for a job, the brain injury patient needs to determine whether or not he wants to return to work. This must be clear and discussed with the family or the rehabilitation providers. The National Resource Center for Traumatic Brain Injury has published a workbook for brain injury patients. It includes several questionnaires and information to help the patients to understand their situation and know which types of services are available to help them [99].

Returning to work or finding a new job is often a challenge for people with brain injury. Even if many communities have specialized employment services, the patient needs help or encouragement to contact such services. A recent article provides an excellent framework of a self-guided therapeutic return to work program [100]. Clinicians will find useful information to discuss with their patients with brain injury when returning to work is planned.

To successfully achieve a vocational rehabilitation program, the neuropsychologist must help the vocational counsellors or the clinicians to clearly identify the patient's aptitudes and to determine the strategies or objectives necessary to obtain the specific vocational goals [101]. This assessment will also guide the counsellor to choose realistic options such as further training, education, job coaching or realistic placement.

Unfortunately a standardized neuropsychological assessment has limited ecological validity, especially for the executive functions. The patient's performances in a controlled assessment situation are different from a natural, unstructured vocational setting, such as a workplace [102, 103]. Therefore, for obtaining more realistic and ecological data for vocational predictions, a situational vocational evaluation is highly recommended [94, 104-110].

Vocational programs and supported employment

Brain injury patients face many difficulties in returning to the workplace. Cognitive deficits especially limit the patient's ability to cope in a work environment and often employers do not have the ability to accommodate the needs of the brain injury patients. Thus, many different vocational rehabilitation programs have been developed to optimise the work potential of people recovering from brain injury. These programs can be divided into either vocational rehabilitation programs or community re-entry programs. They must help the clinician or the counsellor to determine if the patient is able to return to the same job with the same employer, to find and accept a different job in the same workplace or to find a different job using the existing skills.

Community Re-entry Program

This program is proposed to brain injury patients after the period of active rehabilitation. It focuses on remedial and compensatory treatment for cognitive, behavioural and physical deficits in order to increase the integration of these patients in the community and thus to obtain a greater work productivity. In many cases, specific job training is also needed and therefore, some community re-entry programs offer a vocational phase, as job trials or placements [107-109].

In USA, based on a comprehensive-integrated approach, a specified intensive day treatment program is available for brain injury patients with severe cognitive and self-awareness deficits [110, 111]. It aims to improve the cognitive and behavioural modifications, especially anosognosia and the acceptance of deficits by the patient. The features of this comprehensive (holistic) day treatment have been described in a national consensus conference [112].

Among 94 patients who finished this type of training, 53% were still employed, 23% were in sheltered or subsidized employment, and 3% were in academic programs 6 months later [113]. In a review of the data of 15 programs, Malec and Basford report that only 29% of 856 patients were unemployed and over 56% had an independent work or were involved in school or homemaking [37]. This positive effect of comprehensive day treatment program is confirmed in another study where 67% of 66 persons with brain injury were competitively employed 17 months after the end of program [90]. A less favourable outcome at long-term follow-up was reported for patients with more severe self-awareness deficits.

The benefit of such a program is also maintained in long-term vocational follow-up for patients admitted many years post-injury [113, 114, 115]. This program offers a significant improvement in societal participation, especially within the first year post-injury. However, significant gains are also made by patients who entered 2 to over 10 years post-injury [116]. The level of disability before entering the program provides low to moderate prediction of long-term outcomes. It seems that the patients with significant impairments in self-awareness and with multiple cognitive and behavioural deficits are typically recommended to comprehensive day treatment program. *In fact, according to the promoters of this program, it is really important to develop self-awareness and acceptance of deficits to become productive [117]. Self-awareness of deficits is an excellent prognosticator of return to work and it can be measured by a reliable questionnaire developed by Prigatano* [15, 90, 118, 119].

The New York University Head Trauma Program is divided in two phases. The first attempts to increase awareness and acceptance of deficits of survivors of moderate to severe brain injury. In phase 2, the patients engage in vocational trials [120)]. According to the data of 59 patients, all completed the phase 1 and the great majority the phase 2.

Thus the comprehensive day treatment program is very useful for brain injury patients in improving activity and societal participation, even for the persons with a long period of limited participation after moderate to severe brain injury. In the model of Prigatano and colleagues, a cognitive training approach is privileged, meanwhile a holistic approach is chosen by Ben-Yishay and associates [113, 121]. An intensive 24-hour residential program to improve behaviour modifications is also proposed as a means of vocational training [122]. Whatever the model is used, about 50% of patients obtain an employment.

Work re-entry program

For persons with severe to moderate traumatic brain injury, the work re-entry program is an alternative to improve their vocational outcomes [123]. Traditional vocational programs propose sheltered training prior to job placement. The characteristics of these programs are 1) to train the work competencies, work behaviour and productivity of the patient, 2) to place the patient in the institution or the centre to improve his competencies and capacities with a job coach, 3) to place the patient with the support of a vocational counsellor in an real job, 4) to progressively decrease the support. Using such a vocational program, among 130 patients followed over 3 years, 67% were competitively employed [123]. Even given these encouraging results, many specialists consider this type of program ineffective [101, 120, 124]. It is difficult to compare the results of the studies on the effect of vocational rehabilitation process and they point out that the success of a program lies in terms of different program approaches. They do not usually compare programs [50, 118, 121, 125].

Better results are obtained with a supported employment approach, with job placement, followed by job-site training and support [123, 124, 126, 127]. The key feature of this program is the use of an employment specialist (job coach), who will provide training, counselling, and support for the patient at the job site [124]. At any time, the job coach can intervene for resolution of problems either with the patient or the employer. There are different models of supported employment but the usual components of this type of programs can be found in detail in two previous articles [124, 127-130].

Using the model of supported employment, studies showed that patients are more successful in obtaining and maintaining a job. Seventy-one percent of 41 persons continued to work 6 months after initial placement with this model [15]. About 290 hours of employment specialist intervention were necessary to obtain these excellent results. They worked an average 31.2 hr/wk and earned an average hourly wage of $4.61. Moreover, the patients returned to similar jobs that they had preinjury and worked a similar number of hours. Wehman *et al.* estimated the supported employment cost per person at about $8,000 [126]. However, the costs decrease over time from $ 10,198 for the first year to $ 8,614 for the average annual costs. The participant income was an average of $ 17,515 over the 14-year time period of the study [131].

For persons with severe TBI, the supported employment model with job-site training and support is sometimes insufficient to maintain employment [126]. When the behavioural or the cognitive deficits are too significant, a pre-placement activity, such as cognitive retraining, must be proposed.

Over the world, many rehabilitation centres offer these types of vocational training programmes to TBI patients. Each of them has usually its own specificities to train and support people to return to economic work. However, according to a systematic review of Crowther *et al.*, who have compared the efficacy of the different models of vocational programmes, concludes that a supported training with a job-coach on the job site offer a better chance to obtain and maintain a competitive and economic employment [128]. Among the TBI patients who can benefit from a vocational program, 60 to 80% will be able to obtain and maintain an independent job [37, 133].

Vocational rehabilitation in the Clinique Romande

In the Swiss system of insurances, vocational rehabilitation belongs to the disability compensation insurance. It intervenes as soon as the medical situation is stable whatever was the cause of the work disability. However, before this lapse of time, many patients have sufficiently improved to be able to do a few activities. Then it is important to use these capacities and to train them rapidly because the precocious return to work is beneficial when its aim is therapeutic [134].

In our Clinic, at the end of neurological rehabilitation, when the patient is independent in his daily activities and he is ready to re-entry the community, a vocational rehabilitation is progressively introduced as soon as the patient is able to concentrate over 20 minutes on a task. With the support of neuropsychologists and job coaches, the patients are trained in a ecological work environment in order to improve the cognitive deficits or behaviour modifications. The periods of training are adapted according to the fatigue and the cognitive performances of patients. Progressively, the complexity of tasks is increased or new strategies are proposed. Then, this period of observation and training in a professional environment allow to determine the real capacities of patients, especially of learning new knowledge, their endurance, their motivations, and their time allowance [105]. After this first evaluation, the patient can be placed in his usual professional environment and continue the training under the supervision of a job coach and with the support of the employer. Regularly the real work capacities of patients are evaluated to determine the salary according to the performances demonstrated at work by the patients.

When the training in the real work situation is not possible, we must wait for the complete stabilisation of medical situation of TBI patients. Usually 6-12 months later, the patient is admitted to our centre for a vocational evaluation during a minimum of 3 weeks. Again, the capacities of patients are evaluated and especially the cognitive one. This evaluation allows us to determine whether the patient can continue his previous job normally or with adaptations or if it is necessary to learn a new profession. In this case, with the support of the disability insurance, the patients spend 3 or 6 months in a vocational rehabilitation centre, belonging to this insurance company or working in connexion with the insurance, to evaluate band search for a new profession before starting this new professional education, still under the supervision of this insurance. Among the criteria for admission to these vocational rehabilitation centres, a clear description of capacities of patients and his motivation are mandatory. Moreover, the patient must be able to stay at least 4 hours per day at a work place.

Sometimes, the patient will be able to continue his previous job after a period of training but he has no more employment or probably needs some adaptations at the work place. In this case, with the agreement of the disability insurance, the patient will be trained in our centre before a job placement under the supervision of a job coach. When a real capacity of work is obtained, the disability insurance helps the patient find a new employment and maintain it.

Conclusion

Vocational rehabilitation of TBI patients, especially those with severe cognitive deficits or behaviour problems, is a real challenge for the multidisciplinary team of rehabilitation centres. In spite of the encouraging results of numerous studies, the reality in terms of return to work is not always favourable, especially when economic conditions are not good. Economic recession decreases the possibilities of TBI patients finding a new job adapted to their difficulties, above all with a reduced productivity. Moreover, the charges for rehabilitation and employment services for TBI patients are very high. Therefore, vocational rehabilitation is crucial and the best way to obtain success is to increase the motivation of patients and to offer them supported employment as soon as the medical situation allows it.

References

1. Thurman D, Alverson C, Dunn K *et al.* (1999) Traumatic brain injury in the United States: a public health perspective. J Head Trauma Rehabil 14: 602-5
2. Rehabilitation of persons with traumatic brain injury (1998). NIH Consensus Statement 16: 1-41
3. Kreutzer JS, Marwitz JH, Walker W *et al.* (2003) Moderating factors in return to work and job stability after traumatic brain injury. J Head Trauma Rehabil 18: 128-38
4. Johnson R (1998) How do people get back to work after severe head injury? A 10 year follow-up study. Neuropsychol Rehabil 8: 61-79
5. Greenspan AI, Wrigley JM, Kresnow M *et al.* (1996) Factors influencing failure to return to work due to traumatic brain injury. Brain Inj 10: 207-218
6. Brooks N, McKinlay W, Symington C, Beattie A, Campsie L (1987) Return to work within the first seven years of severe head injury. Brain Inj 1: 5-19
7. Hurt GD (2000) Vocational rehabilitation. In: Raskin SA, Mateer CA (eds). Neuropsychological management of mild traumatic brain injury. New York: Oxford University Press, p 215-30
8. Mc Mordie WR, Barker S, Paolo TM (1990) Return to work after head injury. Brain Inj 4: 57-69
9. Humphrey M, Oddy M (1980) Return to work after head injury: a review of post-war studies. Injury 12: 107-14
10. Fraser R, Dikmen S, McLean A (1988) Employability of head injury survivors: first year post-injury. Rehabil Couns Bull 31: 276-88.
11. Kaplan SP (1988) Adaptation following serious brain injury: an assessment after one year. J Applied Rehabil Couns 19: 3-8
12. Rao N, Rosenthal M, Cronin-Stubbs D *et al.* (1990) Return to work after rehabilitation following traumatic brain injury. Brain Inj 4: 49-56
13. Wrightson P, Gronwald D (1981) Time off work and symptoms after minor head injury Injury 12: 445-54
14. Thomsen IV (1989) Do young patients have worse outcomes after severe blunt head trauma? Brain Inj 3: 157-62
15. Wehman PH, Kreutzer JS, West MD *et al.* (1990) Return to work for persons with traumatic brain injury: a supported employment approach. Arch Phys Med Rehab 1047-52
16. Possl J, Jurgensmeyer S, Karlbauer F *et al.* (2001) Stability of employment after brain injury: A 7 year follow-up study. Brain Inj 15: 15-27
17. Vogenthaler DR, Smith KR, Goldfader P (1989) Head Injury, a multivariate study: Predicting long-term productivity and independent living outcome. Brain Inj 3: 369-85
18. Johnstone B, Nossaman L, Schopp LH *et al.* (2002) Distribution of services and supports for persons with traumatic brain injury in rural and urban Missouri. J Rural Health 18: 109-17
19. Office fédéral de la statistique. www.statistik.admin.ch/findex.htm.
20. Johnstone B, Mount D, Schopp LH (2003) Financial and vocational outcomes 1 year after traumatic brain injury. Arch Phys Med Rehabil 84: 238-41
21. Langlois JA, Kegler SR, Butler JA *et al.* (1997) Results from a 14-State Surveillance System. http://www.cdc.gov/mmwr/preview/mmwrhtml/ss5204a1.htm

22. Thurman D (2001) The epidemiology and economics of head trauma. In: Miller L, Hayes R, editors. Head Trauma: Basic, Preclinical, and Clinical Directions. New York (NY): Wiley and Sons

23. Kalsbeek WD, McLaurin RL, Harris BS *et al.* (1980) The national head and spinal cord injury survey: major findings. J Neurosurg 53: S19-S31

24. Chesnut R Traumatic brain injury rehabilitation. The Argentina Project. http://www.ohsu.edu/news/archive/2001/120301brain.html

25. Cifu D, Craig E, Rowland T (1996) Neuromedical considerations affecting return to work in the brain injured adult. J Vocational Rehabil 7: 257-65

26. Annoni JM, Beer P, Kesselring J (1992) Severe traumatic brain injury: Epidemiology and outcome after 3 years. Disability Rehabilitation 14: 23-6

27. Evans RW, Ruff RM (1992) Outcome and Value: a perspective on rehabilitation outcomes achieved in acquired brain injury. J Head Trauma Rehabilitation 7: 24-36

28. Adams D (1993) The economics of return to work for survivors of traumatic brain injury: vocational services are worth the investment. J Head Trauma Rehabil 8: 59-76

29. Spoonster J Defining economic damages in traumatic brain injury cases. Available from Vocational Economics Inc. http//www.vocecon.com.

30. O'Neill J, Hibbard MR, Brown M *et al.* (1998) The effect of employment on quality of life and community integration after traumatic brain injury. J Head Trauma Rehabil 13: 68-79

31. Bell KR, Sandel ME (1998) Brain injury rehabilitation. 4. Postacute rehabilitation and community integration. Arch Phys Med Rehabil 79(Suppl 1): S21-S25

32. Asikainen I, Kaste M, Sarna S (1998) Predicting late outcome for patients with traumatic brain injury referred to a rehabilitation program: a study of 508 Finnish patients 5 years or more after injury. Brain Inj 12: 95-107

33. Burleigh SA, Farber RS, Gillard M (1998) Community integration and life satisfaction after traumatic brain injury: long-term findings Am J Occup Ther 52: 45-52

34. Curl RM, Fraser RT, Cook RG *et al.* (1996) Traumatic brain injury vocational rehabilitation: preliminary findings for the co-worker as trainer project. J Head Trauma Rehabil 11: 75-85

35. O'Connell MJ (2000) Prediction of work following traumatic brain injury: intellectual, memory, and demographic variables. Rehabil Psychol 45: 212-7

36. Traumatic Brain Injury Model Systems. Information section on the database. Available from: http//www.tbims.org.

37. Malec JF, Basford JS (1996) Postacute brain injury rehabilitation. Arch Phys Med Rehabil 77: 198-207

38. Coetzer BR, Hayes NM, Du Toit PL (2002) Long-term employment outcomes in a rural area following traumatic brain injury. Aust J Rural Health 10: 229-32

39. Kraus JF, Rock A, Hemyari P (1990) Brain injuries among infants, children, adolescents, and young adults. Am J Dis Child 144: 684-91

40. Klonoff H, Clark C, Klonoff PS (1993) Long-term outcome of head injuries: a 23 year follow-up study of children with head injuries. J Neurol Neurosurg Psychiatry 56: 410-5

41. Koskiniemi M. Kyykkä T, Nybo T *et al.* (1995) Long-term outcome after severe brain injury in preschoolers is worse than expected. Arch Pediatr Adolesc Med 149: 249-54

42. Nybo T, Koskiniemi M (1999) Cognitive indicators of vocational outcome after severe brain injury (TBI) in childhood. Brain Inj 13: 759-66

43. Ruff RM, Marshall LF, Crouch J *et al.* (1993) Predictors of outcome following severe head trauma: follow-up data from the Traumatic Coma Data Bank. Brain Inj 7: 101-11

44. Ip RY, Dornan J, Schentag C (1995) Traumatic brain injury: factors predicting return to work or school. Brain Inj 9: 517-32

45. Vogenthaler DR, Smith KR Jr, Goldfader P (1989) Head injury, an empirical study: describing long-term productivity and independent living outcome. Brain Inj 3: 325-9

46. Dikmen SS, Temkin NR, Machamer JE et al. (1994) Employment following traumatic head injuries. Arch Neurol 51: 177-86

47. Stambrook M, Moore A, Peters L et al. (1990) Effects of mild, moderate and severe closed head injury on long-term vocational status. Brain Inj 4: 183-90

48. Cifu DX, Keyser-Marcus L, Lopez E et al. (1997) Acute predictors of successful return to work 1 year after traumatic brain injury: a multicenter analysis. Arch Phys Med Rehabil 78: 125-31

49. Crepeau F, Scherzer P (1993) Predictors and indicators of work status after traumatic brain injury: a meta analysis. Neuropsychol Rehabil 3: 5-35

50. Levati A, Farina MA, Vecchi G et al. (1982) Prognosis of severe head injuries. J Neurosurg 57: 779-83

51. Fleming J, Tooth L, Hassell M et al. (1999) Prediction of community integration and vocational outcome 2-5 years after traumatic brain injury rehabilitation in Australia. Brain Inj 13: 417-31

52. Lehmann U, Gobiet W, Regel G et al. (1997) Functional, neuropsychological and social outcome of polytrauma patients with severe craniocerebral trauma. Unfallchirurg 100: 552-60

53. Lubusko AA, Moore AD, Stambrook M et al. (1994) Cognitive beliefs following severe traumatic brain injury: association with post-injury employment status. Brain Inj 8: 65-70

54. Ponsford JL, Olver JH, Curran C et al. (1995) Prediction of employment status 2 years after traumatic brain injury. Brain Inj 9: 11-20

55. Keyser-Marcus LA, Bricout JC, Wehman P et al. (2002) Acute predictors of return to employment after traumatic brain injury: a longitudinal follow-up. Arch Phys Med Rehabil 83: 635-41

56. Gollaher K, High W, Shere M et al. (1998) Prediction of employment outcome one to three years following traumatic brain injury. Brain Inj 12: 255-63

57. Sander AM, Kreutzer JS, Rosenthal M et al. (1996) A multicenter longitudinal investigation of return to work and community integration following traumatic brain injury. J Head Trauma Rehabil 11: 70-84

58. Wehman P, Sheron P, Kregel J et al. (1993) Return to work for persons following severe traumatic brain injury: supported employment outcomes after five years. Am J Phys Med Rehabil 72: 355-63

59. McKinlay W, Brooks D, Bond M (1983) Post-concussional symptoms, financial compensation and outcome of severe blunt head injury. J Neurol Neurosurg Psychiatry 46: 1084-91

60. Thomsen IV (1984) Late outcome of very severe blunt head trauma: a 10-15 year second follow-up. J Neurol Neurosurg Psychiatry 47: 260-8

61. Johnstone B, Vessell R, Bounds T et al. (2003) Predictors of success for state vocational rehabilitation clients with traumatic brain injury. Arch Phys Med Rehabil 84: 161-7

62. Felmingham KL, Baguley IJ, Crooks J (2001) A comparison of acute and postdischarge predictors of employment 2 years after traumatic brain injury. Arch Phys Med Rehabil 82: 435-9

63. Yasuda S, Wehman P, Targett P et al. (2001) Return to work for persons with traumatic brain injury. Am J Phys Med Rehabil 80: 852-64

64. MacKenzie EJ, Shapiro S, Smith RT *et al.* (1987) Factors influencing return to work following hospitalization for traumatic injury. Am J Public Health 77: 329-34
65. Klonoff PS, Lamb DG, Henderson SW (2001) Outcomes from milieu-based neurorehabilitation at up to 11 years post-discharge. Brain Inj 15: 413-28
66. Groswasser Z, Cohen M, Keren O (1998) Female TBI patients recover better than males. Brain Inj 12: 805-8
67. van der Naalt NJ (2001) Prediction of outcome in mild to moderate head injury: a review. J Clin Exp Neuropsychol 23: 837-51
68. Vanderploeg RD, Curtiss G, Duchnick JJ *et al.* (2003) Demographic, medical, and psychiatric factors in work and marital status after mild head injury. J Head Trauma Rehabil 18: 148-63
69. Tennant A, Macdermott N, Neary D (1995) The long-term outcome of head injury: implications for service planning. Brain Inj 9: 595-605
70. McMordie WR, Barker SL, Paolo TM (1990) Return to work (RTW) after head injury. Brain Inj 4: 57-69
71. Burnett DM, Kolakowsky-Hayner SA, Slater D *et al.* (2003) Ethnographic analysis of traumatic brain injury patients in the national Model Systems database. Arch Phys Med Rehabil 84: 263-7
72. Wagner AK, Hammond FM, Sasser HC *et al.* (2002) Return to productive activity after traumatic brain injury: relationship with measures of disability, handicap, and community integration. Arch Phys Med Rehabil 83: 107-14
73. Gomez-Hernandez R, Max JE, Kosier T *et al.* (1997) Social impairment and depression after traumatic brain injury. Arch Phys Med Rehabil 78: 1321-6
74. Corrigan JD, Bogner JA, Mysiw WJ *et al.* (1997) Systematic bias in outcome studies of persons with traumatic brain injury. Arch Phys Med Rehabil 78: 132-7
75. Godfrey HP, Bishara SN, Partridge FM *et al.* (1993) Neuropsychological impairment and return to work following severe closed head injury: implications for clinical management. N Z Med J 106: 301-3
76. Schwab K, Grafman J, Salazar AM *et al.* (1993) Residual impairments and work status 15 years after penetrating head injury: report from the Vietnam Head Injury Study. Neurology 43: 95-103
77. Reynolds S, Paniak C, Toller-Lobe G *et al.* (2003) A longitudinal study of compensation-seeking and return to work in a treated mild traumatic brain injury sample. J Head Trauma Rehabil 18: 139-47
78. Kibby MY, Long CJ (1996) Minor head injury: attempts at clarifying the confusion. Brain Inj 10: 159-86
79. Groswasser Z (1994) Rehabilitating Psychosocial Functioning. In A-L Christensen & BP Uzzell (Eds): Brain Injury and Neuropsychological Rehabilitation: International Perspectives; Hillsdale: LEA
80. Ponsford JL (1995) Returning to the community after TBI. In J Ponsford, S Sloan, P Snow (Eds): Traumatic Brain Injury: Rehabilitation for Everyday Adaptive Living; Hove: Psychology Press
81. Cohadon F, Castel J-P, Richer E *et al.* (1998) Les traumatisés crâniens, de l'accident à la réinsertion. Vélizy-Villacoublay: Arnett

82. Cattelani R, Tanzi F, Lombardi F *et al.* (2002) Competitive re-employment after severe traumatic brain injury: clinical, cognitive and behavioural predictive variables. Brain Injury 16: 51-64

83. Vilkki J, Ahola K, Holst P *et al.* (1994) Prediction of psychosocial recovery after head injury with cognitive tests and neurobehavioral rating. Journal of Clinical and Experimental Neuropsychology 16: 325-38

84. Truelle JL, Brooks DN, Marinescu M *et al.* (1995) Retentissement des troubles cognitifs et du comportement sur le handicap social, familial et professionnel. In C Bergego & Ph Azouvi (Eds): Neuropsychologie des traumatismes crâniens graves de l'adulte; Paris: Frison-Roche

85. Girard D, Brown J, Burnett-Stolnack M *et al.* (1996) The relationship of neuropsychological status and productive outcome following traumatic brain injury. Brain Injury 10: 663-76

86. Mazaux JM, Masson F, Levin HS, Alaoui P, Maurette P, Barat M (1997) Long-term neuropsychological outcome and loss of social autonomy after traumatic brain injury. Arch Phys Med Rehabil 78: 1316-20

87. Sohlberg MM, Mateer AC (2001) Cognitive Rehabilitation: An integrative neuropsychological approach; New York: The Guilford Press

88. Luria AR (1966) Human brain and psychological processes. New-York: Harper and Row

89. Melamed S, Groswasser Z, Stern MJ (1992) Acceptance of disability, work involvement and subjective rehabilitation status of traumatic brain-injured (TBI) patients. Brain Injury 6: 233-43

90. Sherer M, Bergloff P, Levin E *et al.* (19989 Impaired awareness and employment outcome after traumatic brain injury. J Head Trauma Rehabil 13: 52-61

91. Wood RLI (2000) Understanding neurobehavioural disability. In RLI Wood & TM McMillan (Eds): Neurobehavioural disability and social handicap following traumatic brain injury; Hove: Psychology Press

92. Sbordone RJ (2001) Limitations of neuropsychological testing to predict the cognitive and behavioural functioning of persons with brain injury in real-world settings. Neuro Rehabilitation 16: 199-201

93. Shallice T, Burgess PW (1991) Deficits in strategy application following frontal lobe damage in man. Brain 114: 727-41

94. LeBlanc JM, Hayden ME, Paulman RG (2000) A comparison of neuropsychological and situational assessment for predicting employability after closed head injury. Journal of Head Trauma Rehabiloitation 15: 1022-40

95. Parente R, Stapleton MC, Wheatley C (1991) Practical strategies for vocational reentry after traumatic brain injury. J Head Trauma Rehabil 6: 35-45

96. Briel LW (1996) Promoting the effective use of compensatory strategies on the job for individuals with traumatic brain injury. J Vocational Rehabil 7: 151-8

97. Glisky EL, Schacter D (1987) Acquisition of domain-specific knowledge in organic amnesia: training for computer-related work. Neuropsychologia 25: 893-906

98. Rosenthal M, Dijkers M, Harrison-Felix C *et al.* (1996) Impact of minority status on functional outcome and community integration following brain injury. J Head Trauma 11: 40-57

99. Kreutzer J, Kolakowsky-Hayner S (1999) The Brain Injury Workbook: A Guide for Living and Working Productively. Richmond, Virginia: The National Resource Center for Traumatic Brain Injury. www.neuro.pmr.vcu.edu

100. Kolawkowsky-Hayner SA, Kreutzer JS (2001) Return to work after brain injury: A self-directed approach. NeuroRehabilitation 16: 41-7

101. Barisa MT, Barisa MW (2001) Neuropsychological evaluation applied to vocational rehabilitation. Neurorehabilitation 16: 289-93
102. Hart T, Hayden ME (1986) The ecological validity of neuropsychological assessment and remediation. Clinical Neuropsychology of Intervention. Boston: Marintus Nijhoff
103. Stuss D, Mateer C, Sholberg M (1994) Innovative approaches to frontal lobe deficits. Brain Injury Rehabilitation: Clinical Considerations. Baltimore, MD: Williams & Wilkins
104. Velozo C (1993) Work evaluations: Critique of the state of the art of functional assessment of work. Am J Occup Ther 47: 203-9
105. Fraser R(1991) Vocational evaluation. J Head Trauma Rehabil 6: 46-58
106. Roberts R (1992) Vocational evaluation and planning. In: Handbook of Head Trauma: Acute care to Recovery. New York: Plenum Press
107. Fawber H, Wachter J (1987) Job placement as a treatment component of the vocational rehabilitation process. J Head Trauma Rehabil 3: 27-33
108. Haffey WJ, Lewis FD (1989) Programming for occupational outcome following traumatic brain injury. Rehabilitation Psychology 34: 147-59
109. Ben-Ishay Y, Rattock J, Lakin P (1985) Neuropsychologic rehabilitation. Quest for a holistic approach. Seminars in Neurology 5: 252-9
110. Ben-Ishay Y, Prigatano GP (1990) Cognitive remediation. In : Rosenthal M, Griffith ER, Bond MR, Miller JD, editors. Rehabilitation of the adult and child with traumatic brain injury. 2nd ed. Philadelphia: FA Davis, p. 393-409
111. Prigatano GP, Fordyce DJ, Zeiner HK et al. (1986) Neuropsychological rehabilitation after brain injury. Baltimore (MD): Johns Hopkins University
112. Trexler LE (2000) Empirical support for neuropsychological rehabilitation. In : Christensen AL, Uzzell BP, editors. International handbook of neuropsychological rehabilitation. New York, Kluwer Academic/Plenum, p 137-50
113. Ben-Yshay Y, Silver SM, Piasetsky E et al. (1987) Relationship between employability and vocational outcome after intensive holistic cognitive rehabilitation. J Head Trauma Rehabil 2: 35-48
114. Namerow NS (1987) Cognitive and behavioural aspects of brain-injury rehabilitation. Neurol Clin 5: 569-83
115. Malec JF, Smigielski JS, DePompolo RW et al. (1993) Outcome evaluation and predicition in a comprehensive-integrated post-acute outpatient brain injury rehabilitation programme. Brain Inj 7: 15-29
116. Malec JF (2001) Impact of comprehensive day treatment on societal participation for persons with acquired brain injury. Arch Phys Med Rehabil 82: 885-95
117. Ben-Yshay Y, Lakin P (1989) Structured group treatment for brain injury survivors. In: Ellis DW, Christensen AL (eds): Neuropsychological Treatment After Brain Injury. Boston, Kluwer Academic, p 271-95
118. Prigatano G, Klonoff PS, O'Brien K (1994) Productivity after neuropsychologically oriented milieu rehabilitation. J Head Trauma Rehabil 9: 91-2
119. Awareness questionnaire of Prigatano. http://www.tbims.org/combi/aq/index.html
120. Ezarachi O, Ben-Yshay Y, Kay T et al. (1991) Predicitng employment in traumatic brain injury following neuropsychological rehabilitation. J Head Trauma Rehabil 6: 71-84
121. Prigatano GP, Fordyce DJ, Zeiner HK et al. (1983) Neuropsychological rehabilitation after closed head injury in young adults. J Neurol Neurosurg Psychiatry 47: 505-13

122. Burke WH, Wesolowski MD, Guth ML (1988) Comprehensive head injury rehabilitation: an outcome evaluation. Brain Injury 2: 313-22

123. Haffey WJ, Abrams DL (1991) Employment outcomes for participants in a brain injury work reentry program: Preliminary findings. J Head Trauma Rehabil 6: 24-34

124. Wehman P, Wood W, Sherron P (1988) Supported work model for persons with traumatic brain injury: toward job placement and retention. Rehabil Counselling Bulletin 31: 298-311

125. Abrams D, Barker LT, Haffey W et al. (1993) The economics of return to work for survivors of traumatic brain injury: vocational services are worth investment. J Head Trauma Rehabil 8: 59-76

126. Wehman P, West M, Fry R et al. (1989) Effect of supported employment on the vocational outcomes of persons with traumatic brain injury, J Applied Behavior Analysis 22: 395-405

127. Wehman P, Kreutzer J, West M et al. (1989) Employment outcomes of persons following traumatic brain injury: preinjury, postinjury, and supported employment. Brain Injury 3: 397-412

128. Mank DM, Rhodes LE, Bellamy GT (1986) Four supported employment alternatives. In: Kiernan WE, Stark JA, eds. Pathway to employment for adults with developmental disabilities. Baltimore: Paul H. Brookes, p 139-53

129. Moon MS, Griffin SL (1988) Supported employment service delivery models. In: Wehman P, Moon MS, eds. Vocational rehabilitation and supported employment. Baltimore, Paul H. Brookes, p 17-30

130. Wehman P, Kregel J (1985) A supported work approach to competitive employment of individuals with moderate and severe handicaps. J Assoc Persons Severe Handicaps 10: 3-11

131. Wehman P, Kregel J, Keyser-Marcus L et al. (2003) Supported employment for persons with traumatic brain injury: a preliminary investigation of long-term follow-up costs and program efficiency. Arch Phys Med Rehabil 84: 192-6

132. Crowther R, Marshall M, Bond GR et al. (2001) Helping people with severe mental illness to obtain work: systematic review. BMJ 322: 204-8

133. Malec JF, Degiorgio L (2002) Characteristics of successful and unsuccessful completers of 3 postacute brain injury rehabilitation pathways. Arch Phys Med Rehabil 83: 1759-64

134. Malec JF, Buffington AL, Moessner AM et al. (2000) A medical/vocational case coordination system for person with brain injury: an evaluation of employment outcomes. Arch Phys Med Rehabil 81: 1007-15

Vocational rehabilitation and spinal cord injuries

A.T. Al-Khodairy and W.S. El Masry

Introduction

There are an estimated 40 to 60 new cases of traumatic spinal cord injury (SCI) per million population per year in the United States occurring at a mean age of 31 years (median 26 years), that is, the beginning of the period of highest financial productivity [1]. Advances in short-term and long-term management have resulted in a life expectancy after injury that is close to the life-expectancy of able-bodied individuals. Estimated lifetime costs for an individual with SCI often exceed one million dollars and the annual cost of SCI to society, including both direct and indirect costs, is somewhere between $7.3 and 8.3 billion [2-4].

Some suggest that the process of psychological adaptation to a disability is analogous to the psychological stages leading to acceptance of death. With SCI patients, one or more of the five stages of grieving – shock, denial, anger, bargaining, depression and finally acceptance are usually encountered [5]. While persons with SCI do have special needs and deal with problems not faced by non disabled persons following expert treatment and rehabilitation, they are not necessarily burdened psychologically by their disability [6].

Return to work is often used as a measure of overall recovery from injury or illness. It is a particularly relevant measure when examining the individual and societal burden of injury as the majority of those inflicted are young [1, 7]. A working life is generally considered as an ultimate aim of the disabled person, indicating the success of rehabilitation [8]. The ability to return to work after injury not only depends on the physical and emotional well-being but also on non-health related factors such as age, education, previous work experiences and support from close friends and family [9]. The positive links in various studies between the fact of having a job and survival, satisfaction in life and a sense of well-being tend to strengthen the consensus among rehabilitation professionals and the disabled about importance of work [2, 10]. Nevertheless, because of the physical limitations that result, spinal cord injury presents many discouragements to a return to gainful employment and is associated with a significant decline in employment [11]. A large number of studies indicate that only 13% to 48% of those with SCI have a job [12].

Employment after spinal cord injury

The major goal for almost all working age persons is employment. Employment is seen by society as a measure of status and productivity in addition to being a source of income. It helps fulfil hierarchical needs such as those of survival, stimulation, safety and security, love and esteem.

Unemployment and low self-esteem feed upon one another. As a person expects less of himself, there is a coincident rise in medical complications, in drug and alcohol dependence, and in family problems. To accept oneself after the onset of a physical impairment is a vital prerequisite to developing a productive lifestyle. Unemployment results in a loss of purchasing power of money, energy outlet, a source of diversion, temporal structuring, social contacts and status in society. This may lead to depression, anxiety, and decrease in self-esteem [13]. The loss of income among people who do not return to work after a disability is a significant stress factor to the economic well-being of individuals and their families [14].

Work is a core element of our physical, social, and psychological survival. Its significance for spinal cord injured persons is no less than it is for the able-bodied persons. It is especially important for them to attain satisfactory employment status, because their basic living costs are increased and because self-esteem and life-satisfaction may already be significantly lowered by other factors such as a negatively altered body image, a lack of mobility to perform routine tasks, and alienation from family and friends. Employment after disability marks a return to a productive rewarding lifestyle.

Quality of life after spinal cord injury

Quality of life (QoL) is associated with meeting individual needs, controlling one's environment, and having opportunities to make choices. QoL issues for SCI population have been examined and results indicate that it is significantly lower than for a normative population [15-18]. Individuals sustaining SCI are faced with physical, emotional, financial, and vocational changes. These problems are often complex and profound and therefore can have a negative effect on one's QoL and satisfaction especially with community re-entry and employment [19]. There are several variables that affect the degree of QoL of individuals with SCI. Both education and employment have strong association with QoL post-injury [2, 4, 20, 21]. Functional ability is also an important determining factor and it correlates highly with both physical and mental health [22]. The level or the extent of SCI seems not a predictor of life satisfaction [19].

Results from studies which have utilised QoL to measure success of employment services for individuals with disabilities indicated improved QoL for persons participating in competitive employment [17, 23-25]. Since employment is important in our society not just in terms of financial security but also for self-esteem, independence, social relationships, self worth, and personal identity, it becomes critical to provide ongoing assistance in addition to effective rehabilitation programs. This would enable persons with SCI to return to work and as a result enhance their QoL.

Vocational rehabilitation

Improved knowledge in physical medicine and rehabilitation and the setting up of centres specialising in SCI care has allowed a significant increase in life expectancy with a large number of patients getting back home [26]. Interaction between the rehabilitation team and the SCI person can promote the experience of control over environment, a feeling of responsibility for success of the rehabilitation process, the ability to solve functional problems outside the rehabilitation environment, an understanding of the range of behavioural and environmental options available to the individual, and successful performance of job-related tasks in a supportive setting [27]. To develop expectations of a productive life-style, vocational planning must be initiated early in the rehabilitation process.

There are seven measures of vocational development after injury [28]: (1) immediate vocational plans, the choice of vocational objectives immediately following disability; (2) ultimate vocational plans, long-range goals; (3) responsibility for vocational plans, the acceptance of individual responsibility for making plans; (4) work values, the meaning of work to the individual; (5) remotivation, the desire to work following disability; (6) fantasised interests versus realistic interests, the degree of realism attached to work interests; and (7) rehabilitation outlook, the degree of optimism or pessimism about outcome of disability.

Persons with spinal cord injuries do have significant vocational potential. They may have reached a level of vocational identity before and/or after the onset of disability which enables them to be more decisive and confident in decision making [6]. However, problems of vocational decision making are mainly characterised by lack of information about employment opportunities, uncertainty about vocational and educational abilities, lack of knowledge of occupations and uncertainty in many (avocational) areas of life [6]. During inpatient rehabilitation, it is realistic for vocational services to include interviews with patients about previous vocational development for purposes of future planning and sharing vocational information about patients with the rehabilitation team. The vocational goals can therefore be incorporated into the total rehabilitation plan, with provision of vocational counselling and information as needed by patients and their families. Vocational rehabilitation counsellors need to become more sensitive to issues of vocational development and adjustment after spinal cord injury. Considering that more than 95% of total functional recovery after a traumatic SCI will occur by 12 months after injury [29], that development usually begins to plateau after 18 months, and that patients need time to deal with medical needs and adjustment to family and home, it is sometimes not realistic to expect active vocational planning to occur during inpatient comprehensive rehabilitation or during the first months after discharge [30]. SCI victims may be more responsive to vocational rehabilitation services, including vocational testing and evaluation, vocational exploration and counselling, training, job placement, and follow-up after the first six months post-discharge.

Rehabilitation programs aim to enhance adjustment to life following SCI by equipping the individual and his/her family and friends with the skills and resources required for community living. Rehabilitation professionals face several challenges with regard to the employability of their SCI clients [11]. Specialised vocational rehabilitation programs designed to address both generic vocational issues such as skill acquisition and development, as well as transportation options and access issues, may help in reducing the influence of these factors as barriers to post-injury gainful employment. Vocational rehabilitation programs need to be developed with input from individuals who have sustained a SCI. The need for specific vocational counselling; talking with peers who are in the workforce and the creation of special interest groups as means to facilitate the gaining and sustaining of employment post-injury has been highlighted [31]. In Switzerland for example, reinsertion to work and reorientation of the disabled after an injury is subsidised by a federal organisation, the "Assurance Invalidité" [32]. The incorporation of a co-ordinator from that organisation in the vocational rehabilitation team has recently been advocated through a convention between this organisation and the two SUVA (principal Swiss insurance company against accidents) rehabilitation clinics. This has often helped to shorten the usual legal delay for further vocational testing and evaluation, and referrals of appropriate patients to state vocational rehabilitation agencies from 2 years to a few months.

A vocational training and counselling program for SCI individuals is especially effective in improving functional independence and employment rates not only in paraplegics but also in tetraplegics [33]. Individuals with quadriplegia may benefit from additional education or specialised training, because a substantial percentage of these participants successfully return to and maintain employment. The subjective ratings of intensity when performing functional daily activities is judged "with greater ease" by both paraplegics and tetraplegics following a vocational training program [33]. Additional training, no doubt, would increase the sustainability of employment for many of these individuals.

Because the employment prospects are bleak for individuals who are older at injury, particularly in their mid to late 50s, rehabilitation professionals need to provide these clients with realistic information about the probability of returning to work [11]. Unless there is an opportunity to return to pre-injury employment, it may be better to help the individual prepare for a meaningful retirement (including productive activities) rather than retraining [11].

The understanding and portraying of the return to work of persons with severe impairment is complex. The selection and tailoring of the work place is tightly bound with the integration or reintegration of people with disabilities into the work environment. It cannot be said that there is a clear vocational stereotype, or one powerful single factor that permeates the post-accident employment situation of the person with spinal cord injury. Creativity and ability to set goals is related to productive living [34].

Return to work

Many of the individuals sustaining SCI have considerable functional limitation resulting in differences in the qualitative aspects of employment, including job content, job satisfaction, and expectations of future employment. Most people do not return to work after SCI, not even in physically less demanding jobs. There has been extensive research into the general rates of job acquisition and the vocational potential of SCI victims. In two literature reviews, the employment rates ranged from 13% to 48% [35] and 13% to 69% [36]. One reason for the variability may be due to differences in the employment definition being used. While narrow definition includes only those in paid employment or self-employment, the broader definition includes homemaker and students as well. Another reason may be the time after the injury when the study was conducted since employment rates improve with increasing time after injury [2]. Based on a review of 24 studies, the overall return to work was estimated at 39.3% [37].

Employment rates decrease dramatically when comparing pre- and post-injury rates. Return to gainful employment was most likely in minimally disabled, highly educated men whose pre-injury job only demanded light to moderate physical capacities and who followed a retraining program [38]. Of those who return to work, more start new jobs rather than return to their employment and those who returned to previous jobs did so much earlier than those who found new jobs [39]. Those who return to work which involves the same level of physical intensity as pre-injury tend to work part-time [40]. People with heavy or strenuous physical work pre-injury regained work in only 25% and 21% respectively [38]. Those with a low labour force participation rate are likely to be employed part-time rather than full-time, to be less satisfied with their current job, less optimistic about their future prospects, and less likely to report having autonomy at work. A significant change in the type of occupation was observed as almost half of those in paid employment pre-injury fell into the category of unemployed, students or volunteer workers after injury [31]. Levi *et al.* [40] found that SCI subjects were more often working with computers and less often working in (heavy) manual labour. In his study, being male was important to employment, but gender differences were highly dependent on cultural and social norms.

The percentage of unemployed thought to be capable of working is remarkably high. Among those, many report that functional limitations created a major problem in their life, and are less likely to report a desire to work. Only a minority returned to gainful employment after SCI, even to a physically less demanding job.

Our impression is that in many cases people are only ready to think of regaining work when they are at a stable level of functioning and their domestic situation is settled. At that time, they are discharged from the rehabilitation centre so less help with job specific functional training is available and intensive inpatient rehabilitation is less attractive.

In addition to intensive inpatient rehabilitation and long-term support in job seeking/switching to a less demanding job, compensation, sufficient enough but not too much so as not to inhibit the motivation to return to work, may promote return to work. The percentage of individuals entering the workforce after injury was higher for those who were not entitled to any form of compensation compared to those receiving compensation (51% and 23% respectively) [41]. The high financial compensation in Netherlands, which equals to 70% of the last earned wage, might also explain the high number of people who do not return to work post-injury [38].

Obstacles reported by individuals with disabilities that prevent them from returning to or entering the workforce include inability to obtain sufficient health care insurance to enable them to live and work independently, financial disincentives to work in current benefit programs, physical barriers and inability to access effective employment training and placement services. Many who do not have a full time job have to rely on some sort of social benefit as their source of income. Their financial reserves are sparse. In addition, they have difficulty obtaining employment due to lack of knowledge in terms of eligibility and services that would assist them in obtaining employment and to which they are entitled. It is critical that access to medical and rehabilitation services are maintained and ensured.

The effects of secondary morbidities on return to work or work interruption must not be neglected [29]. Return to work after SCI is a dynamic process with the ability to work changing over time.

Predictors of return to work after spinal cord injury

A number of specific individual and injury related factors have consistently been associated with return to gainful employment following SCI. Gender does not seem to be significantly associated with return to work [7, 11, 25, 39]. However, men were twice as likely as women to be in paid employment, whereas women were more likely to be engaged in a non-paid productive role which includes voluntary work, full and part-time students and homemakers [42]. Gender was significantly associated with the number of hours worked per week; men were more likely to be working full-time than women [25]. Two studies pointed out that being a Caucasian woman in the United States played a role in successful employment outcomes [43, 44] in addition to being less than 29 years of age at injury, having an incomplete lesion and having at least 16 years history with SCI [43].

Age at injury onset appears to be most important for return to work and is significantly related to both current employment status and employment status since injury [11]. The highest current employment rate was for those injured before 18 years of age (69%) with the rate decreasing to only 9% for those injured after 45 years. Older age at injury is negatively correlated with post-injury employment with the 16-30 age group having the highest employment rate and the 51 to 60 year group having the lowest [4, 39]. Age is the only statistically significant predictor of poor occupational outcome, with the older patients being worse off irrespective of the extent of the disease and functional anatomy [45].

Level of education pre- and post-injury has been constantly reported to be positively correlated to return to work [40]. Nearly 95% of all persons with 16 or more years of education had worked at some time after injury [2]. Education not only reflects higher socioeconomic status but also increases the range of jobs to which an individual may return. Those with a higher educational status and those who improved their education following injury were more likely to have obtained employment following injury [46]. A higher level of formal education attained prior to injury [25, 47, 48] and pre-injury vocational interests in more cognitive fields [49], have been positively linked to successful vocational outcome. A lower level of pre-injury education was correlated with employment in a lower scale occupation post-injury and by contrast a higher proportion of those with a university degree or diplomas were employed in higher scale occupations [31].

Several studies have examined the relationship between return to work and injury severity (neurological level, completeness). Relationship between return to work and injury severity have not been significantly correlated [11, 28]. Some studies have reported that individuals with paraplegia and/or incomplete lesions were more likely to be employed [33, 39, 46, 50], while other studies have not been able to link injury severity with employment [6]. El Ghatit *et al.* [46] reported that although individuals with quadriplegia were less likely to obtain employment, they were equally able to sustain employment. Conroy *et al.* found that having a complete cervical lesion reduced the likelihood of employment post-injury: Fifty-six per cent of cervical complete injuries returned to work, compared to 70% of incomplete cervical types [31]. Functional independence is highly correlated to the neurological level and injury severity. Any intervention leading to more functional independence is likely to improve employment potential. In patients with tetraplegia for example, a continent catheterisable conduit may enable an individual to catheterise independently, tendon transfers may enable an individual to have greater upper extremity function, and adaptations may make it possible for an individual to drive. The ability of the Motor Index Score in combination with demographic variables was examined to predict return to work during a period of three years for individuals with SCI [51]. Higher score can be associated with higher physical abilities, which therefore increases the likelihood of return to work. Violence at injury was associated with lower employment rates especially among Caucasians [25]. The influence of severity of injury on return to gainful employment has been less clearly defined. It would be intuitively expected that the degree of disability resulting from a complete cervical lesion would impact more severely on all life roles including that of the worker. While Goldberg and Freed [28] proposed a lack of realistic vocational expectations as contributing to lower work rates of individuals who have sustained complete cervical injuries, Castle [39] and Krause [2] indicated the need for career adjustment, change and retraining to re-enter into the workforce. Injury related issues including younger age at onset of injury [52, 53] and increased length of time since injury [54] have been similarly related to successfully securing a job. Issues of adjustment and reintegration into the community have been established as important precursors to vocational re-engagement [55, 56] with the interval 2-10 years post-injury proposed as the key time to assess vocational potential [47]. For some, the only factor affecting self-reported functional independence levels is the level of injury [33]. Consequently, patients with paraplegia are more likely to be employed than patients with tetraplegia. As one might expect individuals with paraplegia to demonstrate higher self-reported independence levels than subjects with quadriplegia [33]. In a sample of 745 male spinal cord injured veterans, post-injury education was not related to level of injury [46]. However, contradictory findings have been reported in terms of the relationship between the level of injury and return to work. While some have noted level of injury as a strong predictor of a return to work [46, 50], others did not support this view [2, 4, 11, 41]. Similarly, completeness of the injury, whether individuals were paraplegics or tetraplegics, was found as a predictor of return to work for some [39], while others reported that the only significant difference between individuals with paraplegia and tetraplegia was that individuals with paraplegia were more likely to return to their pre-injury jobs than those with tetraplegia [2, 41]. These studies suggest that for persons with SCI, barriers to return to work are created by their physical functioning limitations. These limitations prevent full participation and independence at the work site, which may further lead to a low satisfaction level or having to work part-time.

Being an independent driver impacted favourably on return to work or study post-injury, with reduced dependence on the inflexible, inaccessible or unreliable options of taxi services and public transports [31].

Significant relationships between pre- and post-injury marital status and improvement in education were found for those who were single, separated, or divorced [46]. An intact post-injury marriage was associated with improvement in education [46]. The number of children correlated significantly with vocational adjustment [28].

Doing household chores before injury seems to influence employment rates with a higher tendency for full-time jobs especially in men [57].

Individuals who were employed at the time of injury had more clearly defined vocational goals and more positive self-perceptions than those who were unemployed [44]. In general, more problems were reported by those unemployed [6]. Both groups reported accessibility, lack of benefits, transportation and physical limitations as being problems. Those employed reported lack of stamina and confidence, and low morale as problems while those unemployed reported lack of skills, need for retraining, and finding new careers. Persons with tetraplegia felt that they had to rely on others for punctuality and personal care [39]. Being employed at injury was associated with a greater probability of post-injury employment, but only in the first few years after injury [25]. Being a higher scale pre-injury occupation was associated with current employment [31]. Because lower scale occupations generally provide less financial remuneration, people previously employed in these types of jobs may experience less incentive to return to work [31]. Self satisfaction, financial incentives, social interaction, proving one's worth, being a productive member of the society and gaining some sense of normality of life were reasons nominated for working post-injury [31].

In the US, being Caucasian, younger at injury, having lived more years with SCI, having a less severe injury, and having more years of education were all predictive of being employed and were associated with greater likelihood of working [11, 25].

When the relationship between return to competitive employment and the physical intensity of pre-injury employment was investigated [38], it was found that of the 37% who returned to work, 25% had heavy work and 21 % strenuous physical work pre-injury. Persons with less physically intense occupations pre-injury are more likely to return to work. It has been suggested that in returning to physically intense occupations, there may be difficulties in adapting the work site. In addition, they may be less motivated to choose a less physically intense occupation, such as administrative work, which may require a higher level of education. Individuals who are employed reported that functional limitation, such as upper and lower extremity functions and mobility, affected them in terms of moving about in the workplace and getting to and from work [58].

Being male, young at onset of injury in a light to moderate physical job pre-injury, with a high Barthel Index post-injury, high educational level, vocational plans, work interests, work values, remotivation, rehabilitation outlook were important predictors for return to work for some [28, 33], while age, gender, number of medical complications, and time since injury were not related to employment status for others [33].

Why are SCI individuals not working?

A number of authors have examined the characteristics of SCI individuals who do not work, and cite the following as reasons [9, 46, 59-61]: 1) Fear of ending up fiscally less well-off due to loss of compensation and free medical benefits, 2) Inadequate educational opportunities appropriate to the individual's abilities, 3) Inaccessible workplaces and lack of enabling technology to allow competitive work output, 4) No accessible transportation to and from work, 5) Unavailability of consistent attendant care to ensure reliable and punctual work attendance, 6) Negative attitudes of employers and prospective employers about the things a paralysed person can and cannot do, 7) Poor self-image, fear of failure, lack of working peer role models, and generally low self-expectations of potential workers.

Lack of confidence from the employer in one's ability to competently carry out work tasks have gained some support as having a detrimental effect on return to work post-injury [28]. Workplace discrimination due largely to negative or naïve employer perceptions about the potential productivity of individuals with SCI has been negatively correlated with return to employment [39]. A lack of understanding of the nature of SCI may impact on employer selection of candidates for more skilled professional or management occupations. As a result, individuals who have sustained a SCI may seek employment in lower scale, clerical type positions [19, 62].

Early vocational approaches were highly controlled by rehabilitation professionals, but research has shown that high levels of professional support can be intrusive, and that businesses are more able to participate in the support process than was initially assumed [63]. A new generation of partnership that supports and builds the capacity of employers to create opportunities and neutralise the possible impact of employer prejudice to successfully employ individuals with severe disabilities was proposed [11, 63]. The interaction between the rehabilitation team and the employer should be characterised by clear, non-technical communication, an understanding of what functional activities the patient actually does (rather than what the person can do), a willingness to try creative solutions to environmental and performance problems, and a recognition of the employer's need for quantity and quality of production. Challenging employer perceptions and attitudes, and lobbying for improved transport systems and genuine equal access to all public facilities may be required from the broader community. Reducing financial disincentives to working, increasing funding for personal care attendants, and providing modification of workplace equipment to facilitate competent vocational performance may require new policies to be developed on a political front [31]. All these combined are likely to reduce the potential for failure and enhance the likelihood of achieving the highest possible level of vocational potential [27].

Work problems may play a role in preventing the return to work or the decline of achieving the capability to work. Environmental barriers may be factors making it more difficult to work [12, 39], but do not necessarily prevent employment or study opportunities [31]. A survey of a group of 46 SCI individuals revealed the following potentially encountered work problems: using equipment/tools/computers/typewriters/telephones, access to parking/work site/restrooms, getting the job done (working to a fixed schedule, reduced productivity, getting the job done with fatigue), performing tasks, personal care (eating/drinking, toileting), and transportation (commuting/local travel) [64]. The solutions to these problems may take many forms: assistance from co-workers, flexible schedules, modifying work tasks, pacing oneself during the day and rearranging furniture or material. Others include providing special equipment and/or aides, modifying the job or retraining the employee and/or transferring them to a new job. Such accommodations are generally not expensive with 30% costing less than $500 [65]. It has been suggested that persons with SCI are able to engage in competitive employment if appropriate accommodation that meet their needs in eliminating both psychological barriers and the physical barriers of the workplace are provided. Nearly three-quarters of SCI individuals were reported to require some type of accommodation to maintain or improve their productivity [58]. The reason for terminating employment or abandoning study was the perception that the job demands were too difficult or that the personal skill level was inadequate for the satisfactory completion of the job [31].

Transport difficulties were found to be associated with employment in lower scale occupations which tend to pay less and may thus limit the individual's ability to purchase his/her own vehicle, necessitating the use of public transport or dependence on others for transportation [31]. Lack of an independent means of transport has gained some support as having a detrimental effect on return to work post-injury [56, 66]. Addressing transportation needs and providing training so that individuals can get to and from work is critical for ensuring the individual's self-determination in employment, housing and social and recreational outlets [67].

The most frequently reported reasons for not working were: inability to physically perform the same type of work post-injury (60%) followed by poor health, stamina or endurance (28%), loss of benefits (28%), feeling not physically capable of working (27%) and inaccessibility of the workplace (23%) [1,36]. Problems of vocational decision-making included lack of information about employment opportunities, uncertainty about vocational and educational capabilities, lack of knowledge of suitable occupations and uncertainty in many are as of life [6]. Gender, race, age, and level of injury were all associated with these different reasons [20]. Health complications, chronic pain, long hours in the wheelchair causing pressure sores, frequent hospital readmissions, absence of satisfactory wheelchair access, a feeling of not being adequately trained for the job market, inadequate transport, inability to find a suitable job, domestic reasons, lack of motivation, and lack of education figured amongst others reasons for not working [17,

41, 57, 60, 68, 69]. Urinary and skin complications are the two main reasons for hospital readmissions in people with chronic SCI [70]. Risk of readmissions increases with time since injury and with disability and handicap severity with a rate of 74% in tetraplegia [71]. Several implications for therapeutic intervention arise from these findings. Firstly, individuals who were older at the onset of their SCI (above 30 years), those who sustained a complete cervical injury, and those with lower levels of pre-injury education (no more than school level of education), were found to be less likely to return to work/study following their injury [31].

Some individuals with SCI experience health problems and physical symptoms that appear to be related to aging. They tend to be more fatigued, less active, and experience more symptoms and illnesses as they age [72]. Many persons with SCI experience an increased need for medical treatment 10-15 years after injury [49]. The incidence of pain in upper extremity joints, likely caused by wheelchair propulsion and transfers, has been shown to increase with the duration of SCI [72-74]. The effect of aging on functional independence may be significantly accelerated in individuals with SCI. Studying the impact of aging on function revealed that 22% of those who had a duration of SCI of at least 20 years required more physical assistance than they had earlier in their injuries [75]. Those attributed their need for more help to several factors, including fatigue, muscle weakness, pain and stiffness, weight gain, and specific medical problems. The average age when additional assistance was first needed was 49 years for subjects with tetraplegia or tetraparesis and 54 years for those with paraplegia or paraparesis. Even with younger clients, it is important to make preparation for the potential need for early retirement, because employment rates decrease considerably for participants between the ages of 51 and 60 [11]. Individuals with SCI continue to have issues and challenges they have to adjust to. The need for rehabilitation does not end after hospital discharge [17].

The perceived disadvantages of losing social security benefits, which would lead to exclusion from accessing government funded equipment supplies, transport schemes and medical subsidies, may deter people from seeking employment [31].

The role of computers and technology in vocational rehabilitation and return to work

The past two decades are characterised by increasing access to information and technology, together with an employment market dominated by service/information providers rather than the manufacturing industry. Society in general is becoming more educated and previously held negative stereotypes of people with disabilities are being overcome by education programs and policy changes [76].

It is important to examine the impact of information and technology on the employment prospects of the disabled. People with SCI appear to have less access to computers because most people learn how to use computers at work, and only a minority of people with SCI work [77]. The lower rate of use of computers among people with SCI is unfortunate because the steep employment and earnings declines often experienced after a SCI are partially mitigated for those who have computer skills [77]. Computer use and training is of special benefit to people with SCI because computer technology may help lessen the impact of mobility limitations that are inherent with this disability [77].

Level of computer skills and computer training are significant predictors of employment outcomes after SCI. The greater the level of computer training and skills, the higher the probability of a positive employment outcome [76].

Policies and programs aimed at increasing access to computers and computer training for people with severe disabilities are important [77]. Patients should be encouraged to learn the basic use of computer and standard tools such as word processors and spreadsheets as an increasing number of job information is accessible through a computer. Moreover, people with disabilities are able to apply for many of the jobs that are information-based. Depending on their needs, they should be encouraged to learn more advanced skills. Education about careers, their necessary skills and training accordingly is also an important issue that the rehabilitation teams should care about. To take full advantage of future opportunities, SCI patients must be equipped with the skills required in the information age. Some SCI victims believe that the level of computer skills had been a factor in obtaining their current position [76].

The use of assistive devices such as hands-free telephones, environmental control systems and mouth sticks play also a role in half of the patients [76]. The utilisation of effective assistive technology supports is one of the challenges that influence employment success [78].

Spinal cord injury at young age and employment

For health care professionals involved with rehabilitation of children and adolescents with SCI, the ultimate goal is to develop strategies that will lead to better employment outcomes as the patient transitions to adulthood. Instilling expectations in the patient and family that employment is not only possible but also expected is a first step. Targeting efforts toward those at highest risk for unemployment, especially males with high-level injuries or violent origins, would be another important strategy. Because of the important negative impact of medical complications on employment, preventing complications such as pressure ulcers is critical [57].

Keeping young persons with SCI in school is an important objective towards the goal of employment. Two studies have examined the experiences of students with SCI shortly after return to school and give contradictory results. Graham et al. [79] showed that students who returned to school reported positive attitudes among teachers and peers with some reporting receiving little education or vocational counselling beyond scheduling classes. Mulcahey [80] pointed out that students had significant concerns about self-image, teacher expectations, academic expectations, peer reactions and appeal for inclusion of school re-entry planning in acute rehabilitation efforts. Drop out from school after SCI were frequent occasional because of medical reasons (pain and spasticity) and lack of wheelchair accessibility to a required class with the contribution of other premorbid factors [79]. Students with SCI demonstrate adequate participation and performance in educational settings, but may benefit from more vocational counselling and opportunities for paid employment [81].

There are three important barriers against return to work of the young: Low expectations of family, friends, and professionals, societal expectations that the person with a disability will be dependent, and lack of knowledge about resources and vocational services on the part of the individual with a disability and their family have been suggested as causes for the low employment rate of individuals with physical disabilities [82]. One related barrier may be that children and adolescents with disabilities have fewer job experiences while they are growing up than their peers.

Younger people are more likely to be more severely injured at admission and discharge and are more likely to have a wider social support network including parents, siblings, spouses, and friends who are all physically capable to take care of them [83]. This may explain why younger patients are least likely to be discharged to an institutional setting. Spinal cord caregivers experience a tremendous amount of both physical and emotional distress that are ongoing and have long-term effects [84]. It becomes critical to provide support to them as well as to those sustaining SCI. Since young persons with SCI require social support for community re-entry, this will indirectly enhance the likelihood of higher return to work outcomes.

Four factors were associated with employment: education, community mobility, functional independence and decreased medical complications. Other variables associated with employment included community integration, independent driving, independent living, higher income, use of illicit drugs and life satisfaction [57]. Employment in higher scale occupations post-injury is linked to younger age at onset of injury and having a longer duration of injury for two reasons: firstly, vocational plans are less rigid at a younger age, allowing flexibility in vocational adjustment and appropriate future career planning; and secondly, a change in career direction requires more time for vocational exploration, education and training in new fields [2, 31, 55]. The highest current employment rate in a group of individuals injured 6 years previously was seen in those who were injured at the age of 17 years or younger [2]. Compared to peers without disability, adolescents with SCI (mean age 16.2) were significantly less likely to have paid work experience [85]. The level of SCI acquired in childhood was not related to employment later in life [81]. Amongst US individuals who sustained a SCI at the age of 18 years or younger, 48-51% were employed during adulthood 7 or more years later [2, 42, 57], contrasting with the 81% employment rate in the general population of approximately the same age [86].

Sport and return to work

It has been demonstrated that involvement in sports by wheelchair users improves their rehabilitation outcomes and quality of life, and gives them aspiration for their further development [87, 88]. While some authors have stated that active involvement in sports and recreation increases the likelihood employment of SCI victims [89-91], others have failed to demonstrate such a significant link [68]. There seems to be a positive relationship between physical fitness and the gainful employment of paraplegics, but no significant relationship between physical fitness and the acceptance of physically demanding work by such individuals [89].

Employment outcomes after spinal cord injury

Occupations prior to the spinal cord injury were wide ranging throughout all employment categories [26]. Those in employment post injury showed a move towards the administration, clerical and finance categories, with science and engineering also providing some jobs [39]. Athanasou *et al.* demonstrated the diversity in outcomes regarding post-injury employment and vocational achievements of persons with SCI in Australia [36]. One third of the subjects went on to obtain further qualifications since their injury. The majority of subjects utilised informal means of returning to paid work through their previous job or through friends or relatives. Around one-fifth of the sample was employed full-time with a majority in clerical and management jobs. Thirty-one percent were engaged in part-time or full-time work.

Follow-up provided once employment has been gained may need to be monitored for longer periods particularly in older individuals and those who were in lower scale pre-injury occupations as these are the groups which appear to be most at risk of not sustaining employment [31]. Programs would need to adjust their focus once employment was gained to additionally address issues such as workplace discrimination, time management and negotiation skills, which were found to contribute to difficulties in sustaining work.

Best predictors of successful vocational outcomes were educational attainment, educational plans made before injury, and origin of interests in work [30]. A positive relationship has been found between life satisfaction and adjustment after SCI, and employment status [4, 6, 21]. Those employed were behaviourally more active, had fewer medical treatments, completed more years of education, perceived themselves to have fewer problems, were more satisfied with their lives, and rated their overall adjustment higher than those who were unemployed [4, 21]. Termination of employment also seems to be associated with declines in adjustment. The results were more consistent with becoming employed leading to better adjustment, rather than the reverse [92]. Employment and education are two of the main factors that determine outcome after SCI in terms of quality of life with the employed displaying superior adjustment skills as compared to the unemployed [11, 14].

In the US, the least successful outcomes were observed in minority men, participants of 50 years or older at injury, persons with complete quadriplegia, and participants with fewer than 12 years of education [43].

When work satisfaction variables of both employed and unemployed persons with SCI were examined, the majority of persons employed indicated that they would either change jobs or some employment variable such as duties, supervisor, or hours worked [17].

Successful reintegration, which includes return to work, is influenced by the ability of the individual to exercise control of their environment and make personal choices. Their ability to grasp and develop new skills is also an important factor. Participation in community events and activities decreased post-injury, due to lack of support and assistance with transportation, finances and overcoming architectural barriers. As a result of decreased mobility and independence, social integration was negatively affected [93-95].

Conclusion

Return to work after a medullary lesion is a complex process in which the severity of the lesion, the individual's aptitudes, skills and motivation, the working conditions as well as social and demographic aspects each have a significant role [96]. Predicting the return to work is challenging, given that presumably minor logistical factors can hinder or prohibit attempts to work. The principal task of the rehabilitation team is to help the spinal injured individual to discover his new body, ameliorate his quality of life by preventing medical complications, and help him to face his disabilities and handicaps. Socio-professional reintegration will be achieved by determining his interests, by evaluating his capacities and skills and by offering the means to palliate his deficiencies.

High unemployment rates among individuals with spinal cord lesion imply that specialised training and job-finding assistance are essential. Years without employment, the person's skills may become less competitive or even obsolete. Inevitably, self-esteem and confidence in work capability are often diminished. Providing specialised training assistance and guidance in job procurement is essential for improving the quality of life as well as boosting the self-esteem.

References

1. Cifu DX, Wehman P, McKinley WO (2001) Determining impairment following spinal cord injury. Phys Med Rehabil Clin N Am 12: 603-12
2. Krause JS (1992) Employment after spinal cord injury. Arch Phys Med Rehabil 73: 163-9
3. McKinley WO, Jackson AB, Cardenas DD et al. (1999) Long-term medical complications after traumatic spinal cord injury: a regional model systems analysis. Arch Phys Med Rehabil 80(11): 1402-10
4. Krause JS (1990) The relationship between productivity and adjustment following spinal cord injury. Rehabil Couns Bull 33: 188-99
5. Kubler-Ross E (1969) On death and dying. UAB press, Birmingham
6. Crisp R (1992) Vocational decision making by sixty spinal cord injury patients. Paraplegia 30: 420-4

7. MacKenzie EJ, Shapiro S, Smith RT et al. (1987) Factors influencing return to work following hospitalization for traumatic injury. Am J Public Health 77(3): 329-34

8. Cogswell BE (1968) Self-socialization: readjustment of paraplegics in the community. J Rehabil 34: 11-3

9. Kemp BJ, Vash CL (1971) Productivity after injury in a sample of spinal cord injured persons: a pilot study. J Chronic Dis 24(4): 259-75

10. Decker SD, Schulz R (1985) Correlates of life satisfaction and depression in middle-aged and elderly spinal cord-injured persons. Am J Occup Ther 39(11): 740-5

11. Krause JS, Sternberg M, Maides J et al. (1998) Employment after spinal cord injury: differences related to geographic region, gender and race. Arch Phys Med Rehabil 79: 615-24

12. Ville I, Ravaud JF (1996) Work, non-work and consequent satisfaction after spinal cord injury. Int J Rehabil Res 19(3): 241-52

13. Warr P (1982) Psychological aspects of employment and unemployment. Psychol Med 12(1): 7-11

14. Krause JS, Anson CA (1997) Adjustment after spinal cord injury: relationship to participate in employment or educational activities. Rehabil Couns Bull 40: 202-14

15. Clayton KS, Chubon RA (1994) Factors associated with the quality of life of long-term spinal cord injured persons. Arch Phys Med Rehabil 75(6): 633-8

16. Stensman R (1994) Adjustment to traumatic spinal cord injury. A longitudinal study of self-reported quality of life. Paraplegia 32(6): 416-22

17. Wehman P, Wilson K, Parent W et al. (2000) Employment satisfaction of individuals with spinal cord injury. Am J Phys Med Rehabil 79(2): 161-9

18. Westgren N, Levi R (1998) Quality of life and traumatic spinal cord injury. Arch Phys Med Rehabil 79(11): 1433-9

19. De Vivo MJ, Richards JS (1992) Community reintegration and quality of life following spinal cord injury. Paraplegia 30: 108-12

20. Krause JS, Anson CA (1996) Self-perceived reasons for unemployment cited by persons with spinal cord injury: relationship to gender, race, age, and level of injury. Rehabil Couns Bull 39: 217-27

21. Krause JS (1992) Adjustment to life after spinal cord injury: A comparison among three participant group based on employment status. Rehabil Couns Bull 35: 218-29

22. Ota T, Akaboshi K, Nagata M et al. (1996) Functional assessment of patients with spinal cord injury: measured by the motor score and the Functional Independence Measure. Spinal Cord 34(9): 531-5

23. Schalock RL, Keith KD, Hoffman K, Karan OC (1989) Quality of life: its measurement and use. Ment Retard 27(1): 25-31

24. Hall KM, Knudsen ST, Wright J et al. (1999) Follow-up study of individuals with high tetraplegia (C1-C4) 14 to 24 years postinjury. Arch Phys Med Rehabil 80(11): 1507-13

25. Krause JS, Kewman D, DeVivo MJ et al. (1999) Employment after spinal cord injury: an analysis of cases from the Model Spinal Cord Injury Systems. Arch Phys Med Rehabil 80(11): 1492-500

26. DeVivo MJ, Richards JS, Stover SL et al. (1991) Spinal cord injury: Rehabilitation adds life to years. West J Med 154(5): 602-6

27. Kanellos MC (1985) Enhancing vocational outcomes of spinal cord-injured persons: the occupational therapist's role. Am J Occup Ther 39(11): 726-33

28. Goldberg RT, Freed MM (1973) Vocational adjustment, interests, work values, and career plans of persons with spinal cord injuries. Scand J Rehabil Med 5(1): 3-11

29. Waters RL, Adkins R, Yakura J et al. (1998) Donal Munro Lecture: Functional and neurologic recovery following acute SCI. J Spinal Cord Med 21(3): 195-9

30. Alfred WG, Fuhrer MJ, Rossi CD (1987) Vocational development following severe spinal cord injury: a longitudinal study. Arch Phys Med Rehabil 68(12): 854-7

31. Conroy L, McKenna K (1999) Vocational outcome following spinal cord injury. Spinal Cord 37: 624-33

32. Al-Khodairy A (2003) Réadaptation professionnelle et lésions médullaires. Rev Med Suisse Romande 123: 643-6

33. Wang RY, Yang YR, Yen LL et al. (2002) Functional ability, perceived exertion and employment of the individuals with spinal cord lesion in Taiwan. Spinal Cord 40(2): 69-76

34. Trieschman RB (1979) Spinal cord injuries: Psychological, social, and vocational adjustment. Pergamon Press New York

35- Trieschmann R (1988) Spinal cord injuries: The psychological, social, and vocational rehabilitation. Demo publications New York

36. Athanasou JA, Brown DJ, Murphy GC (1996) Vocational achievements following spinal cord injury in Australia. Disabil Rehabil 18: 191-6

37. Murphy G, Athanasou J (1994) Vocational potential and spinal cord injury: a review and evaluation. J Appl Rehabil Couns 25: 47-52

38. Tomassen PCD, Post MWM, Van Asbeck FWA (2000) Return to work after spinal cord injury. Spinal Cord 38: 51-5

39. Castle R (1994) An investigation into the employment and occupation of patients with a spinal cord injury. Paraplegia 32: 182-7

40. Levi R, Hulting C, Seiger A (1996) The Stockholm spinal cord injury: Psychological and financial issues of the Swedish annual level-of-living survey in spinal cord injury subjects and controls. Paraplegia 34: 152-7

41. Engel S, Murphy GS, Athanasou JA et al. (1998) Employment outcomes following spinal cord injury. Int J Rehabil Res 21(2): 223-9

42. Young M, Alfred WG, Rintala DH et al. (1994) Vocational status of persons with spinal cord injury living in the community. Rehabil Couns Bull 37: 229-43

43. Krause JS, Anson CA (1996) Employment after spinal cord injury: relation to selected participant characteristics. Arch Phys Med Rehabil 77(8): 737-43

44. DeVivo MJ, Fine PR (1982) Employment status of spinal cord injured patients 3 years after injury. Arch Phys Med Rehabil 63: 200-3

45. Taricco M, Colombo C, Adone R et al. (1992) The social and vocational outcome of spinal cord injury patients. Paraplegia 30(3): 214-9

46. El Ghatit AZ, Hanson RW (1979) Educational and training levels and employment of the spinal cord injured patient. Arch Phys Med Rehabil 60(9): 405-6

47. DeVivo MJ, Rutt RD, Stover SL et al. (1987) Employment after spinal cord injury. Arch Phys Med Rehabil 68(8): 494-8

48. Pinkerton AC, Griffin ML (1983) Rehabilitation outcomes in females with spinal cord injury: a follow-up study. Paraplegia 21(3): 166-75

49. Lammertse DP, Yarkony GM (1991) Rehabilitation in spinal cord disorders. 4. Outcomes and issues of aging after spinal cord injury. Arch Phys Med Rehabil 72(4-S): S309-311

50. Stover SL, Fine PR (1986) Spinal cord injury : the facts and figures. UAB Press Birmingham

51. Hess DW, Ripley DL, McKinley WO *et al.* (2000) Predictors for return to work after spinal cord injury: a 3-year multicenter analysis. Arch Phys Med Rehabil 81(3): 359-63

52. McShane SL, Karp J (1993) Employment following spinal cord injury : a covariance structure analysis. Rehabil Psychol 38: 27-40

53. Richards B (1982) A social and psychological study of 166 spinal injured patients from Queensland. Paraplegia 1982: 90-6

54. Crisp R (1990) Return to work after spinal cord injury. J Rehabil 56: 28-35

55. Krause JS (1992) Longitudinal changes in adjustment after spinal cord injury: a 15-year study. Arch Phys Med Rehabil 73(6): 564-8

56. Hammell KR (1994) Psychosocial outcome following spinal cord injury. Paraplegia 32(11): 771-79

57. Anderson CJ, Vogel LC (2002) Employment outcomes of adults who sustained spinal cord injury as children or adolescents. Arch Phys Med Rehabil 83: 791-801

58. Dowler D, Batiste L, Whidden E (1998) Accommodating workers with spinal cord injury. J Vocat Rehabil 10: 115-22

59. Dvonch P, Kaplan LI, Grynbaum BB *et al.* (1965) Vocational findings in postdisability employment of patients with spinal cord dysfunction. Arch Phys Med Rehabil 46(11): 761-6

60. El Ghatit AZ (1978) Variables associated with obtaining and sustaining employment among spinal cord injured males: a follow-up of 760 veterans. J Chronic Dis 31(5): 363-9

61. Felton JS, Litman M (1965) Study of employment of 222 men with spinal cord injury. Arch Phys Med Rehabil 46(12): 809-14

62. Greenwood R, Johnson VA (1987) Employer perspectives on workers with disabilities. J Rehabil 53: 37-45

63. Hagner D, Cooney B (2003) Building employer capacity to support employees with severe disabilities in the workplace. Work 21(1): 77-82

64. McNeal DR, Somerville NJ, Wilson DJ (1999) Work problems and accommodations reported by persons who are postpolio or have spinal cord injury. Asst Technol 11: 137-57

65. Berkeley Planning Associates (1982) A study of accommodations provided to handicapped employees by federal contractors, final report: Vol 1. Study findings. Berkley, CA

66. Tate DG, Stiers W, Daugherty J *et al.* (1994) The effects of insurance benefits coverage on functional and psychosocial outcomes after spinal cord injury. Arch Phys Med Rehabil 75(4): 407-14

67. West M, Hock K, W Dowdy *et al.* (1998) Getting to work: Training and support for transportation needs. J Vocat Rehabil 10: 159-67

68. Tasiemski T, Bergstrom E, Savic G *et al.* (200) Sports, recreation and employment following spinal cord injury . a pilot study. Spinal Cord 38(3): 173-84

69. Weidman CD, Freehafer AA (1981) Vocational outcome in patients with spinal cord injury. J Rehabil 47(2): 63-5

70. Savic G, Short DJ, Weitzenkamp D *et al.* (2000) Hospital readmissions in people with chronic spinal cord injury. Spinal Cord 38(6): 371-7

71- Klotz R, Joseph PA, Ravaud JF *et al.* (2002) The Tetrafigap Survey on the long-term outcome of tetraplegic spinal cord injured persons: Part III. Medical complications and associated factors. Spinal Cord 40(9): 457-67

72. Pentland W, McColl MA, Rosenthal C (1995) The effect of aging and duration of disability on long term health outcomes following spinal cord injury. Paraplegia 33(7): 367-73

73. Aljure J, Eltorai I, Bradley WE *et al.* (1985) Carpal tunnel syndrome in paraplegic patients. Paraplegia 23(3): 182-6
74. Sie IH, Waters RL, Adkins RH *et al.* (1992) Upper extremity pain in the postrehabilitation spinal cord injured patient. Arch Phys Med Rehabil 73(1): 44-48
75. Gerhart KA, Bergstrom E, Charlifue SW *et al.* (1993) Long-term spinal cord injury: functional changes over time. Arch Phys Med Rehabil 74(10): 1030-4
76. Pell AD, Gillies RM, Carss M (1997) Relationship between use of technology and employment rates for people with physical disabilities in Australia: implications for education and training programmes. Disabil Rehabil 19: 332-38
77. Kruse D, Krueger A, Drastal S (1996) Computer use, computer training, and employment. Outcomes among people with spinal cord injuries. Spine 21(7): 891-96
78. Inge KJ, Wehman P, Strobel W *et al.* (1998) Supported employment and assistive technology for persons with spinal cord injury: Three illustrations of successful work supports. J Vocat Rehabil 10: 141-52
79. Graham P, Weingarden S, Murphy P (1991) School reintegration: a rehabilitation goal for spinal cord injured adolescents. Rehabil Nurs 16(3): 122-27
80. Mulcahey MJ (1992) Returning to school after a spinal cord injury: perspectives from four adolescents. Am J Occup Ther 46(4): 305-12
81. Massagli TL, Dudgeon BJ, Ross BW (1996) Educational performance and vocational participation after spinal cord injury in childhood. Arch Phys Med Rehabil 77(10): 995-9
82. White PH, Shear ES (1992) Transition/job readiness for adolescents with juvenile arthritis and other chronic illness. J Rheumatol Suppl 33: 23-7
83. Cifu DX, Steel RT, Kreutzer JS *et al.* (1999) Age, outcome, and rehabilitation costs after tetraplegia spinal cord injury. NeuroRehabilitation 12: 177-85
84. Kolalowsky-Hayner SA, Kishore R (1999) Caregiver functioning after traumatic injury. NeuroRehabilitation 13: 27-33
85. Anderson CJ, Vogel LC (2000) Work experience in adolescents with spinal cord injuries. Dev Med Child Neurol 42(8): 515-7
86. Bureau of census (2000) Current population reports. US Department of Commerce, Washington DC
87. Guttmann L (1976) Significance of sport in rehabilitation of spinal paraplegics and tetraplegics. JAMA 236: 195-7
88. Shepard RJ (1991) Benefits of sport and physical activity for the disabled: implications for the individual and for society. Scand J Rehab Med 23: 51-9
89. Noreau L, Shephard RJ (1992) Return to work after spinal cord injury: the potential contribution of physical fitness. Paraplegia 30(8): 563-72
90. Foreman PE, Cull J, Kirkby RJ (1997) Sports participation in individuals with spinal cord injury: demographic and psychological correlates. Int J Rehabil Res 20(2): 159-68
91. Curtis KA, McClanahan S, Hall KM, Dillon D, Brown KF (1986) Health, vocational, and functional status in spinal cord injured athletes and nonathletes. Arch Phys Med Rehabil 67(12): 862-5
92. Krause JS (1996) Employment after spinal cord injury: Transition and adjustment. Rehabil Couns Bull 35(4): 244-55
93. Targett PS, Wilson K, Wehman P *et al.* (1998) Community needs assessment survey of people with spinal cord injury: An early follow-up study. J Vocat Rehabil 10: 169-77

94. Turner E, Wehman P, Wallace JF *et al.* (1997) Overcoming obstacles to community reentry for persons with spinal cord injury: Assistive technology, ADA and self-advocacy. J Vocat Rehabil 9: 171-86
95. Wehman P, Wilson K, Targett *et al.* (1999) Removing transportation barriers for persons with spinal cord injuries: An ongoing challenge to community reintegration. J Vocat Rehabil 13: 21-30
96. Yasuda S, Wehman P, Targett P *et al.* (2002) Return to work after spinal cord injury: a review of recent research. NeuroRehabilitation 17(3): 177-86

Vocational rehabilitation and pulmonary programs

C.F. Donner

Definition of the problem

Chronic broncho-pulmonary diseases represent an important and growing social problem on account of the expected increasing prevalence of these diseases [1] and their negative impact on working capacity. These diseases represent, on a European scale, a frequent motive for work absenteeism and invalidity. For these reasons and considering the positive results that respiratory rehabilitation has yielded over the last few years [2], use of the techniques of rehabilitation should be considered in all patients who are bearers of functional impairment following chronic broncho-pulmonary diseases.

Patients with chronic obstructive pulmonary disease (COPD) tend to seek assistance at a time when breathlessness or other symptoms are at a comparatively advanced stage of the disease. While there is no doubt that the ability to remain gainfully employed could be enhanced if these patients were shifted to a more suitable form of employment, only limited criteria have been set forth to differentiate between those who should apply for disability benefits and those who should be recommended for a vocational rehabilitation (VR) program.

A retrospective analysis of data from the very poor literature concerning long-term vocational rehabilitation in subjects with chronic lung diseases has identified certain physiologic variables, such as forced expiratory volume in 1 sec (FEV1), forced expiratory flow between 25 and 75 percent of the forced vital capacity (FEF 25-75%) and maximum voluntary ventilation (MVV), which seem to correlate with the VR potential of COPD patients selected for a VR program [3].

Current knowledge of the evolution of occupational asthma is based on a few clinical studies in groups of patients sensitized to red cedar, colophony, crab boiling water and isocyanates [4]. Whatever the sensitizing agent, respiratory sequelae appear to be very frequent (in 50% or more of subjects after removal from exposure) and characterized by the persistence of an asthmatic condition with a variable degree of severity. For the greater part of these cases, certain features at the time of diagnostic assessment appear to be of prognostic value for the evolution of occupational asthma: age, duration of occupational exposure, duration of symptomatic exposure, presence of alteration at spirometry, and degree of bronchial hyperreactivity. In all cases, persistence of exposure after diagnosis produces unchanged or worsened symptoms as a consequence.

After removal from exposure the course of occupational asthma may be classified into three groups:

– recovery;
– intermittent attacks lasting more than one month after exclusion of exposure;
– persistence of an airflow obstruction.

Each course has distinctive features which should be considered when evaluating the sequelae: symptoms, degree of bronchial hyperreactivity, presence of airway obstruction, need for long-term steroid therapy, and impossibility to find another employment on account of asthmatic attacks due to effort in cold atmospheric conditions or to atmospheric pollutants. Finally, a specific feature of the course of intermittent attacks which should be taken into consideration is that it does not allow a full appreciation of the severity of sequelae before six months or even one year after allergen exclusion.

Review of the literature

The development of the techniques of pulmonary rehabilitation has benefitted from the very important progress made in the field of early diagnosis of these diseases, in particular concerning respiratory pathophysiology and lung function assessment [5, 6].

Pulmonary rehabilitation programs in patients with chronic pulmonary disease with a view to their reintegration into the working community include the following main steps [7, 8, 9, 10, 11]:

– pulmonary rehabilitation mainly based on exercise training;
– reintegration into the social community;
– job re-training;
– return to work.

Pulmonary rehabilitation is mainly based on exercise training: According to a recent meta-analysis [2] the minimum duration of a rehabilitation program is usually three months, with three sessions of 2.5 hours per week divided approximately into 30 min of health education, 45 min of exercise training, 30 min of physical therapy and relaxation and 45 min of gymnastics and/or outdoor exercise training. Four components [8, 10, 11, 12] play a major role in the rehabilitative phase:

Health education. The main aim of health education is to optimise the patient's compliance with treatment, in order to ensure a long term commitment to regular physical activity. Definitive evidence of the positive influence of education in pulmonary rehabilitation is, however, still lacking [8].

Psychosocial support. Despite little knowledge about its mechanisms, psychosocial support helps in restoring coping skills and in learning how to manage stress. Dyspnea and anxiety are reduced in the short term, but long term results are unknown. As an adjunct to exercise training, psychosocial support is effective in improving compliance, exercise tolerance and health related quality of life [8].

Exercise training. It is well documented that COPD patients feel better and improve their exercise tolerance after exercise training. Psychological as well as physiological changes are the basis of these improvements. Patients become desensitized to the sensation of dyspnea and the limb muscles undergo physiological changes similar to those observed in normal subjects. Many recent studies have focused on the possible role played by the dysfunction of the skeletal muscles of the limbs in COPD patients: this dysfunction may contribute to exercise intolerance. Less is known about anabolic hormones and nutritional supplementation [13]. The first aim of exercise training is to ensure that the exercise intensities determined in the laboratory are used during actual training. Exercise intensity can be monitored with a heart rate monitor and programmed alarm system in order to verify that the correct target heart rate is being followed. Concerning the practical aspects, indoor training, on a bicycle or treadmill, is usually proposed. However, it is important to stress to the patient that they do other activities, especially outdoor activities such as walking. Indeed, outdoor activities are usually more enjoyable, and the more enjoyable the activity the better the compliance should be. Repeated periods of exercise seem preferable to a single long period for the same stimulation duration, at least during indoor training. Indeed, a high level of motivation is well maintained by the first option but actually "best" modalities for training sessions (e.g., repeated periods of exercise vs. a single long period, high intensity/short duration vs. low intensity/long duration training) have not been defined as yet. Exercise training is still considered the best approach in pulmonary rehabilitation in terms of the results achieved, and should be recommended for general application in vocational rehabilitation.

Specific muscle training. There is, at present, little evidence of significant clinical benefit of ventilatory muscle training over general exercise alone. Both aerobic exercise training and local peripheral muscle training has been applied. Lower intensity aerobic exercise for muscle training resulted in modest improvements in submaximal exercise tests, but no increases in maximal exercise performance were observed. In contrast, high intensity aerobic training improved both maximal and submaximal exercise tests and induced both cardio-respiratory and peripheral muscle adaptations, similar to those observed in healthy subjects. Respiratory muscle training has been shown to increase inspiratory muscle strength, quality of life and exercise capacity in patients with inspiratory muscle weakness and a ventilatory limitation to exercise; therefore it should be included in all rehabilitation programs for COPD patients [8].

In this process, follow-up is very important to ensure the readjustment of training intensity and to discuss the improvements with the patient in order to reinforce their motivation. The fundamental goal of the rehabilitation program is to introduce the respiratory patient to a new life-style which includes regular physical activity. To achieve this goal, it is essential to develop and implement exercise maintenance programs that can be followed at home and maintained for the patient's whole residual life.

Characteristics of vocational rehabilitation programs in different pulmonary disorders [14, 15, 16]

A program of vocational rehabilitation for patients with chronic pulmonary disease should aim to meet the following general goals:

– assess upper extremity mobility, strength and endurance;
– develop self-monitored home-based exercise programs;
– evaluate basic and advanced self-care activities;
– provide suitable aids to increase independence in daily life activities;
– train in energy conservation and work simplification techniques;
– carefully evaluate the home and workplace including suggested modifications to provide a safe and barrier-free environment.

Obviously in each single case, not all the above factors are relevant – the specific goals of an individual's vocational rehabilitation program depend on the characteristics and severity of the disease.

In order to gain a meaningful picture of the rehabilitation process it is necessary to know and understand something of the differences in health status and other factors between individual patients at the outset. A very recent Swedish study [17] reported that individual differences in health status, length of sick-leave and unemployment exist at the upstart of vocational rehabilitation. Locus of control was found to exert an important influence on the differences between individuals, with persons with external locus of control having a less favourable point of departure at the start of VR compared to other groups. The authors concluded with the suggestion that rehabilitation programs should be developed and selected to match the specific needs and differences whether they are of an individual or of a social nature.

COPD. COPD patients, assessed by specific quality of life questionnaires, usually show a low level of satisfaction as a whole, in addition to a low level of satisfaction with several domains [19]. This suggests that the majority of the patients are unable to cope successfully with the consequences of their impairment and, therefore, more attention must be given to this in the rehabilitation phase. In mild to moderate COPD, education and psychological support to maintain a correct lifestyle and cope with disability are very important, in particular with regard to smoking habit, nutritional state, and interpersonal relationships. Chest physiotherapy can be considered in the hypersecretive patients. Obese chronic bronchitic patients and underweight emphysematous subjects with loss of muscle mass should be referred to the dietician for assessment and specific treatment when needed. Significant outcomes have been found in terms of improved exercise endurance, reduced dyspnea, better quality of life (QoL) and reduced healthcare utilization [8, 10]. In severe COPD, the components outlined above can also be applied, but the exercise protocols have to be adapted (e.g., self-paced walking instead of bicycle ergometer). Supplemental oxygen should be provided during training to relieve dyspnea when substantial desaturation occurs during exercise.

Asthma. Education is essential to ensure effective prevention, proper adherence to treatment, and correct monitoring [6]. In general, educational interventions in asthmatic patients have demonstrated a series of benefits such as a reduction of wheezing, improved work attendance and performance, less use of healthcare services (e.g. emergency visits and hospitalisations) and improved cooperation/support from families [7, 11]. Asthmatic patients are quite frequently deconditioned for fear of exercise-induced bronchoconstriction. Exercise training is therefore recommended and the same protocols as for COPD can be considered. As a rule, sporting activities should not be discouraged because of asthma. Occupational therapy plays a major role since many asthmatic patients are young subjects of working age.

Cystic fibrosis and bronchiectasis. In view of the fact that secretions clearance represents the basic clinical problem here, chest physiotherapy plays a major role, allowing a more uniform lung ventilation and helping in the prevention of infections. Nutritional support can be combined with substitution therapy with pancreatic enzymes. Education and psychological interventions are pivotal to support patients and family in coping with the heavy burden imposed by the disease, which begins in the early stages of life.

Chest wall disorders. Smoking prevention/cessation, clearance of secretions, prevention of respiratory infections, general exercise, respiratory muscle training, nutritional advice and ergonomic measures are all to be considered in rehabilitation programs.

Respiratory sleep disorders. A full clinical (respiratory, cardiac, nutritional, neurological and otolaryngological) and functional evaluation is mandatory before planning the treatment. Educational and psychological support can help in stopping the deleterious voluntary habits such as smoking, excessive alcohol and food intake. Obese subjects should seek the physician's advice. The main treatment option is nasal continuous positive airways pressure (cPAP) or bi-level positive airways pressure (BiPAP).

The selection criteria for admitting patients to a rehabilitation program [20] are extremely critical. Very few experimental data exist in the literature, and publications tend to be of old date in that most of the research was performed in the seventies. Hence there is a risk of an overly empirical approach regarding selection criteria.

One of the most significant studies carried out in this field, which dates back to 1975 [3], concluded that patients with COPD would be unlikely to benefit from participation in a vocational rehabilitation program if their FEV1 is less than 50% of predicted and their MWW is less than 40% of predicted. The authors believe that some exceptions should be made for patients who are well motivated, possess specialised and/or needed skills, or whose job can be modified to meet the reduction in their pulmonary capacity. It should be emphasized that the factors which lead to the ability to work are very complex. For instance, Petty et al. [21] described several patients who were able, with continuous supplementation of oxygen, to meet the oxygen requirement for the energy expenditure of their job.

Also psychosocial factors play some role in predicting the vocational rehabilitation potential of patients with pulmonary disease. Patients should be carefully screened prior to being admitted to a VR programme if they have shown a recent significant negative change in lifestyle, personality change, or inability to mobilize psychosocial assets.

A recently published paper concludes that it is possible to improve cooperation in vocational rehabilitation by systematic rehabilitation group meetings [22]. The rehabilitation may be viewed as a meeting place for "experts" and clients. This approach differs from the "case management" approach of relatively common use in the rehabilitation field.

In a vocational rehabilitation program for pulmonary patients it is important to take into account the following general suggestions:

– use breathing control while working;
– sit for as many activities as possible;
– use slow, smooth flowing movements: rushing will only increase discomfort;
– take frequent rests;
– organize your activities; establish routines to increase efficiency;
– consider when it is the best time for doing each activity;
– pre-plan activities (daily and weekly schedules); alternate light and heavy activities; eliminate unnecessary tasks;
– organize your work space;
– maintain good posture; use proper lifting techniques; push don't pull; slide don't lift;
– always exhale with the strenuous part of the activity or with the part of the activity requiring motion towards the body.

Some factors related to work capacity should play a major role in planning and carrying out the different steps of the program. It seems reasonable to consider the following aspects [23]:

Rate of work: a) use a slow steady pace with short rest periods , b) fast walking takes 1.5 times more energy than slow walking, c) walking up stairs takes 7 times more energy than walking on level ground.

Rest: frequent short rests are a must and of more benefit than fewer long rests

Distribution of work load: a) peak loads for short periods may call for more energy than can be afforded, b) avoid straining in emergencies, c) don't try to do a two-man job alone.

Weather: a) it is difficult to do as much work on a hot humid day as on a cool one, b) direct sunlight increases strain on the body, c) dress warmly, use scarves or masks on cold winter days.

Physical conditioning: regular moderate activity will help to maintain good physical condition.

Weight: keep weight normal, overweight overworks the lung and heart.

Age: work capacity decreases with increasing age. At 50 years, assuming good health, the capacity will be approximately 70% of what it was at 25 years; at 70 years it will be approximately 50%.

Emotion: worry, fears and/or tension prevent relaxation during rest, placing an extra burden on the heart.

In a study of Bazzini [16] data are reported concerning a vocational rehabilitation program carried out for 3 weeks in 12 stable COPD patients (age 56 ± 7 yrs, FEV1/FVC $57 \pm 14\%$) with $PaO2 > 60mmHg$, $PaCO2 < 48mmHg$. The patients were submitted twice daily to training sessions devoted to an activity specific to their job simulated by a Lido WorkSET dynamometer at the patient's own pace (score 3 on Borg's scale). During the first week, each session consisted of three exercise bouts of 5 min. duration each, with 5 min. intervals in between. During the second and third weeks, each session consisted of three 10 min. exercise bouts. Before and after training patients performed a 5 min. isotonic endurance test and a maximal isokinetic test (10 repetitions) for the usual task and for a similarly energy-demanding task (not trained). Dyspnea was monitored every 30 s with a modified Borg scale and a Visual Analog Scale (VAS). The data assessed on days 1 and 21 of treatment showed, after the training program, that the total work done of the regularly performed task increased significantly ($p < 0.007$). Equivalent levels of work elicited a lesser degree of dyspnea as assessed by both Borg scale and VAS. Figure 1 shows a comparison of the results, after training, on performance of the usual task as opposed to performance of the untrained task. This improvement seems less attributable to an improved muscle strength than to an increased velocity of performance (i.e., increased number of repetitions of the task).

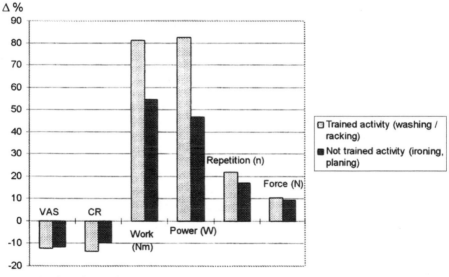

VAS = Visual Analog Scale
CR = Modified Borg scale (0-10 category-ratio)
Both scales measure dyspnea.

Fig. 1 – Changes in 12 COPD patients after vocational rehabilitation exercise training in the performance of the trained task versus an untrained similarly energy-demanding task (modified from 16)

Cost-effectiveness of vocational programs

Despite the magnitude of the public health problem represented by respiratory diseases and their increasing socio-economic impact, few studies have been focused on the vocational rehabilitation (VR) potential of patients with the most diffuse pulmonary diseases.

In reality there does not exist a specific body of literature on this topic, but rather only a few sporadic articles.

For this reason it is practically impossible to make a comparative evaluation of the cost effectiveness of different VR programs in patients with pulmonary disease. I will therefore limit myself to discussing the major points from the few sporadic works which have been published.

Concerning asthma, two German studies can be cited. The first is a study by Kohl *et al.* in 1991 [24] on the efficacy of a special training program for adolescents disabled by asthma or allergic disease who were not able to start an apprenticeship. The program had a duration of 1 year, and besides vocational guidance and try-out of different occupations, medical and psychological diagnostics were performed. Medical service was provided all day and a hospital with emergency unit was available in the area. Though 41% of the participants had left school after the compulsory school age without any qualified graduation, 79% were able to start an apprenticeship after the program.

The second paper focused on the effectiveness of secondary preventive programs for patients with asthma and rhinitis in the baking industry. Since 1992, the German Industrial Professional Association for the Food Industry and Gastronomy (Berufsgenossenschaft Nahrungsmittel und Gaststatten) which is responsible for a statutory accident insurance has offered a specific patient education program to bakers suffering from occupationally-induced obstructive pulmonary disease or allergic rhino-conjunctivitis, who do not quit their jobs and wish to continue working as bakers. The program aims at preventing aggravation of the disease in subjects with a mean duration of illness of 10 years. Participants in the program reported highly significant reductions in the frequency of disease-specific complaints during work and outside the working place, in sleep disturbances and in situations requiring immediate medical intervention. Between 64% and 85% of the patients experienced an improvement in stress, physical and work performance, private and family life, and ability for self management. Lung function did not deteriorate. It was concluded that the program was effective in reducing symptoms and stress and in improving quality of life in bakers with occupational respiratory disease who voluntarily continue to work as bakers (25).

Concerning pulmonary tuberculosis there is only one recently published paper by Russian authors which reported the results of medical and vocational rehabilitation [26]. This study showed a low efficacy of treatment in the long-term period. Of the able-bodied persons, 40% resumed their work activity (58.5% in their previous occupation) and 16.7% of these experienced exacerbation of lung tuberculosis in the course of work.

Conclusions

Functional recovery, even if only partial, enables the disabled person to be reintegrated in society. At the very least, it enables them to conduct their social life autonomously. But functional recovery and reintegration in society are not always associated with the resumption of employment [27].

It can sometimes happen that functional recovery is incomplete and not sufficient to permit the subject to resume his/her former employment because this would demand an energy cost too elevated in relation to the subject's present capacity.

In other cases, functional recovery is complete but it is not possible for the subject to resume former employment on account of environmental risks (e.g. heat, humidity, dust, chemical fumes, gas, smoke).

In conclusion, the opportunities that readjustment offers to subjects with chronic bronchopulmonary disease should be a sufficient stimulus to warrant the promotion and development to the fullest extent possible of this type of assistance. All such patients should be offered the possibility of reintegration in society and, if possible, in their chosen job.

References

1. Murray CJ, Lopez AD (1997) Alternative projections of mortality and disability by causa 1990-2000: global burden of disease study. Lancet 349: 1498-504
2. Lacasse Y, Wong E, Guyatt GH *et al.* (1996) Meta-analysis of respiratory rehabilitation in chronic obstructive pulmonary disease. Lancet 348: 1115-9
3. Kass I, Dyksterhuis JF, Rubin H *et al.* (1975) Correlation of psychophysiologic variables with vocational rehabilitation outcome in patient with chronic obstructive pulmonary disease. Chest 67: 433-40
4. Rosenberg N, Gervais P (1989) Evaluation des séquelles de l'asthme professionel. Rev Mal Resp 6: 35-8
5. Gosselink R, Troosters T, Decramer M (1996) Peripheral muscle weakness contributes to exercise limitation in COPD. Am J Respir Crit Care Med 153: 976-80
6. Ringsberg KC, Wicklund I, Wilhelmsen L (1990) Education of adult patients at an "asthma school". Effects on quality of life, knowledge and need for nursing. Eur Respir J 3: 33-37
7. Clark NM. (1999) Asthma self-management education. Research and implications for clinical practice. Chest 95: 1110-3
8. Ambrosino N, Vitacca M, Rampulla C (1995) Standards for rehabilitative strategies in respiratory diseases. Monaldi Arch Chest Dis 50: 293-318
9. Donner CF, Muir JF (1997) Selection criteria and programmes for pulmonary rehabilitation in COPD patients. Eur Respir J 10: 744-57
10. Donner CF, Lusuardi M (1999) Pulmonary rehabilitation. In: Brambilla C, Costabel U, Naeije R, Rodriguez-Roisin R (eds). Pulmonary Diseases. McGraw-Hill, London, p 577-84
11. Donner CF, Decramer M (eds). (2000) Pulmonary Rehabilitation. Eur Respir Monograph Vol 5, No. 13
12. British Thoracic Society Standards of Care Subcommittee on Pulmonary Rehabilitation. Pulmonary rehabilitation. (2001) Thorax 56: 827-34
13. Lacasse Y, Guyatt GH, Goldstein RS (1997) The components of a respiratory rehabilitation program. Chest 111: 1077-88
14. Patessio A (2000) Exercise training in lung disease. In: Donner CF, Decramer M. (eds). Pulmonary rehabilitation. ERS Monograph 13 (vol. 5), p 90-8

15. Baker NA., Jacobs K (2003) The nature of working in the United States: an occupational therapy perspective. Work 20(1): 53-61
16. Bazzini G (1999) Vocational rehabilitation. In: Ambrosino N, Donner CF, Rampulla C. Advances in rehabilitation. Topics in pulmonary rehabilitation. Maugeri Foundation Books, Pavia, Vol 7. p 279-93
17. Nieuwenhuijsen K, Verbeek JH, Siemerink JC et al. (2003) Quality of rehabilitation among workers with adjustment disorders according to practice guidelines; a retrospective cohort study. Occup Environ Med 60 (Suppl.1): 121-25
18. Millet P, Sandberg KW (2003) Individual status at the start of rehabilitation: Implications for vocational rehabilitation programs. Work 20(2): 121-9
19. Sturesson M, Branholm IB (2000) Life satisfaction in subjects with chronic obstructive pulmonary disease. Work 14(2): 77-82
20. Donner CF, Lusuardi M (2000) Selection of candidates and programmes. In: Donner CF, Decramer M (eds). Pulmonary Rehabilitation. Eur Respir Monograph Vol 5, No. 13 132-142
21. Petty TL, MacIlroy ER, Swigert MA et al. (1970) Chronic airway obstruction, respiratory insufficiency and gainful employment. Arch Environ Health 21: 71-8
22. Jakobsson B, Schuldt Haard U, Bergroth A et al. (2002) Improved cooperation in vocational rehabilitation with systematic rehabilitation group meetings. Disabil Rehabil 24(14): 734-40
23. Woolf CR (1986) Respiratory rehabilitation: a practical guide. Tower Litho Toronto
24. Kohl C, Brill B, Lecheler J (1991) Occupational training measures for adolescents with asthma and allergy: one-year vocational education. Monatsschr Kinderheildk 139 (9): 597-9
25. Grieshaber R, Nolting HD, Rosenau C et al. (1998) Effectiveness of secondary preventive programs for patients with asthma and rhinitis in the baking industry. Pneumologie 53 (7): 656-65
26. Fomicheva NI, Usatiuk AI, Mozgova OV et al. (2003) Medical and social rehabilitation of coal miners suffering from pulmonary tuberculosis, Lik Sprava (1): 77-9
27. Casula D, Sanna-Randaccio F (1975) Possibilités pratiques de réadaptation et de reprise de travail des insuffisants respiratoires. Résultats à long terme. Acta Tuberculosea et Pneumologica Belgica 66: 222-44

Cardiac rehabilitation and vocational reintegration

J.-M. Casillas, H.-J. Smolik and J.-P. Didier

Introduction

Cardiovascular diseases still represent the leading cause of mortality in industrialized nations. What is more, they are on the increase and are placing a major financial burden on the health economy. Their repercussions are not limited to medico-surgical responsibilities but extend to the social and occupational aspects, often translating into a fall-off or a loss of activity. The occupational aspect is particularly worrying since the consequences of cardiovascular disease at this level are severe in terms of disability and aggravating the damage to physical health and the economy. In France, for example, cardiovascular disease represents the third most frequent cause of inability to work [1].

Rehabilitation, which is essential during cardiovascular diseases, has the twin objectives of secondary prevention and of returning to a range of activities that is as complete as possible. Occupational reintegration is thus a part of these objectives, with exercise therapy being essential. However, due to the wide variety of individual situations, the difficulties in evaluating occupational capabilities and work-related risks and the socio-cultural dimension linked with these diseases, this reintegration fails only too often. For instance, elements such as socio-economic conditions, level of job satisfaction, age and the patient's view of the seriousness of his illness are frequently determining factors when returning to a working life whereas objective criteria such as the ability to adapt to exercise are inadequately taken into account.

In France, after an unexpected cardiovascular disease, previously employed patients will sometimes benefit from rehabilitation. Their possible return to work will then be the responsibility of the occupational doctor. However, the regulatory context of social reimbursement for the disease and handicap often interferes, hindering any return to work.

For these reasons, we wish to present the effects and methods of rehabilitation, the specifics of French social law and legislation and the results of rehabilitation at the level of occupational reintegration

Cardiac rehabilitation

Cardiac rehabilitation developed at the end of the 1980s when an average improvement of 25% in the mortality rate was demonstrated among coronary patients following rehabilitation [2, 3]. Rehabilitation structures were progressively organized to meet their dual goal of occupational reintegration and secondary prevention by putting a multidisciplinary team at the disposal of patients (doctors, physiotherapists, nurses, occupational therapists, nutritionists, psychologists, etc.) and a technical platform designed for reconditioning people to physical exertion.

Indications for cardiac rehabilitation have become better defined over time: myocardial infarction, coronary revascularisation (by bypass or angioplasty), stable angina, cardiac insufficiency, cardiac transplant, valve replacement, arteriopathy of the lower limbs. However, the significant prevalence of these ailments makes the integration of all these patients into rehabilitation programmes illusory in view of the inadequacy of specialised rehabilitation infrastructures. Thus, in industrialised countries, only an average of 20% to 30% of patients who warrant rehabilitation can actually take advantage of it. [4, 5]. Patients are selected by those who habitually prescribe rehabilitation, the cardiologists and cardiovascular surgeons. This leads to the relative exclusion of older subjects and women [6], which results in the profile of the type of patient rehabilitated most frequently being a younger man, active at a socio-professional level.

The effects of cardiac rehabilitation have largely been established: the greatest impact is an improvement in physical capacity among patients most often poorly adapted to exercise. This is a decisive element for return to work that is underpinned by an increase in oxidative muscular metabolism [7] and by improved muscular perfusion linked with a reactivation of the endothelium-dependent vasodilatation [8]. The average increase of 20% of the VO2 max bears witness to this mainly peripheral vasculo-muscular improvement caused by exercise therapy [9]. This improvement in bioenergetic efficiency associated with the rebalance of the neuro-vegetative system to the benefit of para-sympathetic tone [10] provides relative myocardial protection, with a decline in the ischemic threshold, less frequent stress during exercise. Rhythm disorders are less frequent [11] and reflex coronary vasomotion is improved with increased coronary diastolic perfusion time [12], but without any noticeable effect on ventricular ejection fraction [13]. These different impacts are even found in cases of cardiac insufficiency [14, 15, 16].

Maintained long term [18], the reduction in cardiac mortality and morbidity [17] is probably linked to a combination of health/dietetic changes and medicinal treatment. It is multifactorial in origin, involving the effects of rehabilitation mentioned above and those of improved control over risk factors [19]: a drop in arterial pressure [20], an improvement in lipid profile [21], a reduction in insulin resistance with improved glycemic balance among diabetics [22], a reduction in excess weight [23], improved blood rheology [24], weaning off smoking [25]. The consequence is a delayed progression of coronary damage [26].

Programmes of cardiac rehabilitation must address the twin objective of exercise reconditioning and an optimum control of risk factors. They are necessarily personalized within objective parameters, which permit quantified evolving monitoring and direct socio-occupational reintegration. In the majority of cases, these are out-patient programmes developed in units specialising in cardiac rehabilitation. When required by the patient's general condition (difficult post-operative effects, precarious haemodynamic state, associated pathologies) or in cases of geographical distance, this is carried out as in-patient care.

Exercise rehabilitation

The level of training is adapted to the capabilities of each patient following a preliminary evaluation.

This evaluation is usually based on standardised exercise tests carried out on an ergometric bicycle or on a treadmill, with electrocardiograph and blood pressure monitoring. In cases of cardiac insufficiency, an analysis of the exhaled breath to measure oxygen consumption is frequently included. This permits a better appraisal of the deconditioning of the oxidative metabolism and allows its development to be followed under the effect of rehabilitation. Sometimes the maximum test is conducted using an upper-limb ergometer when the lower limbs cannot be used for any exercise of sufficient intensity (neurological, orthopaedic, vascular difficulties) or because of job-related severe strain on the upper-limbs. These are tests without any modification to the medical treatment, limited by fatigue and dyspnea symptoms, and involving the classic discontinuation criteria (clinical intolerance, myocardial ischemia, severe rhythmic or conductive disturbances, blood-pressure anomalies, etc.). They provide information on maximum physical capabilities (power developed), and on cardiovascular adaptation, but they are likewise a good indicator of patients' motivation. Where oxygen consumption is concerned, the maximum oxidative performance is quantified (VO2 max) as is sub-maximum aerobic capacity (anaerobic threshold) that show the level of training. In cases of cardiac insufficiency, Weber's classification establishes correlations between VO2 peak values and the functional repercussions of the left ventricular dysfunction [27] (Table 1). Cardiac frequency is of little interest as an absolute value, taking into account the widespread use of bradycardic agents. On the other hand, based on the various exercise levels during the maximum test, it represents the easiest way of determining the level of useful exercise during the exercise sessions. It remains an essential point of reference in the final evaluation of cardiovascular constraints linked with occupational activities.

Table 1 – Weber classification.
Class A corresponds to zero or discrete repercussion of cardiac insufficiency. For Class B, the gene remains moderate. At level C, it is important and becomes severe at level D.

Class	Max oxygen uptake (peak VO2) (ml/kg/min)
A	> 20
B	16-20
C	10-15
D	< 9

Other types of standardised tests have been developed. They are essentially based on the evaluation of different types of walking.

The 6-minute walk test: this consists of measuring the greatest distance covered in 6 minutes on an indoor marked track. The 2nd and 4th minutes are signalled to the patient who need not run but can adjust his walk to suit himself (he can slow down or even take a break if tired). This test is reproducible [28], well tolerated [29], it correlates with aerobic capacity [30], and is an objective measure of functional progress linked with exercise rehabilitation [31].

The fast walk test: conversely, the distance is set (usually, approximately 200 metres) and the time taken to cover it is measured. The patient's instructions are to complete this test within the shortest amount of time but without running. This investigates the sub-maximum capacity, half-way between the results of the 6-minute walk test and the maximum exertion test [32].

During these walk tests, various parameters can be recorded:

Clinical events (faintness, lameness, limping, balance problems, blood-pressure problems, etc.). Dyspnea and fatigue are the most important aspects to be evaluated. These tests allow the data obtained from questioning to be clarified using the NYHA (New York Heart Association) classification (Table 2). The patients' sudden awareness of a feeling of fatigue corresponding to different levels of exertion is of particular interest for the self-management of their physical activity in the mid-term:

– mild exertion corresponding to a warm-up;
– moderate exertion, corresponding to an effective training level;
– extreme, potentially dangerous exertion.

Table 2 – NYHA classification (New York Heart Association).

Classification stage	Appearance of dyspnea
I	Extreme exertion (no functional repercussions)
II	Moderate exertion such as walking quickly, climbing stairs
III	Mild exertion such as getting dressed (usual movements)
IV	With the least exertion or at rest

Among the scales of perceived exertion, the Borg scale is the one most widely used [33]. It is comprised of 15 escalating levels of exertion (Table 3).

Cardiac frequency is a commonly used criterion. Easy to measure (cardio frequency meter, ECG telemetry), it enables the data measured during the walk test to be compared with the maximum frequency achieved during the exertion test. It can be an alternative to VO2 data collection in that it calculates the index of the physiological cost of walking. This index is equal to the relationship of the difference between stabilized cardiac frequency when walking and cardiac frequency at rest to walking speed [34]. It enables measurement of walking efficiency in heartbeats per metre. However, it is not always possible to obtain a truly stabilized cardiac frequency during a walk test. Moreover, cardiac

Table 3 – Borg scale.

6	
7	Very, very light
8	
9	Very light
10	
11	Fairly light
12	
13	Somewhat hard
14	
15	Hard
16	
17	Very hard
18	
19	Very, very hard
20	

frequency at rest is subject to fluctuations, particularly according to environmental conditions. These findings have led to the idea of measuring the "total heartbeat index" during walk tests equal to the sum of heartbeats in relation to the distance covered [35]. The potential interest in this index is to be free of awkward data records and an analysis of exhaled breath during the walk. Its measurement would appear to be facilitated by the possibility of storing and analysing of the cardio frequency meters in future.

The forms of exercise rehabilitation

These are classically based on overall aerobic training. As a general rule, the training level is between 60 to 80 percent of maximum capacity. A target cardiac frequency to be reached during the rehabilitation session is frequently set. The primary aim is to improve aerobic muscular metabolism. Exercises are thus developed on various ergometers (bicycle, arm-crank, rowing machine, etc.) in order to employ as significant a muscular area as possible and to vary the forms. Each type of exercise is preceded by a warm-up phase and followed by a recuperative phase. The length of exercise period should be 20 to 30 minutes on average in order to create sufficient stress at cardiovascular and metabolic level.

Increasingly, segmentary muscular strengthening is added. These are resistance exercises developed with the strongest muscular groups in the limbs (extensors and flexors of the knee, ankle, elbow, arm adductors, etc.). Here again, the main objective is an improvement in aerobic metabolism with a fixed resistance of between 50 and 60% of the maximum voluntary strength [36]. The exercises are comprised of a succession of short static, concentric then eccentric contractions in a regular rhythm. Haemodynamic tolerance is usually good even in cases of heart failure [37]. The aim is to improve the stamina of muscles involved in a patient's habitual movements with particular interest in terms of occupational reintegration [38].

Low-frequency muscular electrical stimulation represents an adjuvant or even an alternative to segmentary muscular strengthening. It entails an increase in strength and volume of the electrically stimulated muscles with the resultant improvement in physical capacity [39]. Usually, these are the muscular masses of the lower limbs (quadriceps, triceps sural, hamstrings) that are integrated into the daily electrical stimulation sessions for a period of one hour.

Monitoring atherosclerosis risk factors

This represents the other basic aspect of cardiac rehabilitation. It has led to the organization of rehabilitation units into multidisciplinary teams, comprising cardiac rehabilitators, cardiologists, specially-trained nurses, occupational therapists, diabetologists, lipidologists, tobacco experts and psychologists, etc. The aim is to implement a personalized intervention programme, ideally to reduce the risk factors simultaneously with exercise-based rehabilitation [40].

Cardiovascular diseases and work

If work in itself does not cause or rarely causes cardiac diseases it can, on the other hand, create a fertile ground for their development or be a source of questioning medical fitness in the workplace.

The role of the occupational doctor. Evaluating occupational risk. Decision on medical fitness in the workplace

First of all, it must be said that the methods of determining fitness for work vary from country to country within the European Union.

In France, the following rules apply:
Role of the occupational doctor:
– The law of 11 October 1946 that created and made occupational medicine compulsory for all employees sets out that occupational doctors are the sole persons with responsibility for determining an employee's fitness for work. This means that the occupational doctor must, first verify that the job is not dangerous for the employee and is thus not likely to cause any alteration in his state of health and, secondly, that the employee is not likely to endanger others in the course of his occupational activities.
– This compels the occupational doctor:
- to be familiar with the restrictions of the job and to assess their impact on the employee;

- to be familiar with the employee, his physiological limits or even pathological limits of adapting, to check that his state of health is compatible with the demands of the job by means of compulsory medical examinations conducted before hiring, at regular intervals each year or after any absence of at least 21 days due to illness [41].

The restrictions linked with work that can have an effect on the fitness of an employee suffering from a cardiovascular disease

Regulatory restrictions linked to the type of job.

Thus, by way of example, cardiovascular diseases such as angina, myocardial infarct, past history of coronary bypass, complex hypertension, cardiac insufficiency, severe valvulopathy, valvular prosthetics, rhythm disturbances, aortic aneurysms, wearing a defibrillator are all barriers to obtaining or holding a licence to drive heavy goods vehicles, public service vehicles or ambulances. Another example: anticoagulant treatment prohibits a sailor from continuing with his job.

Organizational restrictions:

Working alternating hours, at night or unstructured and atypical hours, [42].

Technical restrictions, linked with:

- the workplace (exposure to bad weather while working outdoors, exposure to heat or cold, to humidity, working at heights;

- location of the workplace (working at heights or isolated, generating stress arising from a feeling of insecurity);

- harmful effects of machinery (vibrations, noise) or their form of power supply (electrical risk, exposure to carbon monoxide).

– Products:

- physical: dust, radiation, particularly electromagnetic;

- chemical, particularly substances likely to provoke acute circulatory insufficiency (such as arsenic and halogenic derivatives of aliphatic hydrocarbons), a myocardial attack (such as nitrated derivatives of phenols), modifications to arterial blood pressure (such as lead, anticholinesterase organophosphorus compounds), ventricular rhythm disturbances with the possibility of cardiovascular collapse (such as trichlorethylene), etc.

– Passive smoking:

- the intensity of physical effort linked with occupational movements, with posture (working with the arms below the cardiac axis), handling exertion, wearing protective equipment, etc.;

- psychological restrictions (exposure to a high level of nervous tension) and relational restrictions when they are felt to be aggressive.

Risk evaluation

This depends on the assessment of the level of stress caused by work (cardiac profile of the job determined with the help of a cardiofrequency meter) and on its comparison with the worker's true capacity and limits.

Physiological limits are linked to age, gender, level of fitness, length of service in the profession, training and professional qualifications, intellectual capacity (all elements that enable strategies to be developed that involve less exertion or are beneficial for occupational reclassification), to the psyche (anxiety, depression, adaptation to the illness, negation, sudden awareness of the interested party of his possible limitations, of interest in his treatment and the medical follow-up, etc.).

The pathological limitations in relation to the nature of the cardiovascular disease (severity and extent of the coronary disease), to the associated deficiencies or pathologies, to the secondary effects of the treatment (anticoagulants in case of traumatic risk, beta-blockers in case of intense physical work, etc.).

Conclusions drawn by the occupational doctor

Three different conclusions are possible:
 – The employee is fit for his job.
 – The employee is fit for his job with some reservations: the occupational doctor formulates restrictions on abilities and suggests technical measures to improve working conditions with which the employer must comply (for example, carrying heavy loads might be contraindicated, an arrangement of working hours, a change of job, etc.). If the patient can prove that it is impossible for him to comply with the occupational doctor's instructions, the latter will then stipulate total and final unfitness for the job.
 – The employee is unfit for his job: this decision should be confirmed by re-examination conducted within a minimum of 15 days (law of 26.12.1988). *This period should necessarily be taken advantage of by the occupational doctor to find a reclassification solution within the company. If no reclassification solution proves possible, unfitness for all jobs within the company is declared and results in redundancy.*

The "pre-return" visit

This is an administrative measure aimed at facilitating the return to work. It is a visit to the occupational doctor prior to taking up work again, the aim being to facilitate the necessary measures in case of any change in ability to work. It is not compulsory and can only be conducted at the request of the employee, the general practitioner or doctors of the National Health Service [43].

With regard to rehabilitation, it appears indispensable that this visit should be planned and the occupational doctor be sent, through the patient (to avoid any violation of medical confidentiality), all the information pertaining to the rehabilitation results so that the terms of the return to work are fixed. This visit cannot be concluded by a decision of medical unfitness for the job.

The occupational doctor can prescribe any supplementary examinations that are required to allow a patient's fitness for the job to be better assessed.

The return to work can be part-time.

The patient can request the status of 'disabled worker' at an early stage from COTO-REP (COmmission Technique d'Orientation et de Reclassement Professionnel, created by the directive legislation of 30.06.1975).

From medical unfitness for work to the social undertaking

Cardiovascular diseases and health insurance

Inability to work due to disease entitles patients to receive daily benefits. If this inability to work is prolonged, these daily benefits are paid for 6 months and beyond for three years if the disease is considered to be long-term and as long as a patient's health cannot be considered stabilized. On the other hand, payment ceases as soon as a patient is considered fit for work of some kind or other by the consultant doctor representing Social Security.

An employee cannot be declared unfit for his job by the occupational doctor as long as he has stopped working, with the period of sick leave corresponding to a temporary suspension of the employment contract. A verdict on medical fitness for a job can only be given after the restart visit.

Cardiovascular diseases and handicap

If a cardiovascular disease is the cause of partial or total inability to work, the patient will be directed to COTOREP where a decision will be made on recognizing the status of disabled worker and a financial allowance granted as necessary.

Dependent on the case, this acknowledgement will permit (whether the job is kept or not):

– access to appropriate professional training and/or access to work reserved for handicapped people (6% of jobs in companies);

– arrangements for the workplace as well as relative protection against redundancy.

Cardiovascular diseases and disability

If the cardiovascular disease is not reimbursed as an occupational accident or illness, the patient can benefit during his sick leave from reimbursement within the framework of disability insurance if he has worked for 12 months before the onset of his disease.

The disability rate is fixed by the consultant doctor at Social Security. Dependent on level, it will allow a disability pension to be obtained if necessary. Disability is not final, it can be lost or modified dependent on how the pathology develops.

Cardiovascular diseases, occupational pathology and disability

If the disease is of occupational origin (result of an accident at work or an occupational illness), the victim is taken on by occupational accident or occupational disease insurance. The person concerned thus benefits:

– initially, a daily allowance up to the date of consolidation set by the Social Security consultant doctor;

– secondly, after consolidation, fixed financial compensation dependent on after-effects.

Cardiovascular diseases and responsibilities

Responsibility within the framework of cardiovascular diseases in the workplace lies firstly with the employer, who has social and civil, and even penal, responsibility:

"The employer is obliged to ensure the safety and health of his employees in all aspects associated with work" [44].

Article R.231-54-1 of the Code of Work stipulates that the evaluation of risks is the employer's responsibility.

Responsibility of the doctors:

In the event of an occupational accident or disease as a result of an inappropriate fitness appraisal, the only doctor whose responsibility is involved is the occupational doctor irrespective of any advice given by other doctors. The responsibility on the part of the other doctors can only be investigated in the case of violation of medical confidentiality, which remains absolute and untouchable between them and the occupational doctor.

Responsibility is shared between the rehabilitation doctor, who evaluates physical capacity and stamina, the occupational doctor, who gives his verdict on fitness for the job, the consultant doctor of the health insurance company, who decides on the capacity to work at any job whatsoever and the doctor at COTOREP, who measures the severity of the disability and its occupational repercussions.

The thinking of the different medical disciplines cannot always coincide when it is a matter of putting the right to work and the right to health in perspective with the strictest of respect for medical confidentiality.

Moreover, given different views on the respective responsibilities of the employer and the occupational doctor and recognising of the "principle of precaution", there could be a fear of the occupational reintegration of patients with a cardiovascular disease proving difficult in spite of the patient's known potential at the conclusion of rehabilitation.

Cardiac rehabilitation and return to work

Although superior to the conventional handling of occupational reintegration [45, 46], cardiac rehabilitation does not achieve the anticipated results [47], with the rate of resumption varying between 65% and 85% [48, 49].

Among the factors that influence the resumption of work, there are definitely organic elements: younger patients, after a less severe heart attack, the lack of angina and diabetes [50]. However, the socio-occupational and psychological conditions dominate in terms of features associated with a rapid return to work [51]: fairly high socio-educational level, job considered to be satisfying with limited difficulty, truly motivated to return to work, lack of depression, subjective opinion of state of health and physical capacity, early recourse to occupational medicine [52, 53, 54, 55]. Setbacks concerning the resumption of work are most frequently linked to the patient's perception of a general state that is incompatible with a job considered to be unsatisfying, frequently in a context of claiming financial compensation [56].

These aspects are often given inadequate consideration when preparing for return to work during rehabilitation and more appropriate strategies have been put forward: evaluation of the physical and psycho-social dimensions of the job in comparison with the patient's capability together with suggestions for arrangements in the workplace in order to permit a return under improved and safer conditions [57]. Moreover, more personalized rehabilitation related to the technical characteristics of each patient's workstation (workplace simulation) appears to be more effective than conventional rehabilitation [58].

The impact of the early evaluation by the occupational doctor in terms of shortening the length of time before resumption of work with a reduction in financial costs has been demonstrated [59]. The occupational doctor is the only one able to decide on fitness for the workplace and coordination with the rehabilitation doctor (improves and evaluates physical performance), the cardiologist (quantifies the cardiac risk), the Social Security doctor (decision on the capacity for work of any kind) and the COTOREP doctor (acknowledges the status of disabled worker) should permit an improvement in the rate of resumption, being based on objective criteria such as adaptive physical capacities and stratification of the cardiac risk while limiting the influence of the mental and social conditions.

Early medical coordination should receive high priority with careful management of professional secrecy, which is often a stumbling block to sharing information among doctors with results detrimental to the patient.

Since too few patients benefit from rehabilitation services these need to be made more accessible by developing functional explorations of professional simulations.

Finally, the "principle of precaution" weighs heavily on the employer and the occupational doctor with regard to employees with cardiovascular diseases, who may remain liable to deterioration and relapse in spite of effective medical and surgical treatment and rehabilitation. This remains a barrier increasingly encountered by patients with genuine capabilities attempting to resume work. Thought needs to be given to the definition of the level of acceptable risk for each patient based on medical and functional criteria reached by consensus.

References

1. Omnes C (2003) La médecine du travail face aux maladies cardio-vasculaires. Santé et Travail. 45: 46-7

2. O'Connor G, Buring JF, Yusuf S *et al.* (1989) An overview of randomized trials of rehabilitation with exercise after myocardial infarction. Circulation 80: 234-44

3. Oldridge N, Guyat GH, Fisher MF *et al.* Cardiac rehabilitation after myocardial infarction (1988) Combined experiences of randomized clinical trials. JAMA 260: 945-50

4. Campbell NC, Grimshaw JM, Rawles JM *et al.* (1996) Cardiac rehabilitation in Scotland: is current provision satisfactory? J Public Health Med 18: 478-80

5. Bunker S, McBurney H, Cox H *et al.* (1999) Identifying rates at outpatient cardiac rehabilitation programs in Victoria, Australia. J Cardiopulm Rehabil 19: 334-8

6. Cottin Y, Cambou JP, Casillas JM *et al.* (2004) Specific Profile and Referral Bias of Rehabilitated Patients after an Acute Coronary Syndrome. J Cardiopulm Rehabil 24: 38-44

7. Cottin Y, Walker P, Rouhier-Marcer I *et al.* (1996) Relationship between increased peak oxygen uptake and modifications in skeletal muscle metabolism following rehabilitation after myocardial infarction. J Cardiopulm Rehabil 16: 169-74

8. Gokce N, Vita JA, Bader DS *et al.* (2002) Effect of exercise on upper and lower extremity endothelial function in patients with coronary artery disease. Am J Cardiol 15: 127-27

9. Clausen JP (1976) Circulatory adjustments to dynamic exercise and effect of physical training in normal subjects and in patients with coronary disease. Progr Cardiovasc Dis 18: 459-95

10. Lucini D, Milani RV, Costantino G *et al.* (2002) Effects of cardiac rehabilitation and exercise training on autonomic regulation in patients with coronary artery disease. Am Heart J 143: 977-83.

11. Billman GE (2002) Aerobic exercise conditioning: a nonpharmacological antiarrhytmic intervention. J Appl Physiol 92: 446-54

12. Cinquegrana G, Spinelli L, D'Aniello L *et al.* (2002) Exercise training improves diastolic perfusion time in patients with coronary artery disease. Heart Dis 4: 13-7

13. Adachi J, Koike A, Obayasui T. *et al.* (1996) Does appropriate endurance training improve cardiac function in patient with prior myocardial infarction. Eur Heart J 17: 1511-21

14. Adamopoulos S, Ponikowski P, Cerquejani E *et al.* (1995) Circadian pattern of heart variability in chronic heart failure patients. Effects of physical training. Eur Heart J 16: 1380-6

15. Belardinelli R, Georgiou D, Cianci G *et al.* (1999) Randomized, controlled trial of long-term moderate exercise training in chronic heart failure. Effects on functional capacity, quality of life, and clinical outcome. Circulation 99: 1173-82

16. Hambrecht R, Fiehn E, Weigl C *et al.* (1998) Regular physical exercise corrects endothelial dysfunction and improves exercise capacity in patients with chronic heart failure. Circulation 98: 2709-715

17. Smith SC, Blair SN, Bonow RO *et al.* (2001) AHA/ACA guidelines for preventing heart attack and death in patients with atherosclerotic cardiovascular disease. Circulation 104: 1577-9

18. Hedbäck B, Perk J, Wodlin P (1993) Long term reduction of cardiac mortality after myocardial infarction: 10- year results of a comprehensive rehabilitation program. Eur Heart J 14: 831-5

19. Haskell WL, Alderman EL, Fair JM *et al.* (1994) Effects of intensive multiple risk factor reduction on coronary atherosclerosis and clinical cardiac events in men and women with coronary artery disease: the Stanford Coronary Risk Intrervention Project (SCRIP). Circulation 89: 975-90

20. Church TS, Kampert JB, Gibbons LW *et al.* (2001) Usefulness of cardiorespiratory fitness as a predictor of all-cause and cardiovascular disease mortality in men with systemic hypertension. Am J Cardiol 88: 651-6

21. Durstine JL, Grandjean PW, Cox CA *et al.* (2002) Lipids, lipoproteins, and exercise. J Cardiopulm Rehabil 22: 385-98

22. Hu FB, Manson JE (2003) Walking: the best medicine for diabetes? Arch Intern Med 163: 1397-98

23. Savage PD, Brochu M, Poehlman ET *et al.* (2003) Reduction in obesity and coronary risk factors after high caloric exercise training in overweight coronary patients. Am Heart J 146: 317-23

24. Church TS, Lavie CJ, Milani RV *et al.* (2002) Improvements in blood rheology after cardiac rehabilitation and exercise training in patients with coronary heart disease. Am Heart J 143: 349-55

25. Ussher MH, Taylor AH, West R *et al.* (2000) Does exercise aid smoking cessation? A systematic review. Addiction 95: 199-208

26. Franklin BA, Kahn JK (1996) Delayed progression of regression of coronary atherosclerosis with intensive risk factor modification. Effects of diet, drugs, and exercise. Sports Med 22: 306-20

27. Weber KT, Janicki JS (1985) Cardiopulmonary exercise testing for evaluation of chronic failure. Am J Cardiol 55: 22-31

28. Demers C, McKelvie RS, Negassa A *et al.* (2001) Reliability, validity, and responsiveness of the six-minute walk test in patients with heart failure. Am Heart J 142: 698-703

29. Enright PL, McBurnie MA, Bittner V *et al.* (2003) The 6-min walk test: a quick measure of functional status in elderly adults. Chest 123: 387-98

30. Harada ND, Chiu V, Stewart AL (1999) Mobility-related function in older adults: assessment with a 6-minute walk test. Arch Phys Med Rehabil 80: 837-41

31. Hamilton DM, Haennel RG (2000) Validity and reliability of the 6-minute walk test in a cardiac rehabilitation population. J Cardiopulm Rehabil 20: 156-64

32. Oh-Park M, Zohman LR, Abrahams C (1997) A simple walk test to guide exercise programming of the elderly. Am J Phys Med Rehabil 76: 208-12

33. Borg A (1970) Perceived exertion as an indicator of somatic stress. Scand J Rehabil 2: 92-7

34. MacGregor J (1979) The objective measurement of physical performance with long term ambulatory physiological surveillance equipment. In: Stott FD, Raftery EB, Goulding L, editors. Proceedings of 3rd International Symposium on Ambulatory Monitoring. London: Academic Pr. 29-939

35. Hood VL, Granat MH, Maxwell DJ *et al.* (2002) A new method of using heart rate to represent energy expenditure: the total heart beat index. Arch Phys Med Rehabil; 1266-73

36. DeGroot DW, Quinn TJ, Kertzer R *et al.* (1998) Lactic acid accumulation in cardiac patients performing circuit weight training: implications for exercise prescription. J Cardiopulm Rehabil 79: 838-41

37. Karlsdottir AE, Foster C, Porcari JP *et al.* (2002) Hemodynamic responses during aerobic and resistance exercise. J Cardiopulm Rehabil 22: 170-7

38. Pollock ML, Franklin BA, Balady GJ *et al.* (2000) Resistance exercise in individuals with and without cardiovascular disease: benefits, rationale, safety, and prescription. Circulation 101: 828-33

39. Maillefert JF, Eicher JC, Walker P *et al.* (1998) Effects of low frequency electrical stimulation of quadriceps and calf muscles in chronic heart failure. J Cardiopulm Rehabil 18 (4): 277-82

40. Ades PA, Balady GJ, Berra K (2001) Transforming exercise-based cardiac rehabilitation programs into secondary prevention centers: a national imperative. J Cardiopulm Rehabil 21: 263-72
41. Code du Travail (1989) art. R 241-51, Dalloz, p 893
42. Lang T, De Gaudemaris R (2003) Quand l'organisation du travail pèse sur le cœur. Santé et Travail 45
43. Code du Travail (1989) art. R 241-51, Dalloz, p 893
44. Code du Travail (1991) art. L 230-2, Dalloz
45. Dumont S, Jobin J, Deshaies G et al. (1999) Rehabilitation and the socio-occupational reintegration of workers who have had a myocardial infarct: a pilot study. Can J Cardiol 15: 453-61
46. Simchen E, Naveh I, Zitser-Gurevich Y et al. (2001) Is participation in cardiac rehabilitation programs associated with better quality of life and return to work after coronary artery bypass operations? The Israeli CABG Study. Isr Med Assoc J 3: 427-9
47. Danchin N, Goepfert PC (1988) Exercise training, cardiac rehabilitation and return to work in patients with coronary artery disease. Eur Heart J 9: 43-6
48. Boudrez H, De Backer G (2000) Recent findings on return to work after an acute myocardial infarction or coronary bypass grafting. Acta Cardiol 55: 341-9
49. Monpère C, Rajoelina A, Vernochet P et al. (2000) Réinsertion professionnelle après réadaptation cardiovasculaire chez 128 patients coronariens suivis pendant 7 ans. Arch Mal Cœur 93: 797-806
50. Mulcahy R, Kennedy C, Conroy R (1988) The long-term work record of post-infarction patients subjected to informal rehabilitation and secondary prevention programme. Eur Heart J 9: 84-8
51. Mark DB, Lam LC, Lee KL et al. (1992) Identification of patients with coronary disease at high risk for loss of employment. A prospective validation study. Circulation 86: 1485-94
52. From P, Cohen C, Rashcupkin J et al. (1999) Referral to occupational medicine clinics and resumption of employment after myocardial infarction. J Occup Environ Med 41: 943-7
53. Engblom E, Hämäläinen H, Rönnemaa T et al. (1994) Cardiac rehabilitation and return to work after coronary bypass surgery. Qual Life Res 3: 207-13.
54. Maeland JG, Havik OE (1987) Psychological predictors for return to work after a myocardial infarction. J Psychosom Res 31: 471-81
55. Soejima Y, Steptoe A, Nozoe SI et al. (1999) Psychosocial and clinical factors predicting resumption of work following acute myocardial infarction in Japanese men. Int J Cardiol 72: 39-47
56. Myrtek M, Kaiser A, Rauch B et al. (1997) Factors associated with work resumption a 5 year follow-up with cardiac patients. Int J Cardiol 59: 291-7
57. Shrey DE, Mital A (2000) Accelerating the return to work chances of coronary heart disease patients: part 2 – development and validation of a vocational rehabilitation programme. Disabil Rehabil 22: 621-62
58. Mital A, Shrey DE, Govindaraju M et al. (2000) Accelerating the return to work chances of coronary heart disease patients: part 1 – development and validation of a training programme. Disabil Rehabil 22: 604-20
59. Dennis C, Houston-Miller N, Schwartz RG et al. (1988) Early return to work after uncomplicated myocardial infarction. Result of a randomized trial. JAMA 260: 214-20

Vocational integration
in cancer rehabilitation

H. Delbrück

Tasks and goals

In cancer rehabilitation, influencing the illness is less of an issue than the reduction of subsequent problems caused by tumours and therapies. Negative effects on patients' professional lives are additional elements in rehabilitation apart from somatic, psychological and social problems. Assistance designed to promote vocational integration is thus part and parcel of the tasks involved in oncological rehabilitation [1, 2]. Vocational inactivity not only means financial and existential disadvantages for those concerned as well as for society, but also involves a risk of social isolation and a reduction in self-esteem. In short, it leads to a reduction in the quality of life [3].

Epidemiology

The prevalence of cancer patients living in Western Europe who are capable of gainful employment can only be estimated – in contrast to mortality. Among civil servants in Germany, the percentage of cancer patients under the age of 60 is put at 30%. Additionally, the percentage frequency of people taking early retirement following cancer can only be estimated. In Germany, neoplasia (8%) is in fourth place as a cause for early retirement in civil servants following mental illnesses 47%, musculoskeletal diseases 15.4% and cardiovascular diseases 11% [4].

Cancer is a collective term for a very heterogeneous group of malignant diseases with differing prognoses and differing therapeutic requirements. Special cancer diseases occur with different degrees of frequency in infancy and adolescence, in adulthood and in old age.

Cancer diagnoses most frequently involving a need for vocational rehabilitation in the past 20 years include malignant haematological and lymphatic system diseases, testicular tumours and sarcomas, which have very good lifetime prognoses thanks to the introduction of more recent chemotherapy. As a result of the temporal shifts of certain tumour diseases and thanks to improved precautionary diagnostics, rehabilitation doctors are, however, currently faced to an increasing degree by the vocational problems suffered by patients with gynaecological, gastro-intestinal and pulmonary tumours. Whereas, today, improved therapy strategies and possibilities result in certain tumour diseases either being cured more frequently than before or being converted to a chronic stage, this is, however, often at the cost of considerable side-effects that also affect patients' vocational abilities.

What cannot be disputed is the fact that there have been considerable changes in the prevalence of cancer diseases among patients in employment as well as in vocational issues in the last 20 years. Changes in environmental influences are less responsible for this than improvements in early diagnostics and the improvement in treatment possibilities. In future, it can be assumed that there will be a further increase in the prevalence of cancer patients in gainful employment and thus an increase in the need for vocational rehabilitation.

Due to changing attitudes to work, not to mention the job situation, the need for vocational rehabilitation, the willingness to undergo rehabilitation as well as the likelihood of the success of vocational rehabilitation assistance for cancer patients have changed, not only quantitatively, but also qualitatively.

Tasks involved in the vocational rehabilitation of cancer patients

The following tasks are of major importance. They are commented on in detail below:

– assessment, i.e. identification of any vocational limitations. Statement on the negative as well as the positive performance prospects of the person undergoing rehabilitation (sociomedical opinion);

– measures designed to improve general physical and mental performance;

– measures designed to safeguard and to maintain workplaces;

– introduction of measures for vocational reintegration;

– assessment, evaluation and quality assurance of vocational rehabilitation measures.

Assessment of any vocational limitations. Statement on the negative as well as the positive performance prospects of the person undergoing rehabilitation (sociomedical opinion)

The assessment, the identification of a need for rehabilitation, primarily refers to the identification of dysfunctions and restrictions associated with vocational activities. It describes both the "actual status" as well as the "nominal status" of the performance required to carry out vocational activities. It represents the basis for rehabilitation planning, rehabilitation therapies and evaluation.

Vocational limitations can be conditional *a) on the cancer disease itself, b) on the vocational environment and c) on the effects of therapy*. A summary of the assessment with a description of the negative and positive performance status of the person concerned is given in *d) the sociomedical statement.*

Table 1 – Assessment at the start of the vocational rehabilitation of a cancer patient.

Does the patient have a job?

Does the patient carry out a skilled trade? Did he or she pursue this most recently or was it a semi-skilled activity?

Is the patient expected to be able to resume the vocational activity most recently pursued at some time in the future?

What problems might arise on resumption of work? Can problems be expected when carrying out work?

Is any form of job reallocation meaningful?

Is a gradual resumption of work possible or meaningful?

Does some form of vocational reorientation appear meaningful?

How does the patient view his or her vocational future?

Should an invalidity pension be considered?

Should a temporary invalidity pension be considered?

Are any vocational-rehabilitation related aids meaningful, possible and promising?

Have any vocational-rehabilitation related aids been introduced? (severely-disabled pass, company physician, workplace transfer, pension application?)

Cancer and limited ability to work

Incurable cancer for which there is no treatment generally involves an incapacity to work. However, there are numerous exceptions. For many cancer patients, work represents the only opportunity for self-affirmation and contact with their surroundings. For psychological considerations alone, an incurable tumour should basically not be equated with vocational inactivity. Patients afflicted with chronic cancer can work to a limited degree if the vocational activity pursued is not accompanied by discomfort and a drop in performance.

In a palliative situation, there is an obligation to enable the dying person to live until he dies, at his own maximum potential, performing to the limit of his physical and mental capacity with control and independence whenever possible [5]. This can also include aids to assist in the continuation of his or her work. Apart from this possible human obligation to promote the resumption of vocational activities, an R1 resection (indication of residual tumours) or incomplete remission following chemo- or radiotherapy should not necessarily be equated with working incapacity and the granting of a pension even after an extensive metastisation and despite widely held opinions. Some tumours cause no discomfort or have no effect on people's capacity to work for many years; there may be no requirement for any therapy for many years; some therapies cause so little strain and partial remissions can be so stable that the vocational performance of those concerned is barely affected despite an obvious tumour problem. (Table 2). These patients are frequently capable of work for a long time despite tumour activity. In the case of these patients, however, vocational rehabilitation aids are restricted to aids designed to maintain workplaces.

Table 2 – Cancer disorders that frequently do not involve any discomfort.

Chronic myeloid leukaemia in the chronic phase
Chronic lymphatic leukaemia in the stages Rai 0-II (Binet A)
Indolent non-Hodgkin's lymphoma of low malignancy
Early-stage prostate carcinoma
Early-stage thyroid carcinoma
Localised carcinoids
MALT lymphomas of the stomach (low malignance)
Renal carcinoma without any impairment of kidney functions
Early-stage bladder carcinoma

Restrictions on working capacity in the case of potentially curably treated cancer patients

In the case of a potentially curative therapy (R0 situation), all macroscopically and microscopically visible tumour tissue could be removed, residual tumour tissue can no longer be traced with imaging detection procedures (sonography, computer tomography, NMR and PET) and the tumour markers are in the standard range. If there are any indications of residual tumours, this is called an R1 or even an R2 resection. In the case of palliative therapies, we are frequently dealing with patients according to R1 and R2 therapies respectively.

Incapacity to work is generally encountered during tumour therapy and in the subsequent recovery phase. Dependent on the type of treatment and dependent on individual disposition, (WHO, ECOG and/or Karnofsky index), the recovery phase can differ in duration. The times for working incapacity given in the Table 3 are average values that may be subject to considerable deviations in individual cases.

Table 3 – Average duration of working incapacity following potentially curative treatment and uncomplicated progress (without the help of chemotherapy and/or radiotherapy).

Tumour diseases	Treatment	Months of working incapacity
Stomach carcinoma	Gastrectomy	6-8
Stomach carcinoma	Partial stomach resection	3
Colon carcinoma	Hemicolectomy	3
Rectal carcinoma	Rectal resection	4
Rectal carcinoma	Rectal amputation	6
Bronchial carcinoma	Pneumonectomy	6
Bronchial carcinoma	Lobectomy/bilobectomy	3
Prostate carcinoma	Radical prostatectomy	5
Renal carcinoma	Nephrectomy	2
Bladder carcinoma	Partial resection	2
Bladder carcinoma	Cystectomy with orthotopic neo-bladder	6
Bladder carcinoma	Cystectomy with ileal conduit	4-6
Breast carcinoma	Tumorectomy	2
Breast carcinoma	Breast amputation with axillary lymph node resection	3

In the case of adolescent patients with good prognoses, working motivation and compliance, consideration can be given to measures both designed to retain workplaces as well as promote jobs – including those involving a vocational reorientation.

Vocational environment and restrictions in working capacity

Doctors involved in rehabilitation investigate the vocational environment of cancer patients for any physical and mental stress, for employers' and colleagues' attitudes to cancer diseases, not to mention for the possible level of exposure to carcinogenic materials at work. Even if most of the carcinogenic substances concerned with problems listed in Table 4 and Table 5 have a long induction period, cancer patients should discontinue any activities in which they are exposed to carcinogenic substances. It is presumed that potentially carcinogenic substances have a stronger carcinogenic effect in the case of "cured" cancer patients than is the case with healthy people. A workplace transfer or even a vocational reorientation may be necessary.

Table 4 – Vocational activities with frequent exposure to asbestos.

Shipbuilding activities
Construction industry activities
Asbestos mine activities
Fuel-trade activities

Table 5 – Professional groups exposed to respirable quartz dusts.

Ore and uranium ore miners
Tunnelers
Casting fettlers
Sandblasters
Furnace bricklayers and moulders in the metalworking industry
Personnel in fine-china companies
Personnel in dental laboratories

Effects of cancer therapies and restrictions of working incapacity

A difference must be made between:
- the acute or reversible effects of tumour therapy and
- the long-term or irreversible effects of tumour therapy.

The acute or reversible effects of tumour therapy

Early and reversible post-operative problems include physical weakness, problems with wound healing, anaemia from bleeding, scar weaknesses, reversible problems caused by chemotherapy (e.g. tiredness, nausea, diarrhoea, anaemia, fatigue), reversible side-effects of radiation (e.g. radiation sickness, enteritides). Work is impossible during these acute side-effects. In this phase, rehabilitation therapies predominantly consist of toughening measures and measures designed to strengthen functions so that those affected are fit to resume their original jobs as early as possible. Given physical as well as mental invigoration, a full restoration of working capacity can usually be expected after the acute side-effects have receded.

The long-term or irreversible effects of tumour therapy

This includes consequential disorders, some of which appear many years after the conclusion of treatment. As a result, they are also called late sequelae.

Irreversible disorders include syndromes after the removal of organs (e.g. after gastrectomies conducted on stomach carcinoma patients, with intestinal carcinoma patients with short bowel and/or artificial anus, with bronchial carcinoma patients after pneumonectomies, with bladder carcinoma patients after cystectomies, etc.). These also include undesirable side-effects after radiation therapy (e.g. lymph oedema, pulmonary fibrosis, cardiovascular disorders, etc.) or after chemotherapy (e.g. blood count problems, bone marrow and pulmonary fibrosis, etc.). The effects of irreversible late sequelae can only be relieved and/or compensated for. These patients need rehabilitation measures that go beyond physical and mental invigoration.

Some disorders such as coronary heart disease in the case of lymphoma patients after mediastinal irradiation or cardiac insufficiency in the case of patients with leukaemia or mamma carcinoma treated with anthracycline only appear very late on. These anticipated disorders following therapy must be prevented or at least reduced.

To reduce vocational handicaps, preventive measures are required. Vocational advisory services are very important, in particular for adolescents who have been cured. For example, leukaemia patients treated with meningeal-irradiation should avoid vocational activities that require a high degree of concentration and fast reactions. Following chemotherapy involving anthracycline or mediastinal irradiation, no jobs involving physically strenuous activities should subsequently be attempted due to cardiac risks.

The Tables 6 to 10 list the possible vocational restrictions to which cancer patients with irreversible late disorders may be subject.

Table 6 – Workloads that cured patients with malignant lymphatic and leukaemia diseases should avoid.

Restrictions	Reason for the restrictions
No physically strenuous activities	Frequency of chemotherapy and radiation therapy side-effects on the circulation (e.g. anthracycline, mediastinal irradiation)
No activities in surroundings involving a risk of infection	Frequent immune deficiency syndrome due to illness and therapy
No activities requiring particular concentration and attentiveness	Only after meningeal irradiation
No activities with particular physical and mental stress	Frequent lapses in concentration, effects on the immune system?

Table 7 – Workloads that cured stomach carcinoma patients should avoid after a total gastrectomy (R0).

Restrictions	Reason for the restriction
Jobs connected with frequent bending	Danger of gastro-oesophageal reflux
Physically tough jobs, no lifting or carrying heavy loads	When underweight, danger of gastro-oesophageal reflux
Jobs that presuppose a good head for heights (e.g. roofers)	Dumping symptoms with pains caused by hypoglycaemia
Jobs that require continuous attention	Dumping symptoms with pains caused by hypoglycaemia
Activities in the first six post-operative months	Fairly slow adaptation to the modified stomach-bowel passage
Activities involving unpleasant odours or acrid fumes	Provocation of vomiting, nausea and diarrhoea
Absolutely no night work or shift work	Lower stress threshold
Jobs in which more frequent breaks unusual for the business are possible	More frequent intake of small meals necessary
Unsuitable as a full-time truck driver	More frequent breaks unusual for the job, mental and physical stress, risk of a dumping syndrome with lapses in concentration

Table 8 – Workloads that cured rectal carcinoma patients should avoid after an abdomino-perineal rectal resection (R0).

Severe physical workloads
(This includes lifting, working above head-height, jobs connected with severe vibrations and in which more than 5 kg have to be frequently lifted.)
Unfavourable working posture (e.g. squatting or lying)
Extreme climatic situations (e.g. working in the heat)
Unfavourable working hours (shift and night work)
Unfavourable working breaks
(In order to be able to eat meals regularly and in peace, regular breaks of adequate length are required.)
Rhythmic jobs
(It must be possible to take individual breaks in the case of irregular evacuation of the bowels without interfering with colleagues' work flow.)

Table 9 – Workloads that cured bronchial carcinoma patients should avoid after a pneumonectomy (R0).

Heavy physical loads (these include lifting, working above head-height)
Jobs connected with strong vibrations.
Unfavourable working posture (e.g. doing jobs when squatting or lying)
Activities connected with extreme or frequently fluctuating temperatures
Unfavourable working hours (shift and night work)
Rhythmic jobs: an individual break has to be able to be taken without interrupting fellow workers' workflow.
Piece-work
Activities in dusty professions, with serious air pollution, dry air or powerful and irritating odours.
Activities in chemical laboratories

Table 10 – Workloads that cured breast carcinoma patients with manifest lymph oedem (R0) should avoid.

Work done by clerks, workmen and cleaners
Activities carried out under unfavourable heat radiation or lengthy exposure to the rays of the sun
Activities accompanied by an excessive load on the affected arm
Activities involving a possible risk of injuring the affected arm
Easy, monotonous activities with the affected arm lasting several hours
Activities in which restrictive clothing is required or shoulder straps have to be placed on the shoulder on the affected side
Activities in a water bath or thermal bath higher than 33°C

Sociomedical opinion

A rehabilitation oncologist is required to assess a negative and positive performance status. He must form an opinion on the current ability of the person undergoing rehabilitation with regard to the specific, existing workplace; what prospective working capacity with regard to vocational alternatives exists, just how his or her ability to perform is in the trade learnt, in semi-skilled jobs or on the general labour market and how the chances of success of any vocational rehabilitation measures can be estimated (Table 11).

Table 11 – Criteria involved in the sociomedical assessment among cancer patients.

Comparison of requirements and working capacity
Description of particular vocational stresses
Information on the possible duration of work
Description of positive "activity profiles"
Description of negative "activity profiles"
Recommendations for job-promoting measures
Patient's self-assessment on his or her vocational ability

For the assessment of the vocational performance of potentially cured patients, the same principles apply as those for the assessment of patients with acute or chronic benign diseases and disabilities. Theoretically, a more or less poor prognosis has no influence on a sociomedical assessment [6, 7] in practice, however, it influences at least the type and the scope of any rehabilitation measures that may possibly be introduced. Consequently, in the case of young patients with small-cell bronchial carcinoma in an R0-situation or patients with acute myeloid leukaemia in complete remission, one would be satisfied purely with job-retaining measures due to the poor long-term prognosis evidenced by experience and dispense with vocational reorientation.

Measures designed to improve general physical and mental performance

Measures designed to improve vocational ability to work under pressure. Increase in general physical and mental capacity

Physically strengthening as well as mentally stabilising measures designed to promote motivation for work are frequently required. A range of different in- and outpatient methods are available for this purpose.

In Germany, every cancer patient old enough to be in gainful employment has a statutory claim to in- and outpatient rehabilitation measures that have been specially designed to meet their requirements [8]. They extend from general, illness-unrelated physically strengthening and mentally stabilising measures to illness-related, individually adapted rehabilitation therapies. The aim of regimens designed to invigorate or promote recovery is to facilitate the resumption of work [6]. In Germany, these toughening rehabilitation measures are therefore not financed by medical insurance companies, but by pension funds. It is in their interest for contributors to their schemes to resume their professional activities as speedily as possible. They should remain in their jobs as long as possible instead of depriving the pension fund of benefits and pensions. Outpatient sports and swimming courses designed to maintain vocational abilities as long as possible are promoted. With regard to promotion, these out- and inpatient measures are conditional on their being carried out by a qualified rehabilitation team. Apart from medical oncological skills, sociomedical experience and expertise are essential in an oncological rehabilitation team (Fig. 1). It is often necessary to address a cancer patient's specifically

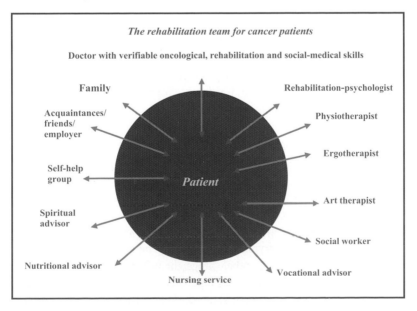

Fig. 1

vocational problems. His or her remaining capacity must be assessed and recorded and vocational rehabilitation measures introduced and documented (Table 6 to 10).

Up to now, Germany is the only country in Europe in which pension schemes conduct these rehabilitation measures specially designed for cancer patients, the aim being to promote vocational reintegration. Roughly one-third of all gainfully employed cancer patients in Germany take advantage of the opportunity of this kind of rehabilitation measure. In all other countries in the European Community, it tends to be medical or social reasons that lead to the introduction of in- or outpatient rehabilitation in the case of cancer patients.

Tumour patients frequently suffer from resignation, fears and depression. These influence patients' vocational willingness to work and, alongside a lack of motivation, are a substantial reason for frequent early pensions. Some authors consider that fatigue symptoms are the most frequent reason for the unsuccessful vocational reintegration of cured cancer patients [9, 10]. Help in coping with the disease, the reduction of fears, depression, helplessness and hopelessness as well as the boosting of compliance and motivation are important. These are the main tasks of a psycho-oncologist. He or she has a vital position in the rehabilitation team for cancer patients (Fig. 1) – in particular, where vocational rehabilitation is concerned. The purpose of intensive psychological care is to influence a patient's resigned attitude and to promote their desire to perform.

Self-help groups fulfil an important role in terms of motivation for self-assistance, help towards self-help and in dealing with tendencies to retreat from society. They exert an activating influence on those concerned and thus contribute towards a willingness to resume work.

Training and medical advisory services are prerequisites for an active and independent approach. For example, some patients are unaware of the numerous vocational protective measures and benefits that are granted in many countries both to chronically handicapped employees in the pursuit of their profession as well as to employers when hiring those affected. What cannot be disputed is that well-informed cancer patients have greater opportunities for social and vocational reintegration than uninformed patients.

Here, too, self-help groups make an important contribution in the fields of advisory and information services.

Measures designed to improve resistance to vocational pressure and to increase specific physical and mental performance

In the case of *stomach carcinoma* patients, it largely consists of training sessions to prevent and reduce postgastrectomy symptoms, in particular, postprandial discomfort. Good nutritional advice can help to reduce the numerous vocational restrictions resulting from gastrectomy when carrying out one's job. The appearance of post-prandial dumping problems prevents, among other things, the pursuit of jobs that require a head for heights (e.g. roofers) or jobs that require permanent attentiveness (e.g. bus drivers, production line workers or pieceworkers). A workplace transfer is necessary in these cases and in physically demanding activities [1].

In the case of *bronchial carcinoma* patients, the restrictions imposed by lung function prevent or restrict all physically demanding activities. By means of breathing exercises, inhalations, accompanying therapies involving medicaments and anti-obstructive physical therapy measures, it is possible to improve patients' ability to handle physical demands. Workplace transfers are frequently required.

In the case of *rectal carcinoma* patients with an artificial anus, it is a mastery of irrigation that makes patients independent of dealing with pouches, which reduces the adverse effect of noises and thus opens up to them so many vocational activities that would otherwise be impossible. Non-irrigating colostomy wearers are frequently unable to conduct any activities involving customer contact. However, almost all activities are possible for irrigating rectal carcinoma patients.

The restoration of the ability to communicate using speech is a cardinal task of rehabilitation after laryngectomy in the case of patients *suffering from laryngal carcinoma*. It is a basic prerequisite for the resumption of work in many professions. Vocational rehabilitation planning is a multidisciplinary task for these patients as the missing larynx not only affects vocal functions and sensitivity to smell and taste but also the absence of any closing of the glottis seriously affects the normal abdominal prelum, and social as well as mental problems frequently occur as a result of physical disfigurement [11].

Measures for the protection and maintenance of workplaces

Irrespective of the symptoms of their problems, cancer patients must fundamentally be considered severely disabled, no matter whether treated potentially curatively or palliatively. In the first years, at least, after the diagnosis of cancer, they enjoy improved protection against dismissal at their workplaces (Table 12) and, after the conclusion of therapy,

Table 12 – Vocational protective measures for cancer patients in Germany [2].

Increased protection against dismissal in the workplace. Dismissal is exceptionally difficult.
Assistance in keeping or acquiring a workplace appropriate for a disabled person, e.g. technical aids or wage subsidies
Acceleration of pension provision
Exemption from overtime and exemption from night-shifts if so desired
Right to 5 days additional holiday per year with a 5-day working week

enjoy particular vocational protective measures in the first 5 years at least that are, however, regulated differently from country to country. In France, cancer is considered one of the "maladies de longue durée" that grant all civil servants and employees concerned the right to workplace retention and vocational functions for up to three years. The government even guarantees their reemployment for up to 5 years after the disease has been diagnosed whereby those concerned can draw a full salary for the first three years, followed by only half of this [12].

Introduction of aids and measures for vocational reintegration

Theoretically, people with cancer who are undergoing rehabilitation are not considered to be a special group in the field of occupational promotion. However, their integration in Germany is the goal, as it is with other persons undergoing rehabilitation according to the type and severity of their functional limitations [6]. A specific form of vocational rehabilitation designed for cancer patients does not therefore exist. Nevertheless, all benefits in the job-promotion field are open to people undergoing rehabilitation.

There are numerous forms of assistance both for employees as well as for employers that are intended to facilitate vocational reintegration. Primarily, these are measures designed to keep jobs. Retraining is rarely considered and – if it is – it is only for younger patients with good lifetime forecasts. Many cured cancer patients of advanced age no longer have the mental flexibility, the stamina and the ability to adapt that are required for successful retraining. In Germany, the only retraining measures that are financed by sponsors – if at all – are for patients under the age of 40.

For the retention or acquisition of workplaces, support and assistance are granted both to the employee as well as to the employer. Integration assistance amounting to between 50 and 70% of remuneration is granted for six months. In justifiable, individual cases, as much as 80% can be paid and its duration can be extended to as much as two years. Pension insurance companies are willing to participate in the financing of ergonomic working chairs, height-adjustable worktables, lifting equipment, access ramps, sanitary fittings and other aids as well as technical working aids if these measures guarantee that cancer patients will keep their workplaces.

Workplace-retaining aids and benefits that promote jobs for cancer patients in Germany include [2]:
- benefits for the maintenance or acquisition of workplaces;
- equipment and technical aids;
- qualification through short courses;
- integration assistance for employers;
- measures to pinpoint jobs and work trials;
- vocational adjustment;
- further training and retraining;
- job and professional promotion;
- supplementary benefits (interim assistance, travelling expenses, household help, workclothes, tools, examination fees, text books, training allowances).

Gradual reintegration into the work process is one vocational rehabilitation measure that is frequently practised. Resumption of work can, for example, be done with the person concerned initially only working two to three hours every day; after a certain time, this is increased to four to six hours and then to six to eight hours until work returns to full working hours. In Germany and France, cancer patients receive their full wages from the medical insurance for the full period of this increasing workload although they are not working full shifts.

Assessment, evaluation and quality assurance. Predictors for occupational reintegration

No quality assurance is possible without assessment and without any progress documentation. Many evaluation parameters are available to examine rehabilitation targets. These not only include the start of vocational activities but also the change in risk factors, the change in obstructions and limitations, the introduction of benefits designed to promote jobs, implementation within companies, job creation, the reorganisation of workplaces to suit disabled people, training and further training in a new professional field.

The rates for the successful vocational reintegration of cancer patients given in the relevant literature vary widely from 30 to 93%. This is not simply attributable to the different quality of the rehabilitation opportunities or to differences in attitude among those affected or to financial possibilities, but is also attributable to the different consideration given to disabled people in society. The fact that the likelihood of successful vocational reintegration is very much greater in the USA than in other countries is not merely due to improved rehabilitation for cancer patients but is also a consequence of their having to earn a living. Financial security in the case of chronic diseases and working incapacity is very differently regulated in individual countries.

In the case of patients with head and neck carcinoma [11], the vocational reintegration quota is very much lower than with testicular and Hodgkin's patients. All investigations consistently showed a close correlation with the patients' age, the type of work they did as well as the type and degree of severity of their tumour disease [3, 11, 13, 14, 15, 16]. According to our own experience which is, however, only covered to some extent by statistics, the factors mentioned in the table as well as vocational ability and the quality of the rehabilitation conducted are important (Table 13).

Table 13 – Factors that can influence the introduction, implementation and the result probability of vocational rehabilitation measures in the case of cancer patients, independent of their vocational performance and the quality of the rehabilitation measures conducted as well as the type and scope of the tumour disease.

Risk of relapse
Lifetime forecast
Age and gender of the patients
Social status
Unemployment prior to falling ill
Level of education, earning status
Patient's motivation and willingness to participate
Patient's desire to be given a pension.
Time elapsed since primary therapy
Sponsors' expectations
Employer's motivation and willingness to participate
Attitude of the workforce and close colleagues
Pressure on workforce in the company
Previous time-limited pensioning
General and special labour market

Whether and to what extent the intended goals are reached or not depends not only on the quality of the vocational rehabilitation measures but also on many predictors (Table XIII). Humanitarian and political labour-market reasons must also be added to these.

Apart from somatic reasons and legal reasons relating to social insurance as well as financial aspects, the decision for or against early pensioning must also give consideration to the positive psychological aspects of dealing with a disease. For many people, their profession and work mean more than just a way to meet their existential requirements. To many people, work is the only possibility for social contact and is a confirmation of their self-esteem. It represents a form of diversion, distance and suppression of the feeling of a constantly threatening Damocles' sword. It can therefore be perfectly legitimate to support cancer patients - even those with greatly reduced working capacity - in resuming their previous jobs.

The demand that the quality of vocational rehabilitation measures must be judged solely by the frequency of successful vocational reintegration must be assessed critically. The rapid introduction of a pension for those unable to pursue gainful employment in the face of an irrefutable and well-documented reduction in their ability to work can also point to good vocational rehabilitation work.

Structures and organization of vocational rehabilitation for cancer patients

The structural and process quality of vocational reintegration measures for cancer patients differs in various EC countries. In Europe, different sponsors are responsible for vocational rehabilitation. In comparison with Germany, other countries frequently do not view sociomedical assessments, the introduction and implementation of vocational rehabilitation measures to be tasks for rehabilitation medicine and most definitely not tasks for rehabilitation oncologists.

Whereas, in Germany, inpatient rehabilitation is at the focus of rehabilitation measures and statements on the ability to work, on the question of vocational forecasts, on the need for vocational rehabilitation, on the capacity for rehabilitation and on the willingness for rehabilitation on the part of those concerned are demanded and initial vocational assistance is also introduced, rehabilitation in the other EC countries is largely outpatient in nature. Rehabilitation oncologists do not consider the clarification of further vocational activity as well as the introduction and implementation of vocational assistance to be their main duties. In these countries, patients are forced to apply to the labour market authorities; a large amount of personal initiative is expected of such patients if they intend to resume work.

Unfortunately, there is no information on the important issue of whether the vocational reintegration quota is increased in Germany by its costly and time-consuming inpatient and outpatient rehabilitation measures. This deficit is attributable not only to a lack of prospective studies and to the selection of patients looked after during rehabilitation but is also a result of the rapidly growing call in recent years for the need for rehabilitation research [17, 18].

References

1. Delbrück H, Haupt E (1998) Rehabilitationsmedizin. Urban Schwarzenberg, Munich
2. Delbrück H (2003) Krebsnachbetreuung. Nachsorge, Rehabilitation und Palliation. Springer, Heidelberg
3. Maunsell E, Brisson E, Lauzier S et al. (1999) Work problems after breast cancer: An exploratory qualitative study. Psycho-Oncology 8: 467-73
4. Lederer P, Weltle D, Weber A (2003) Evaluation der Dienstunfähigkeit bei Beamtinnen und Beamten. Gesundheitswesen 65 (1): 536-40
5. Cheville A (2001) Rehabilitation of patients with advanced cancer. Cancer 92: 1039-48
6. Pannen II (1997) Standards und Qualitätssicherung sozialmedizinischer Maßnahmen im Rahmen der onkologischen Rehabilitation. In Delbrück H (Hrsg.) Standards und Qualitätskriterien in der onkologischen Rehabilitation. Zuckschwerdt W, Munich
7. Verband Deutscher Rentenversicherungsträger (ed.) (1995) Sozialmedizinische Begutachtung in der gesetzlichen Rentenversicherung. Gustav Fischer, Stuttgart Jena New York
8. Tiedt G (1998) Rechtliche Grundlagen der Rehabilitation. In Delbrück H, Haupt E (Ed.) Rehabilitationsmedizin, Urban & Schwarzenberg, Munich: 45-68
9. Curt G (2001) Fatigue in cancer; like pain, this is a symptom that physicians can and should manage. Br. Med. J. 322: 1560
10. Spelten ER, Verbeek J, Uitterhoeve A et al. (2003) Cancer, fatigue and the return of patients to work – a prospective cohort study. Europ. J. Cancer 39: 1562-7
11. Cady J Laryngectomy (2002) Beyond loss of voice – caring for the patient as a whole. Clin. J. Oncol. Nurs. 6(6): 347-51
12. Fédération nationale des centres de lutte contre le cancer (1997) Prévoir demain Guide de la réinsertion des patients traités pour les cancers, Centres de lutte contre le cancer, Paris
13. Spelten ER, Sprangers M, Verbeek J (2002) Factors reported to influence the return to work of cancer survivors: A literature review. Psycho-Oncology 11: 124 –31
14. Heckl U (1996) Gesunde Kranke – Kranke Gesunde. Der Umgang mit einer Tumorerkrankung im beruflichen Umfeld. Europäischer Verlag der Wissenschaften, Frankfurt
15. Fobair P, Hoppe R, Bloom J et al. (1986) Psychosocial problems among survivors of Hodgkin's disease. Journal of clinical Oncology 4: 805-14
16. Schwiersch M, Stepien J, Schröck R. (1995) Inwieweit beeinträchtigen psychosoziale Belastungen den Wiedereintritt ins Berufsleben bei Mammakarzinompatienten. In Delbrück H. (Hrsg.): Der Krebskranke in der Arbeitswelt. W. Zuckschwerdt, Munich (1995)
17. Koch U, Weiss J (1998) Forschung in der Rehabilitationsmedizin. In Delbrück H, Haupt E. Rehabilitationsmedizin. Urban & Schwarzenberg, München pp 150-66
18. Hensel M, Egerer G, Schneeweiss A et al. (2002) Quality of life and rehabilitation in social and professional life after autologous stem cell transplantation, Annals of Oncology 13: 209-17

SECOND PART

SOME EXAMPLES OF VOCATIONAL REHABILITATION MANAGEMENT IN EUROPE

Vocational rehabilitation in Austria

V. Fialka-Moser, M. Herceg, M. Milanovic, D. Czamay and E. Hartter

Presentation of the situation in Austria

The need for vocational rehabilitation arises from persistent impacts on somatic and/or psycho-mental health, affecting the working ability of a person at his/her workplace or occupation. Typical indicators of the problem are early retirement, prolonged sick leave, reimbursement in case of occupational accident or disease, and persistent unemployment. The high incidence and/or severity of accidents and diseases associated with some occupations, as well as of those of non-occupational origin add to the problem.

Early retirement

In Austria, early retirement due to disability or inability to work accounts for about 19% of all retired persons (see Fig. 1a). Disorders of the musculo-skeletal system are the

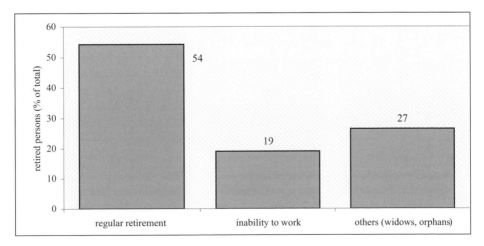

Figure 1a – Prevalence of different reasons for retirement.

leading problem (Fig. 1b; data are from [1], chapter 3.2.). Retirements at <55 years of age result from being widowed, orphaned, or disabled. The work-capacity or earning capacity of the person applying for early retirement due to disability should be less than 50% of the ability of a healthy worker/employee. Applications are processed by the retirement insurance as being equivalent to an application for vocational rehabilitation, i.e., the retirement insurance makes a choice, based on medical expertise, between offering vocational rehabilitation and early retirement (see [2] for more details).

Figure 2 shows that retirements due to disability rise sharply in the age range from 30-40 years, to a rather constant relative figure of more than 50% of the total number of

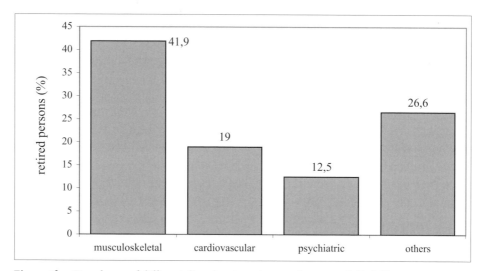

Figure 1b – Prevalence of different disorders in retirement because of disability.

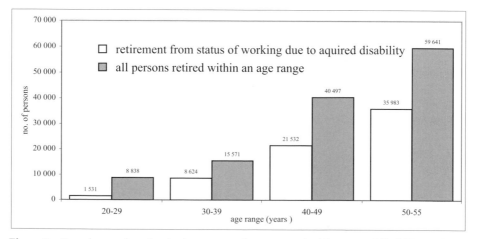

Figure 2 – Prevalence of total retired persons and persons retired because of disability within a specific age range (from [1], Table 3.11).

retired persons lower than 55 years of age. The virtually constant rate of early retirement due to disability from a former status of an employee over the entire age range from 30 to 55 years indicates the need for more effort in vocational rehabilitation for those in the early and middle phase of their working life.

Sick leaves

Figure 3 shows that about 36% of sick leaves in Austria are of more than 36 days' duration, while only about 40% are lower than or equal to the mean duration of 12-14 days. Sick leaves of long duration may be due to serious and chronic disease, ineffective medical treatment might add to the problem. The fact that special work place situations may induce sickness or "feeling of illness" is well established within occupational medicine. Thus, sick leave of long duration certainly needs intervention, which in many cases means vocational rehabilitation. In the year 2001 about 120.000 persons (approx. 4% of all employees) were on sick leave of more than 42 days' duration (from [1], 2.24).

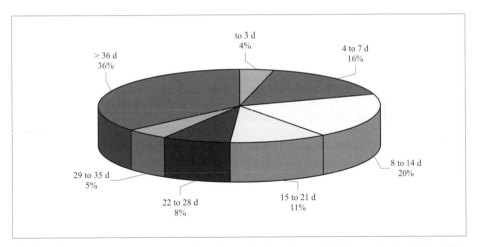

Figure 3 – Relative prevalence (% of total cases) of employees' sick leave in Austria in 2001, depending on the duration (in days) (taken from [3], p 55).

Occupational and occupation – associated accidents and diseases

The incidence of occupational injuries and occupational diseases has been either constant or decreased slightly during the last 5 years. At first glance this fact is suggestive of an enhancement of occupational safety and healthy work conditions. However, a more careful look reveals that this interpretation is biased. The list of occupational diseases contains selected entities. By far the most common health complaints associated with working conditions are psychological/psychosomatic impairment and musculo-skeletal problems. Together they account for about 60% of all cases of premature retirement because of inability to work. Both are not listed as occupational diseases although there is a large body of evidence to show that these entities are clearly associated with specific occupation, either directly or indirectly.

From the data presented in Table 1 it can be seen that "occupational" accidents and diseases (prevalence: 10.417 cases with disability >50%) account for only 2.7% of disabilities accompanied by the inability to work (prevalence: 385.594 cases). The remaining about 97% of cases of disability are exclusively acquired during private life. The incidence (cases per year) of early retirement is twice as high as the prevalence (sum of all cases) of reimbursement in cases of occupational accidents resulting in >50% disability.

The distribution and incidence of occupational injuries in relation to numbers of employees is shown in Figure 4 (data obtained from AUVA, department for rehabilita-

Table 1

Type of pension or reimbursement	No. of persons	% of total
Prevalence of early retirement due to disability (2002)	385.549	100
Applications for early retirement because of disability (2002)	62.384	16.2
Incidence of early retirement due to disability (2002)	23.344	6.1
Data from [3], pp 68-69		
Prevalence of reimbursement after occupational accident/ disease in 2001; (disability >50%; from [1], 4.3.)	10.417	100
Incidence of reimbursement after occupational accident/ disease in 2001 (disability >50%; from [1], table 4.20)	356	3.4

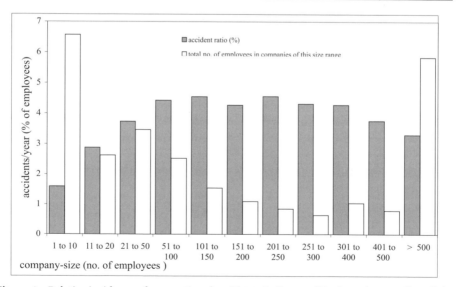

Figure 4 – Relative incidence of occupational accidents & diseases (% of employees affected) in relation to number of employees in a company (data from AUVA)

tion). Surprinsingly, the relative number of accidents is lowest (1.5-3%) in companies with up to 20 employees, rises to a plateau of about 4.5% for companies with 50-300 employees, and then slightly drops to about 3% in companies with more than 500 employees. A possible interpretation of this finding will be given later.

Responsibilities of insurance institutions and other organisations in providing rehabilitation and reimbursement in Austria

Insurance institutions

Personal insurance is compulsory in Austria and is provided by governmental insurance institutions. Three main branches of insurance are defined within each institution: *health insurance* (Krankenkasse), *accident insurance* (Unfallversicherung), and *retirement insurance/pension fund* (Pensionsversicherung).

In Austria about 8 million persons (99% of the total population) are health insured [1, chapter 2.0] . Insurance contributions have to be paid by/for actively working persons (either as private entrepreneurs or employees), by retired persons, and persons out of work with earnings-related benefits. Family members not in the labour market (children, spouses) are co-insured at no additional cost.

Contributions to the pension fund have to be paid by/for all occupationally active persons and persons with earnings-related benefits. Occupationally inactive family-members (children, spouses) are not pension-insured, and are not entitled to benefits (for instance, a pension in case of disability due to an accident or disease). Benefits can be claimed only if contributions to the pension fund have been paid for at least 15 years.

Accident insurance is obligatory for all persons working in the labour market, including those with earnings-related benefits, as well as for schoolchildren and students. Only occupational accidents (but not "private" ones) or diseases or accidents on the way to or from work/school/university are covered by this insurance. In these cases the accident insurance covers the entire spectrum of benefits: medical, occupational (including workplace adaptations) and social rehabilitation, as well as payment of reimbursement in case of reduced working ability. The insurance contribution for the accident insurance of employees is paid by the employer. Consequently, all claims of employees are passed on from the employer to the insurance company.

The insurance system is very diverse in respect of its legal base as well as its services. It is regulated by at least four basic laws for different groups of insured persons (see Table 2 for details).

Not all of the insurance institutions provide all three services (health, accident, pension). Accident insurance is "outsourced" to the AUVA by some institutions (nos. 2, 7 and

8 in Table 2). Therefore, the AUVA is by far the most important accident insurance institution in Austria.

The BVA (for government employees) does not run its own pension fund; the pensions are paid by the government (Ministry of Finance). The same is true for some insurance institutions in certain communities (no. 3 in Table 2). Vocational rehabilitation in case of "private" accident or non-occupational disease is a rare event for government employees, early retirement is the much more common offer.

Table 2 – Health, accident, and retirement insurance in Austria (2001)

Persons employed by	Law	Health ins.	Pension ins.	Accid. ins.
1. (Private) Companies	ASVG	GKK	PV	AUVA
2. Special companies	ASVG	Betriebs-KK		AUVA
3. Special communities	ASVG	Fürsorgeanstalt (FA) Gouvernm.		
4. Governmental employees	B-KUVG	BVA	Ministry	BVA
5. Austrian Railway Company	BK-UVG	VA-E	Ministry	VA-E
Private railway company	ASVG	VA d. Österr. Eisenbahnen (VA-E)		
6. Austrian Mining & Oil Industry	ASVG	VA d. Österr. Bergbaus		AUVA
7. Private entrepreneurs	GSVG	SVA Gew. Wirtsch.,		AUVA
8. Agriculture & forestry	BSVG	SVA der Bauern		

List of abbreviations:
Insurance institutions
AUVA = Allgemeine Unfallversicherungsanstalt (general accident insurance institution)
GKK = Gebietskrankenkasse (regional health insurance)
SV = Sozialversicherungsanstalt (social insurance institution)
VA = Versicherungsanastalt (insurance institution)
BVA = Versicherungsanstalt Öffentlich Bediensteter (insurance institution for government employees)
PV = Pensionsversicherung (retirement insurance/pension fund)
Betriebs–KK = Betriebskrankenkasse (insurance run by selected companies)
Fürsorgeanstalt = insurance run by certain communities (e.g.: City of Vienna, Upper-Austrian teachers' insurance, ...)
Laws
ASVG = Allgemeines Sozialversicherungsgesetz (general social insurance law)
B-KUVG = Beamtenkranken- und Unfallversicherungsgesetz (health and accident insurance law for government employees)
GSVG = Gewerbliches-Sozialversicherungsgesetz (social insurance law for commercial enterprises)
BSVG = Bauern-Sozialversicherungsgesetz (social insurance law for farmers)

Responsibilities of the insurance institutions

Accident insurance companies have to provide rehabilitation and reimbursement in cases of work-related accidents and occupational diseases (including schoolchildren and students). However, the insured person is not legally entitled to a specific type of rehabilitation or reimbursement.

Reduction of one's working ability or disability, resulting from "*private*" accidents, is excluded from the benefits of accident insurance. In these cases rehabilitation measures are provided by the *retirement/pension insurance* because the latter is interested in keeping people involved in the work process, financing their insurance contribution, and discouraging premature retirement. The insured person is not legally entitled to a specific type of rehabilitation. Reimbursement is not provided.

An indirect economic burden arises for *health insurance institutions* in cases of unsatisfactory or low-effect vocational rehabilitation: unemployed persons with earnings-related benefit ("Arbeitslosengeld"; unemployment benefits) pay less for their health insurance. Prolonged sick leave (eventually culminating in unemployment) is a common feature in persons whose working ability is reduced or who are unable to meet the demands of the workplace. At least after 10 weeks of sick leave the health insurance institution has to pay the earnings as long as the person is officially employed by the employer. Sick leaves raise the expense of health insurance because of higher consultation rates of doctors, prescriptions for medication, and diagnostic measures. Nevertheless, the health insurer is not directly involved in vocational rehabilitation.

Financing and organisation
of vocational rehabilitation in Austria

The main institution involved in decision-making and the coordination of vocational rehabilitation in Austria is a governmental institution known as the *Arbeitsmarktservice* or *AMS* (Labour Market Service; website: http://www.ams.or.at). Vocational rehabilitation is an integral part of the endeavour of this organisation to prevent and eradicate unemployment. Following medical rehabilitation in cases of occupational or non–occupational accident or disease, the AMS together with the accident insurance, retirement insurance or the *Bundessozialamt* (federal social welfare agency; see later), counsels and informs the individual about returning to an adequate job or workplace. The AMS finances vocational rehabilitation at least in part.

A team of experts, including social consultants (SozialberaterInnen), specialists with knowledge of the work market and the required professions (Arbeitsmarktservice-BeraterInnen), career advisers, and psychologists, provides advice concerning the content and procedure of vocational rehabilitation in an individual case. The medical expertise on the working ability or disability, the possibility of reintegrating the individual in the work process at the original place of work or within the original work environment (in some cases with the need for adaptation of the workplace or re-training), the status of vocational training and/or education, and last but not least the preferences and aptitude of the affected person, are the basic aspects of this process of counselling and decision-making. Work-related assessment is gaining more and more relevance as a part of this process.

Vocational rehabilitation in the case of occupational accident and/or disease

In the case of an *occupational accident* (including accidents on the way to or from one's place of work) and/or *occupational disease*, the accident insurer takes on all costs of medical, vocational and social rehabilitation. A so-called "Rehabilitationsausschuss" (rehabilitation board) is responsible for decision-making.

189.795 occupational accidents and 1.569 cases of occupational disease were registered by the Austrian accident insurance institutions in 2001 [1, chapter 4.2] (see also Fig. 5). About 17% were enrolled for medical rehabilitation following hospitalisation. The incidence of occupational injuries and diseases in 2001 according to the type of workplace is shown in Figure 6 (data from [4], p 36).

Occupational injuries causing more than three days of sick leave or inability to work must be reported to the accident insurance within 5 days by the hospital or by the physician treating the patient, and also by the employer. This allows the health insurance experts to evaluate the potential need for vocational rehabilitation during the individual's medical rehabilitation, which in the majority of cases is managed by rehabilitation centres run by the accident insurance. A team of experts from the accident insurance company

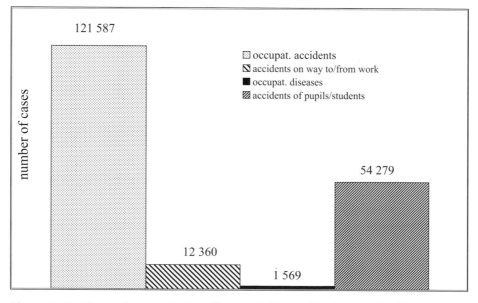

Figure 5 – Incidence of occupational accidents and diseases (absolute numbers) in Austria in 2001 (from [1], Chapter 4, p 3)

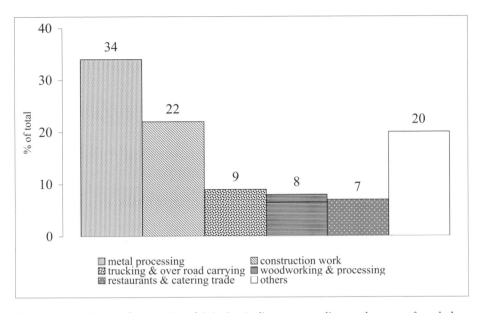

Figure 6 – Incidence of occupational injuries & diseases according to the type of workplace (from [4], p 36)

helps to develop the vocational future of the patient, based on the prospective outcome of medical rehabilitation, the person's abilities, education, preferences and interests.

If the individual is able, or chooses to return to his/her original workplace or work environment (same company, same colleagues), the accident insurance finances measures such as workplace adaptation, re-training, easy access to the place of work, personal technical aid (wheelchair, a specially equipped car, etc.) or education in another field of work within the same company. The same is true for educational courses to obtain new qualifications in case the individual decides to change his occupation or type of work/profession.

Because vocational rehabilitation is continued during the period of unemployment, the accident insurance provides a so-called intermediate benefit (Übergangsgeld) during this time, which amounts to at least 60% of the person's former salary/income, and also pays the contribution to the pension fund. In cases of limited working ability, especially during the initial phase of occupational reintegration, a part of the benefit is paid by the accident insurance.

In addition to the support outlined above, several other possibilities of financing expenses in the course of vocational rehabilitation exist. These are organised by the accident insurance, mainly together with the *Arbeitsmarktservice* (Labour Market Service) and the Bundessozialamt (federal social welfare agency); in special cases organisations for the handicapped may be involved. Detailed information is provided by the *Bundessozialamt* (http://www.basb.bmsg.gv.at).

Independent of the success of vocational rehabilitation and reintegration into work, every individual whose health is impaired by an occupational accident is evaluated for additional reimbursement, wich is paid independently of any other earnings or pension; it may amount to a full pension. Medical experts evaluate the person's condition in percentages of impairment (% Minderung der Erwerbsfähigkeit). Nevertheless, a person suffering from an occupational accident or an occupational disease is free to continue working, even on a full-time basis, in a different profession or at another work-place that is conducive to the disability (for more details see also [5, 6]).

Vocational rehabilitation after non-occupational ("private") accidents and impairment by non-occupational diseases

Medical rehabilitation and the treatment of these persons is managed and paid for by *retirement insurance* and *health insurance* institutions. The retirement insurance institution offers medical as well as vocational rehabilitation to prevent inability to work resulting from progression of the disease or disability. The health insurance pays for continuation of the required medical treatment after hospitalisation as well as during an ongoing disability or disease, with the goal of promoting recovery and preventing chronic disease or aggravation of the disability [3, p. 55].

Nevertheless, the need for vocational rehabilitation is realised rather late in the majority of cases because, in contrast to occupational accidents, no systematic attention is devoted to the individual's future vocational perspectives during his hospitalisation and medical rehabilitation. In many cases, hospitalisation is followed by more or less prolonged sick leave and various treatments given by practising doctors who are not specifically trained or paid for counselling the individual about the impact of accident or disease on the work situation or for initiating vocational rehabilitation.

The employees rarely report early to the employer and dismissals after prolonged sick leave are common. Typically, the issue of vocational rehabilitation is confronted only at this advanced stage, i.e. when the now unemployed person seeks help and advice at the Arbeitsmarktservice.

Alternatively, the health insurer reports prolonged sick leave to the retirement insurance or the individual applies for vocational rehabilitation, and the latter is started.

The retirement insurance organisation also offers vocational rehabilitation to working persons who are at considerable risk of losing their ability to work at their current workplace in the near future because their health is likely to worsen.

Applications for early retirement secondary to disability are common when the unemployment is caused by a disease of long duration. At least in such cases the retirement insurance evaluates the possibility of vocational rehabilitation instead of retirement.

Procedures and measures of vocational rehabilitation provided by the retirement insurance are analogous or identical to those offered by the accident insurance. Accident insurance as well as retirement insurance act in union, mainly with the Arbeitsmarktservice (AMS).

Where the person is offered re-training or education, the expenses are shared equally by the retirement insurance and the AMS. During vocational re-training the AMS pays the same amount as the unemployment benefit; the purpose of this payment is to finance the individual's cost of daily living. Several complex programmes of financial aid for employees as well as employers are available. Detailed information can be obtained from the AMS, the retirement insurance and the Bundessozialamt.

Vocational rehabilitation of handicapped persons

The term "handicap" is used to denote reduced working ability and reduced prospects in everyday work life due to a health problem, disability, or disease. The Austrian social system provides certain services in terms of vocational rehabilitation, especially for handicapped persons. The legal base is the *Bundesbehindertengesetz* (federal law for the handicapped); the main governmental executive organ is the Bundessozialamt (federal social welfare agency). The Bundessozialamt is a well accepted institution in the job market for handicapped persons. It is specialized in working with those who can be reintegrated into the job market, but need targeted, specific and prolonged measures and support. The main partners of the Bundessozialamt are the Arbeitsmarkservice, the association of the handicapped, accident and retirement insurance, and governmental institutions. Detailed information and data can be obtained from [7, 8].

Several institutions offer services relating to vocational rehabilitation, such as re-training, developing new vocational perspectives, special education and qualification, individual training to adjust to a workplace situation, etc. These include the *Berufsförderungsinstitut* (bfi; Institute for Vocational Advancement), the *Wirtschaftsförderungsinstitut* (WIFI; Institute for Economic Advancement), and many others. The leading institution in Austria with a wide range of programmes is the *BBRZ* (Berufliches Bildungs- und Rehabilitationszentrum; Professional Education and Rehabilitation Centre).

BBRZ – Vocational Rehabilitation and Education Centre

When individuals are no longer able to work because of an accident or a disease, they may be confronted with the problem of basic survival and the question of their immediate future existence. In order to ensure that their professional career is not unnecessarily terminated, the BBRZ (Vocational Rehabilitation and Education Centre) aims to help such individuals to gain a firm foothold in their occupation despite their impairment.

BBRZ Austria was established in 1975. With its three business offices in Linz, Vienna and Styria (Kapfenberg) and an external office in Carinthia (Klagenfurt), BBRZ Austria is the largest provider of vocational rehabilitation measures. Individuals with physical and/or psychological impairment can be trained here in very well equipped training and working premises, furnished with modern technologies and new methods, in accordance with a unique occupational orientation and training concept, and can be subsequently reintegrated in the labour market.

Services

The BBRZ offers vocational rehabilitation for disabled persons from the age of 18 years; occasionally also for younger individuals. The training is related to the employment market and focused on completion. It is offered in modules, tailored to the individual abilities, knowledge, and aptitudes of the candidates. Depending on the required knowledge and qualification, it has a maximum duration of 24 months.

The main aims are: *developing new vocational perspectives; qualification and additional specialised training in technical and commercial professions such as EDP technology, informatics, accounting and book-keeping, each with a completed apprenticeship, and short specialized training, e.g. in office communication, staff reimbursement calculation and medical administration; tailored training followed by individual completion certificates; support in procurement.*

Course attendees with incomplete school knowledge who need to be prepared for a proposed educational measure may undergo a general preliminary promotional phase. The BBRZ offers parallel support for persons who wish to complete a course or take an examination for vocational graduation or admission to university.

The course candidates may also avail themselves of a wide range of services relating to parallel support in case of individual issues or problems in various aspects of life. Social consultants provide support in the event of social problems that prove to be a liability and may endanger the individual's successful completion of vocational rehabilitation. Furthermore, candidates are offered a primary counselling session on legal matters.

In addition to counselling and care, those with psychological problems are offered a wide range of mental training programs to prepare for examinations, programs focused on learning techniques, stress coping techniques and relaxation and concentration training, either individually or in groups.

In the medical arena, attention is mainly devoted to identifying those factors which limit the spectrum of potential work areas. The findings of medical studies are major factors used to make decisions about an individual's future occupation.

Parallel to education, the course attendees are assisted in their search for practical training. At the end of the training they are given assistance in finding a job, job applications are written, and job interviews can be rehearsed in a role-playing setting by video training. In many cases the course attendees complete the training, undergo an intermediate practical training, and then become employees of a company.

Partners and Sponsors of the BBRZ

Vocational rehabilitation in Austria is mainly financed by the Arbeitsmarktservice (Labour Market Service), social insurance companies like the Allgemeine Unfallversicherungsanstalt (General Accident Insurance Company), the retirement insurance company, and the provincial governments. The federal social welfare agencies are also significant sponsors of projects, especially in the sector of work integration and qualification. During their training the clients receive financial support from the respective sponsors who bear the course fees.

Specific offers of the BBRZ

Neuro network

Since 1991 the Occupational Training and Rehabilitation Centre offers specific rehabilitation and integration measures for persons who have suffered brain injury. The NeuroNetzWerk Austria (Neuro Network Austria) is an Austrian-wide initiative aimed at networking the medical and occupational-social rehabilitation of persons who have suffered cranial or cerebral injury.

Rehabilitation and integration of those with poor vision and late blindness

Blindness or highly impaired vision signifies massive limitations in the daily life of the individual. BBRZ Linz is the only facility in Austria which offers comprehensive rehabilitation for this group of individuals since 1998.

Occupational diagnosis Austria

Based on several decades of experience, a new approach to occupational diagnosis has been developed. The approach is integral, comprehensive, and oriented towards the individual and the available resources. BerufsDiagnostik Austria (Occupational Diagnosis Austria) is a business unit of BBRZ Austria with offices in Linz, Vienna and Kapfenberg.

Range of services: *Diagnosis of physical performance; workplace simulation with the ERGOS® system; assessment of key qualifications; workplace analysis and expert evaluation; vocational analysis and statement; rehabilitation technology and ergonomics.*

Work and Health Service

A project for early identification of individual occupational limitations (early intervention) has been established within Occupational Diagnosis Austria. BBRZ Austria in Vienna and Styria have set up an office known as "Service Arbeit und Gesundheit" (Work and Health Service) for individuals with health problems at their place of work. Work and Health Service is a form of assistance for the affected individual and his/her employer. The service is closely networked with other institutions involved in rehabilitation, such as the retirement insurance company and other social insurance providers.

A counselling office is supported by the Equal Development Partnership known as the *AEIOU* (Arbeitsfähigkeit erhalten für Individuen, Organisationen und Unternehmen; Maintaining Working Abilities for Individuals, Organisations and Companies) within the occupational initiative of the Austrian Federal Government and the European Social Fund.

Summary

The Occupational Education and Rehabilitation Centre contributes significantly to emancipation and equal chances for individuals with psychological and/or physical impairment by enhancing the opportunities for every course attendee in the labour market through a range of proven training measures. The efforts of the Centre are focused on enabling the person to re-enter his/her professional life by means of vocational rehabilitation. The individual is always viewed from a comprehensive, solution-oriented perspective.

Since the BBRZ was founded in 1975, a large percentage of candidates have been able to achieve their training goals and have been successfully integrated in the work process. According to a study of the Institute of Education and Adult Research in 2001, on a specific day 79% of the graduates were employed at 12 months after completion of the training.

More information is available at the following Internet sites: www.bbrz.at; www.berufsdiagnostikaustria.at; www.servicearbeitgesundheit.at

Problems to be solved and future aspects

Early retirement due to disability – a substitute for vocational rehabilitation

The main challenge in vocational rehabilitation in Austria is early retirement due to disability of "non-occupational" origin, closely associated with preceding unemployment of long duration and a prolonged career of illness or chronic disease. A more in-depth investigation reveals several factors contributing to the problem.

In case of a non-occupational accident or disease, no systematic assessment of the person's occupational environment and situation and the potential implications of his disease on his future working ability is performed either during outpatient care given by a practicing physician or a hospital, or during hospitalisation. Appointments for diagnostic and therapeutic measures, and even decision-making in terms of the strategy of recovery, are left to the patient. Physicians are paid by the health insurance or by the institution that runs the hospital; their responsibility being to provide the best medical service in their field. Networking the different specialists with the goal of optimising diagnosis and treatment is not well established. In contrast to occupational accidents and/or diseases, no systematic advice is provided for dealing with imminent workplace problems relating to the accident or the disease. The problems are usually recognised only when advanced, after the person has lost his/her job following repeated or prolonged sick leave. In the majority of cases the retirement insurance organisation only comes to know about the health problems when a person applies for premature retirement on account of disability.

The situation of occupational and work-related health care and prevention

In 1999 about 83% of a total of 197.419 Austrian firms had less than 10 employees. Approximately 44% of all employees work in "small sized" companies/firms with less than 50 employees (see also Table 3). Private companies are obliged to run a department of occupational safety and health (a safety engineer and an occupational medicine specialist) at their own expense if they employ more than 50 persons (before 1994 only companies with more than 250 employees were subject to this obligation). For smaller facilities, occupational safety and health service is provided free of charge by the accident insurance company (AUVA) and by the so-called *"Begehungsmodell"* ("walk-through" model). The time schedule for occupational medical care is one walk-through per year for enterprises with 11-50 employees; firms with less than 10 employees get a walk-through once every two years [9].

In 97% of all Austrian companies, i.e., those with less than 50 employees, occupational safety and health care is, in practice, not available for establishing and providing continued programs of occupational health care and prevention, registering occupational accidents, managing vocational rehabilitation, and the crucial work of returning to employment and reintegrating the person at his/her workplace. Therefore, the number of occupational accidents in small enterprises with less than 50 employees is very likely to be underestimated. The data shown in figure 4 have been compiled from "raw data" obtained from the department of rehabilitation at the AUVA. An enhancement of quantity as well as of quality of occupational safety and health care to allow the real needs to be addressed, as well as greater attentiveness on the part of the occupational safety and health team focusing on occupational accidents and diseases in small companies, are strongly recommended for the future.

Table 3 – Overview on the distribution of firm sizes in Austria versus persons employed in each firm size range in 1999 [10].

Firm size (employees)	Number of firms		Number of employees	
	absolute	relative (%)	absolute	relative
1 - 9	164,112	83.1	487,223	21.2
10 - 49	27,916	14.1	424,238	23.3
50 - 249	4,494	2.3	452,880	20.1
>250	897	0.5	798,828	35.4
total	197,419	100	2,254,169	100

The scope of action for the employer

The employer is not entitled to obtain information about the prospective duration of his employee's sick leave and its possible consequences on the employee's working ability at his/her workplace. The earnings have to be paid by the employer in case of sick leave for up to 10 weeks duration, in dependence from type of working-contract and time of employment (detailed information can be obtained from the health-insurance institution). It is now well known that the time until an individual returns to work after an accident or disease is considerably reduced if the employee maintains contact with his workplace and the employer is informed about the future prospects of the employee's ability to work [11-13]. In most cases this is not done, and the majority of employees loose their job following repeated or prolonged sick leave.

Special obstacles for efficient vocational rehabilitation

About 77% of the clients referred for vocational rehabilitation to the BBRZ have been unemployed for more than 7 months; about 32% for even more than 2 years. Seventy-two per cent of the clients of the BBRZ are between 21 and 40 years of age, approximately 43% of these persons show up with severe health problems. Seventy-four per cent no longer receive unemployment benefit. Unemployment benefit is usually limited to 30 weeks' duration. This time limit is extended to 39 weeks for those >40 years of age, and to a maximum of 52 weeks for persons >50 years of age, depending on the overall duration of employment. Persons who exceed this period of unemployment may receive a so-called "Notstandshilfe" (emergency aid), a small amount of money barely sufficient to live on. The later the vocational rehabilitation is initiated, the poorer is its outcome [14, 15].

Work-related assessment has been established throughout the world as a helpful tool for making decisions concerning professions or jobs conducive to a person with a distinct disability, as well as for information in respect of those workplaces at which the handicapped person will be unable to work.

In Austria, decisions relating to a person's ability to work are largely based on the individual competence of the accident insurance or retirement insurance expert; general guidelines and consistent quality management in this field are not established. Work-related assessment is used in specific cases by some institutions, such as the AUVA and the BBRZ. There is no institutionalised education on the assessment of the disabled person's ability to work or the assessment process.

Outlook

Effective prevention, early intervention, competent management of the diagnosis and treatment of disease, a statement concerning the need for occupational rehabilitation at the earliest time possible, and cooperation between employer and employee would be straightforward strategies to resolve the problem. Recent approaches in this field by organisations like the Österreichische Arbeitsgemeinschaft für Rehabilitation, the "Arbeitsassistenz Österreich", the initiative "ways-to-work" and last but not least the BBRZ, are very promising.

A medium term improvement in the present Austrian health care system's ability to address these problems would be gained if a statement on the future prospects of a patients' ability to work was an integral part of every medical report of a hospital or a practicing physician. Ideally physicians, psychologists, social consultants, as well as other professional personnel with special training in the field of work-related assessment and vocational rehabilitation should be obliged to contribute their expertise in a cooperative manner to the medical report of a hospital or rehabilitation centre.

The reporting of a prospective need for vocational rehabilitation should be the trigger for the practising physician as well as for the health insurance, to arrange vocational rehabilitation for the patient. The University Department of Physical Medicine and Rehabilitation at the General Hospital of Vienna plans to run a "pilot" project to test the practicability of this approach.

Cooperation with and integration of the occupational health care service – whenever available and possible – should also occur. However, it is not available for about 45% of the working population or 97% of companies in Austria at time (see tab. 3). Under these circumstances establishment of centres for "occupational consulting" which could be run analogous to a doctor's office, could be meaningful options. Financing of such centres might be provided by the insurance institutions due to their interests in maintaining health and employment of their clients.

Acknowledgements

The authors gratefully acknowledge the substantial support by the persons to follow to the generation of this article, by providing data, information and intensive discussions: Prof. Peter Pils, head of the medical staff dept. for rehabilitation, deputy medical head of the AUVA, and Mag. Franz Preßlmayer, head of the dept. for rehabilitation, AUVA; Herbert Fritz, head of the AMS Vienna, Schönbrunnerstraße; Dr. Emmerich Jires, director BVA; Mag. Roman Pöschl, head of the office of the BBRZ in Vienna.

References

1. Statistisches Handbuch der Österreichischen Sozialversicherung 2002
2. Die Invaliditäts- bzw. Berufsunfähigkeitspension (Information 5 Pensionsversicherungsanstalt. Download: *www.pensionsversicherung.at*)
3. Handbuch der Österreichischen Sozialversicherung 2003
4. AUVA Jahresbericht 2001: 36
5. Richtlinien für die Gewährung von beruflichen und sozialen Massnahmen der Rehabilitation (2002). Available from AUVA
6. Rat und Hilfe nach Arbeitsunfällen und Berufskrankheiten (2002). Available from AUVA (www.auva.net)
7. Bericht über die Lage behinderter Menschen in Österreich. Bundes-ministerium für soziale Sicherheit und Generationen (Hrsg.). 14 März 2003
8. Arbeit *und Behinderung* (download: http://www.arbeitundbehinderung.at)
9. Bundesgesetz, mit dem das ArbeitnehmerInnenschutzgesetz, Artikel VI des Bundesgesetzes BGBl. Nr. 450/1994 und das Allgemeine Sozialversicher-ungsgesetz geändert werden. BGBl. I – Ausgegeben am 12. Jänner 1999 – Nr. 12
10. Zach Sabine (2001) Produktion und Dienstleistungen. Leistungs – und Strukturerhebung 1999. Statistische Nachrichten 8: 600-6

11. Winkelhake U, Schutzeichel F, Niemann O *et al.* (2003) Occupationally Orientated Medical Rehabilitation (BOR) for disabilities caused by orthopedic diseases. Rehabilitation (Stuttg) 42: 30-5

12. Haase I, Riedl G, Birkholz LB *et al.* (2002) Verzahnung von medizinischer Rehabilitation und beruflicher Reintgration. Arbeitsmed. Sozialmed. Umweltsmed 37(7): 331-5

13. Seidel HJ, Neuner R, Schochat Th (2003) Betriebsarzt und medizinische Rehabilitation – eine Befragung von Betriebsärzten in Baden Württemberg. Arbeitsmed. Sozialmed. Umweltsmed. 38(4): 228-34

14. Personal communication by BBRZ (internal report 2000)

15. BBRZ. Report about the project WorkAbility Oct. 2001 - Dec. 2002

Social security and vocational rehabilitation: the Belgian model

W. Brusselmans and K. Delplace

To fully understand social security and vocational rehabilitation in Belgium we need to have an idea of the political organisation of that country. Some aspects will be common to all Belgians and others will be different because they depend on the regulations of the regions or the community to which the person belongs.

The federal state of Belgium: the four state reforms

The revision of the constitution in 1970 resulted in the setting-up of three cultural communities. From the legal viewpoint that meant the start of the state reform process.

The establishment of the three cultural communities is, as the name suggests, a sign of a certain autonomy in relation to culture. However, the powers of these cultural communities were still extremely limited.

In 1980, the second state reform took place. The work that had started in 1970 was continued.

Since then the cultural communities have become known just as the Flemish, the French and the German-speaking community, because the communities decided not only on cultural matters but also on matters "relating to the individual", in other words health and social services.

These communities each had a council (their parliament) and a government.

With the state reform of 1980, two regions were also established: the Flemish Region and the Walloon Region.

During the third state reform of 1988-89, it was mainly the Brussels-Capital Region that took shape. Like the other two regions it had its own institutions, and in particular a council – its parliament – and a government. Also, the communities were given more power and the regions were consolidated.

The state reform process, which had started in 1970, was completed with the fourth state reform in 1993. Since 14th July 1993 Belgium is a fully-fledged federal state. The communities and the regions, which were set up under previous reforms, now received their full powers.

When a person becomes ill or disabled and is in need of rehabilitation or professional reintegration, the legal framework and the circumstances will be partly the same and partly different depending on whether they are governed by the federal legislation or the legislation of the communities or the regions. We will explain the most essential elements, which are relevant to our topic: illness, disability and rehabilitation. Firstly we describe the federal elements which are the same for all the Belgian citizens, secondly we address the aspects which can be different because they belong to the action field of the communities or the regions. The following description is based on the state model as it exists in Belgium in 2004. We will not consider measures at the international, provincial or municipal levels.

Social security: a federal matter

Because social security in Belgium is a federal matter, it is the same for all the Belgian citizens regardless of the community or the region to which they belong.

Social security is largely financed by the professionally active population. In the salaried persons' system, both employees and employers have to pay contributions to RSZ-ONSS. The self-employed pay their social security contribution to the social insurance fund they are affiliated with. In case of a deficit, the federal state will also contribute.

We will only describe the most essential elements of the system, details have to be consulted elsewhere (see websites on the Internet [1-6]).

We distinguish two systems in our social protection system: the "classical sectors" of social security and "social assistance".

The classical social security contains seven sectors:

– old-age and survivor's pensions;
– unemployment;
– insurance for accidents at work;
– insurance for occupational disease;
– family benefits;
– sickness and disability insurance;
– annual vacation.

When we refer to "social assistance" or the "residuary systems" we mean:

– minimum subsistence;
– guarantee of income for the aged;
– guaranteed family benefits;
– benefits for the disabled.

The entire classical social security system is divided into a system for salaried persons (such as bank employees, workers in a car assembly plant...), one for self-employed persons and one for civil servants (of the Belgian federal government).

We will only address the social security elements that are relevant to rehabilitation.

The entire Belgian population is entitled to medical care, with a few exceptions. However, a number of conditions have to be met to ensure access to health insurance benefits:

– all those entitled to health insurance must join or register with a health insurance fund;

– the entitlement to health care requires the payment of contributions equalling a minimum amount;

– in principle, there is a six-month waiting period before medical care can be reimbursed.

Medical care is divided into 23 different categories of medical dispensations, the most important of which are:

– ordinary medical care, among others visits and consultations of general practitioners and specialised practitioners, and the care provided by physiotherapists;

– dental care;

– deliveries;

– dispensation of pharmaceutical products (chemist's preparations, pharmaceutical specialities, generic drugs);

– hospital care;

– assistance with rehabilitation.

Just like salaried persons and civil servants, self-employed people are entitled to medical care, but only so-called large risks are covered. These large risks include health care during delivery, hospital admission for observation and treatment, medical drugs provided during a hospital stay, palliative care, etc. A self-employed person who wishes to insure himself against small risks (consultation and visit to a general practitioner or specialised practitioner, consultation of a dental specialist, etc.) can take out a specific insurance with a mutual insurance fund, called "voluntary insurance". This insurance requires the payment of specific contributions. At the beginning of 2004 the discussion on the medical care for the self-employed is ongoing.

Refunding of the cost of medical treatment varies primarily with the nature of the treatment and the status of the insured. In most cases, medical expenses are not entirely refunded. Generally, the personal share or patient share amounts to 25%.

A scheme of higher reimbursement also exists, known as "preferential scheme" for the category of widows, widowers, disabled, retired, orphans, beneficiaries of the subsistence minimum, recipients of OCMW – CPAS support, beneficiaries of guaranteed income for the elderly (IGO – GRAPA), beneficiaries of a disability benefit, people entitled to higher family benefits, unemployed persons aged at least 50, those who have been unemployed for at least one year and being single or with dependants, as well as the dependants of the categories, mentioned up here (WIGW – VIPO category).

Pharmaceutical dispensations include pharmaceutical specialities (brand products) and magistral preparations, i.e., drugs prepared by the chemist himself. On the basis of their social and pharmaceutical utility, pharmaceutical specialities are divided into five reimbursement categories.

The share of costs for handicapped persons is lower than that for ordinary benefi-ciaries.

Hospital costs

In the case of a hospital stay, the patient share will be substantially lower for handicap-ped persons.

To avoid situations in which the rise of the personal share of costs during the past few years would increase medical costs to such an extent as to render medical care unaffor-dable and out of reach for the less well-off categories in the population, a system of social exemption from the patient share was introduced.

Social exemption is aimed at specific categories of people (often in a socially less favourable position) and exempts them from any patient share if the annual amount of personal shares in the costs of reimbursable medical care exceeds 450 euros.

Rehabilitation centres

Rehabilitation centres are part of medical care. There are specific rehabilitation centres for persons with musculo-skeletal and/or neurological impairments, cardiac impair-ments, speech, language and hearing impairments, visual impairments, and psychologi-cal impairments.

With the exception of the visual rehabilitation centres the network of rehabilitation centres is dense. For musculo-skeletal injuries alone there are 48 rehabilitation centres over the country. Most general hospitals have a special service for physical rehabilitation which are allowed to rehabilitate all kinds of pathologies. The specialised centres deal only with those pathologies which are indicated in their agreement with RIZIV-INAMI, but they are entitled to provide more extensive rehabilitation programs for up to 6-8 hours a day, of limited duration. A rehabilitation program for paraplegic patients e.g. can take maximally 9 months, for severe TBI-patients 24 months.

Maintenance therapies are sometimes provided by general rehabilitation centres, but usually by private physiotherapists or speech therapists. Theoretically physiotherapy can be continued permanently after discharge from the rehabilitation centre; speech therapy can be continued for up to two years. Occupational therapy at home after discharge from the rehabilitation centre is not possible.

The need for the whole range of rehabilitation procedures, in a rehabilitation centre as well as at home, must always be approved by a medical adviser.

Compared to other European countries the number of private physiotherapists is extremely high in Belgium. In the last year, the government has tried to control overcon-sumption of physiotherapy.

Sickness benefits

Sick people will not only obtain reimbursement of their medical expenses, but they will also be entitled to benefits covering income losses. Such regulations only apply to diseases and accidents in the private life. Occupational diseases or accidents at work have their own specific regulations.

For sickness benefits, a distinction should be made between salaried persons, civil servants and self-employed persons.

Generally, an employee who is entitled to reimbursement of medical costs is also entitled to benefits in case of disease.

Incapacity for work is divided into two periods: the primary incapacity for work and the period of disability. During the week (labourers) or month (clerks) preceding the primary incapacity period the employee will receive his normal pay.

Primary incapacity for work lasts maximally one year and starts from the first day of sick leave. During the first thirty days of primary incapacity for work, people will receive 60% of their salary from the insurance company (salary ceiled to 101.21 euros a day). From the 31st day the amount remains the same, but only for salaried persons with dependants or for persons who would lose their sole income. Other beneficiaries receive 55%.

The period of disability begins after one year of primary incapacity for work. The disability is established by the RIZIV – INAMI medical disability council.

To establish the level of disability benefits, the family situation and the possible loss of sole income are taken into account. A beneficiary with dependants is entitled to an indemnity rate of 65% of his income ceiled to 101.21 euros. For beneficiaries with no dependants, the indemnity rate is 50% or 40% of the same ceiled income, depending on whether or not they suffer a loss of their sole income.

In the self-employed persons' scheme, three periods of incapacity for work are distinguished:

– a non-indemnified period of one month;
– an indemnified period of primary incapacity for work of eleven months;
– a disability period, starting after one year of incapacity for work.

Rates will be different from and lower than those for salaried persons.

The sickness scheme for civil servants is specific in that it deals with incapacity by means of sick leave days. During his sick leave, the civil servant continues to receive 100% of his salary.

When all the days of sick leave have been used up, the civil servant will be withdrawn from service because of his sickness (disability). In that case, he receives a reduced pay equal to minimum 60% of his last "active salary".

Accidents at work

All salaried persons, including domestic staff, are covered against accidents at work and accidents on the way to and from work. Self-employed persons are not subject to these regulations. Civil servants have their own specific scheme.

Every employer should have a contract against accidents at work with an acknowledged insurance company or with an acknowledged common insurance fund. The Fund for Accidents at Work (FAO-FAT) supervises the insurers.

Risks covered

Both accidents on the workplace and accidents to and from work are subject to the legislation for industrial accidents.

An accident at work in the strict sense of the word is every accident occurring to an employee during, and because of, the execution of his labour contract and causing injury. The cause of such an accident must be a "sudden event".

A victim of an accident at work is entitled to hospital care, physiotherapy, medical, surgical, dental and pharmaceutical care as well as orthopaedic equipment. Care costs are reimbursed according to the applicable fares of sickness insurance and hospital day care prices. The insurance company has to pay the full cost and no costs can be charged to the victim.

Indemnity for loss of income

Medical costs are not only costs that can be reimbursed. During the period of incapacity for work caused by an industrial accident at work, people are entitled to benefits. We must distinguish between two periods: temporary incapacity for work and permanent incapacity for work.

During the first period of temporary full incapacity for work, a victim receives 90% of his average day salary. This average day salary corresponds to 1/365th part of the basic salary. The basic salary is the salary the employee was entitled to during the complete year preceding the accident at work. Since 1st January 2004, this basic salary fluctuates between a minimum of 5,178.85 euros and a maximum of 25,894.27 euros being related to the consumer price index every year.

Temporary partial incapacity for work is also reimbursed. The victim will receive an allowance equal to the difference between the salary he earned before the accident occurred and the salary he obtains by resuming his work.

The period of temporary incapacity for work can end in two ways: the victim is declared either cured or in a state of permanent incapacity for work. The period of permanent incapacity for work starts at the moment of "consolidation". Consolidation is the assessment that the injury caused by the accident at work shows some degree of stability. The incapacity for work is expressed as a percentage indicating to what extent the victim's capacity to work has decreased as a result of the accident (the victim is reimbursed for the loss of economic abilities, not for the physical injury.) The consolidation must be endorsed by both the insurance company and the victim (and this agreement must in turn be ratified by FAO-FAT).

The annual allowance is raised if the victim requires the regular help of a third person ("a third party"). The maximum allowance amounts to twelve times the average minimum monthly salary.

Occupational diseases

Schemes for occupational diseases are often similar to those for accidents at work.

A victim or one of his family members may give notice of an occupational disease using an official form. This form has to be sent to the Fund for Occupational Diseases (FBZ-FMP).

Contrary to the Fund for Accidents at Work, the Fund for Occupational Diseases plays more than just a role of control, co-ordination and organisation. FBZ-FMP is an institution of public utility, responsible for insuring against occupational diseases and taking care of the indemnification of victims. All employers have to contract with FBZ-FMP, so there are no private insurance companies as there are for accidents at work.

An occupational disease is not easy to define, because the link between the exposure to a risk and a disease is often not so clear and the disease might commence after exposure has ended.

This explains why a list of acknowledged occupational diseases was drawn up, making it easier for a victim to prove his occupational disease. If the disease is on the list and the employee works in a sector where there is exposure to some risk, his disease will be acknowledged as an occupational disease. The burden of proof does not lie with the victim, because there is an irrefutable assumption in his favour.

For diseases which are not acknowledged as occupational, victims have the possibility to prove exposure to a risk, and to demonstrate the causal link between the disease and the exposure.

In this field, some degree of parallelism exists between occupational diseases and accidents at work concerning the reimbursed risks.

The specific systems for occupational diseases in the private sector also apply to the public sector.

Self-employed persons are not insured against occupational diseases.

Social assistance

Social assistance does not belong to social security in the strict sense, but it is part of the overall social protection for the Belgian population.

The purpose of social security is to provide a minimum income to the entire population. Social assistance consists of the following provisions:

– benefits for the disabled;
– minimum subsistence;
– guaranteed income for the elderly;
– guaranteed family benefits.

Benefits for disabled people

Benefits for disabled people replace or complete their income where, due to handicap, they are unable to provide themselves with a sufficient income or they have extra financial burdens.

For the non-elderly, two benefits can be distinguished: the income substitution benefit and the integration allowance.

Some administrative or medical requirements have to be met and not everyone can obtain such an indemnity.

For entitlement to an income substitution benefit, it has to be established to what extent the disabled person, due to his handicap, has diminished potential for working in the regular labour market. The benefit then depends on the family situation. The maximum annual shares are (on 1st January 2004): for an entitled person with dependants are: 9,529.93 euros; for an entitled single person: 7,147.44 euros; for cohabitants without dependants 4,764.96 euros.

For the integration benefit, the reduction of autonomy is taken into account. To this end, a medical-social scale is being used to evaluate the person's abilities to:

– self-mobility;
– eat and prepare food by oneself;
– take care of one's personal hygiene and to dress;
– maintain and run the house;
– live without supervision;
– communicate and have social contact.

Every criterion is allocated marks. Depending on the total of these marks the indemnity is as follows (maximal annual amounts on 1st January 2004):

– category I: 7 to 8 points: 942.34 euros;
– category II: 9 to 11 points: 3,211.12 euros;
– category III: 12 to 14 points: 5,130.98 euros;
– category IV: 15 to 16 points: 7,475.18 euros;
– category V: 17 to 18 points: 8,480.13 euros.

The right to this allocation is coupled with existing revenues from other sources.

In addition to the income substitution and the integration allowance, several other benefits exist that will not be discussed here, such as family help, taxi cheques, parking facilities, etc.

The regional funds for the disabled

So far we have described federal matters, applying to the entire Belgian population. What follows can differ according to the region or the community to which one belongs.

During the last few years the different communities and regions have developed somewhat different systems for vocational rehabilitation although they are all based on the legislation of the previous National Fund for the Resettlement of the Disabled which was active from 1963 until 1992. Because the different regional services derive from the same service, many similarities still exist between the different regions. Nevertheless, after some ten years of regionalisation, regional differences are emerging, particularly concerning the models for vocational training and the organisation of the guidance and pathways to work.

The activities of the National Fund are now distributed over the following services:

– the Flemish Fund for the Social Integration of Disabled Persons with a Handicap (Vlaams Fonds voor Sociale Integratie van Personen met een Handicap – VFSIPH). The Flemish Region has about 6,000,000 inhabitants;

– the Walloon Agency for the Integration of Disabled persons (Agence Walonne pour l'Integration des Personnes Handicapés – AWIPH). The Walloon Region has about 3,350,000 inhabitants;

– Service of the German-speaking Community for Disabled Persons with Disabilities (Dienststelle der Deutschsprachigen Gemeinschaft für Personen mit Behinderung). The German-speaking Community has about 70,000 inhabitants;

– French-speaking Brussels Service for Disabled Persons (Service Bruxellois Francophone des Personnes Handicapés). The Brussels Region has about 1,000,000 inhabitants.

Flemish-speaking persons in the Brussels region are covered by the services of the Flemish Fund.

Among these different services there are cooperation agreements allowing persons living in one region to have access to services in another region. Especially persons living in the border area of a certain region will sometimes make use of services in the other region.

To enjoy the opportunities provided by one of the regional Funds one has to be registered as a person with a handicap. Even the conditions for this registration differ from region to region. The conditions to being registered for the Walloon inhabitants and for the Brussels French-speaking inhabitants being 20% mentally handicapped or 30% physically handicapped, which are the same conditions as during the National Fund period. The Flemish Fund in its decree of 27st June 1990 defined disability as follows: "Any major long-term restriction of a person's ability to integrate into society as a result of an impairment of his/her mental, psychological, physical or sensory capabilities". The elements "long term" and "severe" are essential conditions for being accepted into the Flemish Fund. A person can only be admitted to the Flemish Fund if he has one or more needs, which are covered by this Fund. Registration without such a need in terms of activities or participations is impossible. From the beginning The Flemish Fund was strongly inspired by the ICIDH-model, and now the ICF-model [3].

The administrative procedures that have to be undertaken differ, but are beyond the scope of this paper. We further address the vocational training and guidance, subsidies to the employer, interventions for the self-employed, the sheltered workshops and employment/quota for persons with a disability.

Wage cost subsidies for the employer

Following Collective Agreement no. 26, persons with disabilities have to be paid a normal wage, even when they can not work as efficiently as their able-bodied colleagues. The different wage cost subsidies serve to compensate the employer for this limited efficiency. This regulation has been known in Belgium as "CAO 26" and has often been used. Currently this regulation is only used in the Flemish region under this name.

The different measures for wage cost subsidy vary by the region or community where the handicapped persons live (see overview). In addition to the wage cost subsidies, the different regions also seek to compensate for costs of work tools or clothing required because of the disability, and make grants for alterations to the workplace.

Overview of wage cost subsidies

Region	Name (original)	Period	% intervention in wage cost	Sector
Flemish Region	CAO-26/CCT-26 (1)	1 year/ renewable	Max 50%	Private
	Vlaamse Integratie Premie (VIP) (2)	Unlimited	30% (fixed)	Private
Walloon region	Prime à l'intégration (3)	1 year	25% (fixed)	Private + Public
	Prime de compen- sation (4)	1 year/ renewable	Max. 50%	Private + Public
Brussels Capital region	Prime d'insertion (5)	1 year/ renewable	Max. 65%	Private + Public + sheltered workshop
German community	Beschäftigung im Betrieb (6)	1 year/ renewable	Max. 50%	Private + Public

In the Walloon region and in the Brussels Capital region, disabled people who are or become self-employed can receive a limited grant to start their own business. In the Flemish region a grant for modifications to the workplace can be allocated.

Specialised vocational training centres

In Belgium there are about 20 specialised centres for vocational training of persons with disabilities. Previously vocational training centres were specialised in only one or a limited number of occupations. Programs were nearly individualised. There was no or only limited recognised training and job placement was nonexistent or dependent on mainstream procedures. In the last decade vocational training centres have tried to develop highly individualised training programs, including on the job training and job placement. Some programs take place entirely in the workplace in collaboration with the employer.

In the Flemish Region every measure to promote the vocational integration of handicapped persons has to be covered by a "pathways to work service" (Dienst voor Arbeidstrajectbegeleiding). A pathways to work service follows the principles of supported employment and can assist in job finding, job analysis, assessment, job matching and job coaching. The assessment, however, is mainly done in collaboration with specialised vocational orientation centres.

Vocational rehabilitation is usually paid for as services depending on the communities and regions, but some rehabilitation centres, which depend on the federal Ministry of Health funding also try to provide occupational rehabilitation. However, rehabilitation practitioners, especially when they work with severely injured patients, will always need the regional services: in fact, the rehabilitation centres and the administration of the regional funds are strongly intertwined.

Sheltered workshops

Sheltered workshops were also established by the Social Rehabilitation Act of 1963. There are now about 160 sheltered workshops in Belgium (17 in the Brussels region, 66 in the Walloon region and 78 in the Flemish region) with a total of about 20,000 handicapped employees. Since 1992 the number of sheltered workshops has been fixed, but at the same time different programs (e.g., the social workshops), have been started for hard-to-employ people. These initiatives are primarily directed to people who have been unemployed for a long time, but many handicapped persons can also find a job using these initiatives.

Specialised study
and occupational counselling centres

These centres give specialised advice on schooling and vocational matters. They perform also the necessary psychological evaluations and work closely with the different services and institutions for disabled persons.

Non-labour market-related activities

These are aimed at people who have been recognised as disabled by the Flemish Fund who need personal support in the workplace, and who can work with only minimal efficiency. This measure is mainly directed at persons who spend some days every week at a day activity centre and do some additional useful, but unpaid work in a normal occupational environment (usually in the social sector) for one or more days a week.

The "personal assistance budget"

The "personal assistance budget" (PAB) is allocated by the Flemish Fund to persons with a handicap. At the beginning of 2004 this budget varied from 7,436.81 euros to 34,705.09 euros for one year. The number of applicants and the total budget are limited. On 31st December 2003 there were 608 PAB-users in Flanders. The allocated budget can be used for different reasons, e.g., assistance with vocational activities or school activities. J. Huys [2] sees PAB as one element in a larger evolution to self determination and empowerment of the person with a handicap living in the Flemish Community.

Employment regulations

E. Samoy [4] gives a global description of the interventions by regulations.

The Social Rehabilitation Act of 1963 provides the basis of the legal obligations to employ people with disabilities. Although this Act laid down that public and private bodies must employ a certain number of disabled people, the necessary decree to implement the provisions relating to the private sector is still lacking. In 1972 a Royal Order established for the first time that 600 civil service posts (in the federal administration) should be reserved for people covered under the 1963 Act. In a later Order the number was increased to 1,200. In 1977 and 1978 the obligation was extended to provinces and local authorities, which have to employ one disabled person for every 55 employees. The latter obligation still stands although no one knows to what extent it is implemented. However, the obligation for the federal administration is currently outdated because the obligation in the 1963 Law was replaced by an obligation in a new law of 22 March 1999 on "Matters concerning civil servants", but there is no Royal Order yet to implement this. One of the reasons that the law of 1963 had to be revised is the institutional reform of Belgium (from 1980 on), whereby legislative and executive powers have been redistributed. Large parts of what was formerly the federal administration are now administrations of regions and communities. New decrees for the regions and communities stipulate that a certain number of people with disabilities have to be employed in the administrations (e.g., 2% in the Flemish administration and 2.5% in the Walloon administration). Due to a lack of registration it is hard to tell whether the targets are being met. In summary, there are quota obligations in the public administrations (at all levels) but there is no follow-up on the implementation (and no sanctions!), and the private sector escapes all obligations.

There is only limited protection of people with disabilities against dismissal. In general, compensation is payable to employees if the grounds for dismissal are neither economic nor urgent reasons which prevent the continuation of the contract. Some protection also applies during the first six months of work incapacity, during which the labour contract is suspended and no dismissal allowed (although, in practice this is subject to court decisions). Moreover, when the work incapacity is of such a nature that the employee is considered to be permanently unable to work, the labour contract can be terminated on the grounds of "force majeure".

In Belgium, people with disabilities do not have preferential access to specific occupations, and are not entitled to extra leave.

The only protection against discrimination, which is already prevailing, is the Collective Agreement no. 38 ter of 17th July 1998 (made applicable to the whole of the private sector by Royal decree), which stipulates (in article 2 bis) that any discrimination by an employer on personal grounds (including disability) is prohibited at the stage of selection and recruitment. Violations can be contested before the labour courts.

Awareness campaigns and "good practices"

Obligations such as quota or antidiscrimination law are 'hard' interventions, persuasion policies such as information campaigns and positive action plans are 'soft' interventions. In the last decade many small-scale campaigns have been conducted, often initiated by the regional Funds in conjunction with private organisations of disabled people and employers' organisations as well as unions, to improve the employment position of disabled people. The approach consisting of asking for positive action plans is favoured but is still limited to the public sector (regional ministries).

The Flemish Fund, together with two training centres for disabled people and with the cooperation of the Flemish Economic Union has drawn up a "Guide to Good Practice" based on 10 companies that have positive experiences of employing personnel with a handicap. Those companies that usually receive financial support belong to a very wide range of sectors: IT, insurance, temporary staff, the food industry, etc. They employ people with physical or mental handicaps as executives, white-collar workers or blue-collar workers.

On 1st January 1998 the Flemish Fund started up the Consultance project, with support from the European Union. This project has emerged from the need for information to increase the employers' awareness of the employment of handicapped people. The project is mainly intended to offer support to employers in developing a differential personnel policy for people with a handicap. At the same time, work is also being done on structural cooperation with representative employer organisations such as the Flemish Economic Union.

The Institut Wallon d'Etudes, de Recherches et de Formation (FGTB – Belgian General Federation of Labour) and Formation, Education, Culture (CSC – Confederation of Christian Trade Unions) have drawn up a "union manual" to make trade union delegates aware of the fact that disabled people at work are a reality and that they must be retained and integrated. Practical advice is offered in this respect.

The future of service delivery to the disabled

Social security as well as vocational rehabilitation will have to rid itself of the remains of outdated historical structures both in Belgium and elsewhere in Europe.

Several elements are promoting change. First of all there is a growing consensus on health and handicap. E.g. the WHO "International Classification of Functioning, Disability and Health", known as ICF, provides a conceptual basis for the definition, measurement and policy formulations for health and disability.

ICF "mainstreams" the experience of disability and recognises it as a universal human experience. This mainstreaming effect is becoming more pronounced, as evidenced in different services within the Belgian communities.

The Standard Rules on the Equalisation of Opportunities for Persons with Disabilities (UN resolution 48/96) is another inspiring document, promoting equalisation and participation, also with regard to vocational rehabilitation. The CAO 26 in Belgium and the income regulations for persons working in sheltered workshops, are clear examples of an equalisation policy.

The effect of a growing demand for "good quality services" is also already noticeable, the Flemish Fund in its decree of 29st April 1997 described the need for qualified services. Qualified service delivery can be seen as the totality of qualities and the characteristics of the help and services which are relevant to the explicitly formulated or the implicitly existing needs of disabled persons. From 2003 the Flemish services depending on the Flemish Fund have to develop a "quality policy" with a classified quality system and a planning clearly described in a "quality handbook" [1]. For the writing of a quality handbook inspiration can been found in the ISO 9000 norms. The demand for quality is an ongoing process.

Our justified hope is that these different dynamics which are influencing our society today will lead to better services and especially a better quality of qualified vocational rehabilitation of persons with a disability based on the principles of equality and participation.

References

1. Brandt G, Slembrouck H (2000) Kwaliteitszorg in de voorzieningen voor personen met een handicap, Acco

2. Huys J (2002) Revolutie in het Vlaams beleid ten aanzien van personen met een handicap? Een commentaar bij de nieuwe regeling van het persoonlijk assistentiebudget en bij de voorstellen tot invoering van het persoonsgebonden budget; in: Arbeid in gezondheid en ziekte, ed. Donceel P., Masschelein R, Acco p 453-75

3. International Classification of Functioning, Disability and Health, Bohn Stafleu Van Loghum, 2001

4. Samoy E (2002) Active labour market policies for people with disabilities; country profile for Belgium, Vlaams Fonds voor Sociale Integratie van Personen met een Handicap, Brussel

Internet

1. Agence Wallonne pour l'Integration des Personnes Handicapés (AWIPH): Internet: http://www.awiph.be

2. Dienststelle der Deutschsprachigen Gemeinschaft für Personen mit einer Behinderung sowie für die besondere sociale Fürsorge; Internet: http://www.dglivc.be

3. Ministerie van Sociale Zaken; Internet: http://socialsecurity.fgov.be

4. Service bruxellois francophone des personnes handicapés (COCOF-SBFPH); Internet: http://www.cocof.be/sbfph

5. Vademecum van de maatregelen voor de tewerkstelling van gehandicapte werknemers, Nationale Arbeidsraad, Internet: http://www.cnt-nar.be

6. Vlaams Fonds voor Sociale Integratie van Personen met een Handicap; Internet: http://www.vlafo.be

Vocational rehabilitation: the British model

C.W. Roy

Introduction

Vocational rehabilitation in the United Kingdom is in a state of flux. After decades of uncertainty, confusion, and at times, apathy, there is renewed interest in the topic, with initiatives from central government and independent agencies, both in research into better models of vocational rehabilitation, and in provision of help. How have we arrived at this point?

As in many countries, the roots of organized vocational rehabilitation in this country may be traced to disabled ex-servicemen, especially after the Second World War [1]. The solution then was to establish Employment Rehabilitation Centres, to which ex-servicemen would travel to be re-trained to new skills, often in light engineering, commensurate with their residual abilities. This model worked well at a time when there was expanding manufacturing and service capacity and a relative shortage of suitably skilled workers, and a number of well motivated disabled ex-servicemen. The pattern of impairments present included many for which it was relatively easy to make adjustments and provision for employment.

As times changed, both the prevailing economic climate, and the characteristics of the population unable to work through disability or illness, prompted review of the process. By the early 1980s it was clear that more flexible approaches were needed. Employment services appointed Disability Employment Advisors, who worked with potential employers at least as much as the re-employment candidate. There was less emphasis on retraining workers, partly because it was acknowledged that previous schemes had often retrained workers for trades which were shrinking, providing few re-employment opportunities. More and more, the employment service's response was in placing and matching candidates who were "work ready" into jobs, rather than rehabilitation of people not yet ready for work. This was exemplified by "Placement, Assessment, and Counselling" teams.

During this period, there was a diminishing availability of pre-vocational rehabilitation opportunities for those not deemed "work ready". At the same time health services, in many cases, concentrated purely on treating impairments, with pressure increasing to treat more patients for shorter periods of time. There was an increasing tendency to consider vocational aspects only after "treatment" was completed [2]. The scene was set, therefore, for a growing hiatus between the end of health care treatment and the onset of attempts at placement. Health and vocational resettlement became disconnected. More importantly, those who were struggling to return to employment after illness or accident received little practical assistance [3].

The benefits system showed change also. The number receiving incapacity benefit or its predecessor invalidity benefit (a long-term sickness benefit usually awarded to those unable to work for at least six months) rose sharply from 690,000 in 1979 to 2.7 million in 2002 [3]. It certainly appeared that some of this growth was due to individuals transferring from unemployment benefit (where the individual had to be available for work) to Invalidity, which, in certain circumstances, could be more rewarding financially. It is likely that social factors such as finance were more important than health factors in this change of benefit. Effectively, such individuals were often dropping out of the population seeking employment. Medically, certification for invalidity benefit (later replaced by Incapacity Benefit) was carried out largely by general practitioners, often without specific training in how to assess capacity for work.

In an attempt to promote a standardized approach to assessment of long-term incapacity for work, Government agencies produced an "all-work" test, designed to identify those in whom it was unreasonable to expect return to work [4]. This test had a careful, rigorous development, building on the meticulous methodology of the OPCS disability scales. However, it attempted to ensure that capacity was assessed for any work, and, using the former WHO ICIDH terminology, sought to assess impairment and disability only, and specifically excluded taking handicap into account. It is arguable that this is unsound at best, and impossible at worst. The test was not well received by many disabled people and particular questions were raised over the test's ability to assess fairly those with intermittent or invisible disabilities, especially for chronic pain.

At any rate, the numbers on long-term incapacity benefit have continued to rise. New methods of assessment were produced, but realisation that a more fundamental revision of the structures for assisting return to work, and financial support for those not yet able to return, prompted more interest in alternatives. The needs for change have been well presented in two recent documents [2, 3]. The mood now is to encourage early intervention with good multi-agency involvement. The remainder of this chapter will illustrate current and projected provision, and conclude with analysis of how far the current aims listed above have been, or will be, realised.

Insurance companies

Accident and Health Insurance is not compulsory in the UK, nor does "no-fault" compensation exist. Some employers include subscription to private insurance companies as a benefit of employment, but in most cases clients have to make their own decisions to take out insurance, and pay their own premiums.

Traditionally companies dealing with accident insurance have had little impact in the health insurance market; the reverse is also true. This distinction is perhaps blurring to a degree, particularly with mergers between some large insurance companies, but it is convenient to report the two kinds of insurance separately.

In the case of accident insurance, the most usual form of compensation would be lump sum payment for specific injuries. Thus companies may specify the amount the policy would return for a limb fracture, loss of an eye, death, etc. The scale of payment probably bears relationship less to the severity of the injury than to the financial consequences – loss of income, costs of care, etc. Thus the return for death may be less than an impediment leading to life-long disability with high care requirements. To this, some policies would add additional amounts for time spent in hospital, and, in some cases, a contribution towards loss of income. For the majority of claims, the only evidence required of entitlement to claim would be the client's own report, and, often, a report from the attending medical practitioner. Where accident policies cover loss of income, however, more detailed information may be sought where the injury is likely to result in long-term inability to work.

Although private medical costs to treat the injury may be included in the policy, in practice this is less common, partly because the client injured in the UK is almost certainly entitled to free treatment under the National Health Service. Strictly, injuries arising from motor vehicle accidents are outwith the scope of the National Health Service, which may charge costs to the injured person's insurer. In fact the normal recompense is an agreed fee paid by the insurer to the NHS, not to the client. This is often a standard amount unrelated to the complexity of treatment; in practice, Audit Commission reports have drawn attention to the fact that many hospitals do not claim from insurance companies as often as they could. The limitation of NHS treatment does not apply to other forms of accident, solely motor vehicle accidents.

Health Insurance, whilst sometimes paying out lump sums for specific illnesses, is more likely to reimburse health costs for the client suffering from an illness which is covered under the scheme. This may well include private medical costs, or, if the client is treated in NHS hospital, an allowance per day spent in hospital (within the limits of the policy).

Such coverage is not necessarily comprehensive. Policies may exclude specified diseases (e.g. dementia, or some progressive diseases), and may well not cover treatment for conditions pre-existing before insurance cover was taken out – or at any rate only covering pre-existing illnesses with special policies or additional premiums. Some workers however feel that this type of scheme may allow greater choice of when to undergo elective treatment, which can thus be planned to minimize disruption to work or lifestyle. This is one of the reasons why employers may choose to purchase insurance for their staff. Another is that, where a wait for relevant investigations or treatment is prolonging an employee's absence from work, health insurance may be able to purchase these interventions from a private health care supplier, hopefully aiding an earlier return to work.

In this respect, insurance companies are contributing to vocational rehabilitation, but historically there has been no clearer link between insurance schemes and rehabilitation than that. This may now be changing – clearly it should be of particular importance for companies offering income support during absence from work to try to assist the client's return to work if possible. Whereas previously one of the main vehicles for this assistance was by sponsoring appropriate research, some companies are now trying more directly to be involved in their clients' rehabilitation. Whilst the main impetus for this may be efficient claims management, in practice the client may benefit considerably from such an approach. This is discussed in more detail below.

There may be difficulty in identifying which clients need this type of intervention. Studies have been done trying to identify accident insurance clients who would benefit most from vocational rehabilitation, but, although tools are available for this, they may only be reliably applicable after prolonged absence from work. This problem was recognized in the current early intervention Job Retention Pilots, which are described below. Although these are sponsored by government and not insurance companies, one of the aims is to develop an assessment tool separating those who would probably return to work early in any event, and those who would require specific additional assistance to achieve this. It is likely, if the aim is accomplished, that the tool would be of assistance to insurance companies also.

Many employers take out Employers' Liability insurance. In the context of workers injured in the course of their job, a claim against this insurance may result. If successful, this will also result in financial compensation for the employee. These insurance companies may also be interested in ways of increasing return to work.

Thus although the link between insurance reimbursement for injury or illness and vocational rehabilitation has been weak in the past, there is considerable interest in strengthening the link in the future.

Compensation for loss of earnings

Provision for loss of earnings is a combination of state and employers' responsibilities. Most employed people would have a varying amount of "sickness pay" entitlement as part of their employment. Thus, short-term absences would normally receive their normal basic pay. In most cases, entitlement for this for the first seven days is based on the employee self-certifying that their absence is due to sickness, but longer periods require medical certification; normally provided by the worker's family practitioner. There has been interest recently in whether these doctors are best placed to make this determination – both from a training point of view, and a potential conflict of interest [5] – and recently mass media have suggested that many such certificates are provided on flimsy grounds [6]. It is for this reason that the Department of Work and Pensions (DWP) is investigating alternative methods of certification using trained practitioners, or perhaps allied health professionals [3]. Entitlement to employers' sick pay is usually time-limited, with the duration often depending on length of service with the company. When this has expired, or in the case of employees who have no employers' scheme available, the state benefit, Statutory Sick Pay, becomes the method of financial assistance. To receive this, claimants must be unfit for their own work. The same certification system as that of the employers' sick pay is used, but Statutory Sick Pay in many cases would yield a smaller financial amount. After a maximum of 28 weeks on this, if the employee remains absent on sickness grounds, they may transfer to a longer term benefit, Incapacity Benefit. Depending on the worker's circumstances these may be more beneficial than Statutory Sick Pay. Incapacity benefit, however, is a contributory benefit, dependent on the claimant having paid sufficient National Insurance contributions previously. Those who have not may claim Income support. The normal length of time on Statutory Sick Pay before Incapacity Benefit is shortened in cases of terminal illness, and some other specified conditions, where the claimants may proceed directly onto Incapacity Benefit. Those receiving Incapacity Benefit may also receive certain other benefits and entitlements, such as Disability Living Allowance (DLA).

The most common causes of requiring Incapacity Benefit are Mental Health Issues, or musculo-skeletal painful complaints [2, 3, 7]. Critics of the existing certification system point out that these are areas which often depend on the patient's self-report of symptoms, with formal objective signs being less prominent than in some other forms of illness. It is this point, and the well-recognized variability of symptoms such as chronic pain or anxiety, that has called into question the validity of the current certification system. Typically, requests for such certificates are based on a very brief interview and examination, albeit that a face-to-face contact with the certifying practitioner is mandatory. Guidance has been issued on certifying [8], but it is uncertain if this has changed matters greatly.

Whilst many of those who start to receive Incapacity Benefit expect to return to work within a year, in practice many do not, and for those who remain on Incapacity Benefit for one year, the prospect of return to work within five years is poor, with only twenty per cent achieving that [3]. Much effort and investigation therefore is now addressing the issues of preventing people entering a "long-term dependency" situation; and of identifying the reasons causing long-term continuation on Incapacity Benefit. Some of these are undoubtedly clinical, and the potential for Health Service treatment to reduce these factors within a timescale to avoid a prolonged period of Incapacity Benefit, is receiving attention [2]. Some, however, are cultural, social or financial [5, 9]. Claimants may fear that if they try to take a job, or even seek one, which they then find they cannot maintain, they may lose their entitlement to Incapacity Benefit; they are unlikely to qualify for more than a short period of employers' sickness pay due to a short duration of service with that firm; and thus may only have recourse to benefits with a lower financial reward for a further six months. Thus there is a legitimate feeling that they cannot risk trying to return to work unless they have considerable confidence of maintaining this [3, 10].

Recognizing this perverse incentive, there are a number of work trial schemes available within the Work Preparation, and Job Introduction, schemes of the DWP, under which the employee can maintain their Incapacity Benefit whilst attempting to return to work. Travelling expenses to and from work can be another disincentive, and under work trial schemes, these may be reclaimable also. Thus the intention is to ensure that the worker is not disadvantaged by a work trial. Such schemes are also useful in encouraging employers to give a trial of employment to the worker, as the employer may have assistance for salary costs. After a period of time (up to 13 weeks), if the trial is successful, the worker then returns to normal salary and ceases claiming benefit, with both the employer and the employee having confidence in the situation working in the longer term. Job Introduction schemes are predicted to help 3,000 people per year [3]. It is probably true that schemes such as this are not known about by workers who might take advantage of them, employers, and certifying practitioners.

Recognizing this, and in attempts to look at and deal with other perverse incentives, the DWP is proposing a number of other measures to try and assist earlier return to work. Many of these measures, such as work-focussed interviews, are considered below. Employers are also being encouraged to review their policies towards their workers who have been absent for a considerable time, and introduce earlier interventions to try to assist return to work before their employee becomes eligible for Incapacity Benefit – in other words, at a time when work habits and a culture of attending work are likely to be maintained.

As explained in the introduction to this chapter, the criteria for entitlement to Incapacity Benefit have also been revised. Recognizing that what may be a somewhat cursory examination by the claimant's family practitioner is insufficient for such a potentially expensive benefit as Incapacity Benefit, an "All Work Test" was introduced [4]. This was a self-report questionnaire, concentrating on whether the claimant was not only unfit to return to their previous work, but also unfit for any reasonable work. It concentrated on functional activities. In selected cases, the claimant would also be examined by a medical practitioner employed by the Benefits Agency.

This has now changed. In the early stages of absence, the client is required to satisfy an "Own Occupation Test": i.e., can they return to their previous work? If proceeding to Incapacity Benefit, they undergo a "Personal Capability Test"; this examines not only fitness for their own work, but also other employment possibilities. The Personal Capability Test addresses both functional impairment and mental stress. It is not intended to identify those incapable of any work, but rather those in whom it is not reasonable to insist that they seek work. It is administered by DWP staff (including medical practitioners in those cases requiring examination). Those who satisfy the test remain on Incapacity Benefit, but those who do not are required to transfer to Job-seekers' Allowance. Although some concerns have been expressed regarding this process [10]. In general this has been accepted, partly since these clients will continue to receive specific support in seeking a job. A Capability Assessment is expected to aid their Job Centre Plus adviser to discuss future possibilities. The clients also will be eligible for New Deal Initiatives immediately, schemes designed to give unemployed people special assistance in regaining work.

The UK does not have a direct equivalent of the Workers' Compensation Schemes present in many countries. Those suffering injury are therefore treated in the same way as those absent through illness, unless the injury or illness was caused as a result of their work. If the latter is true, they may be entitled to Industrial Injuries Benefit, described below.

Insurance companies have a rôle to a degree in compensation for loss of earnings. Such schemes are voluntary, but may be taken up most frequently by self-employed people. Membership of schemes aimed at private medical treatment may provide some loss of earnings compensation, but income protection policies, paying in the event of sickness or injury resulting in prolonged absence from work, are the main vehicle of this type of payment. Schemes may include a deferral of payment so that entitlement only commences after employers' sickness pay schemes end, for example. Since most workers return to work during the duration of employers' sick pay, the number of potential claims is therefore reduced, resulting ultimately in lower premiums for the members of the schemes. Entitlement to compensation under these schemes normally rests on reports from medical practitioners attending the ill claimant.

Finally, in some cases there may be legal claims taken out by workers who feel that their injury (or occasionally illness) has been caused by acts or omissions of their employer. The UK does not enjoy the "no-fault" compensation for injury schemes prevalent in some countries, and a claimant's redress under this heading relies on litigation. This requires proving fault of another party, and is inevitably adversarial to a degree. Where liability is proven, sums awarded can seem large, although the intention of the process is merely to return the parties financially to the state they would have enjoyed had their career not been interrupted. However most awards come in the form of a lump sum, which may be invested to produce income. Some "structured settlements" are now appearing, where a more detailed long term scheme of regular payments is preferred. This depends on precise functional assessments. Unfortunately, media headlines highlighting large single awards may encourage other claimants to pursue litigation, which is frequently protracted. This may impact on their ability to benefit from rehabilitation, and is thought by many to mitigate against return to work. Conversely, for some very severely injured people, legal settlement may aid rehabilitation [11]. In cases where liability is agreed but quantum of claim is not yet established, it would be regarded as good practice by experienced personal injury lawyers to seek interim payments to provide necessary care, relief, or equipment for the claimant, and in some cases to purchase rehabilitation [2, 11]. As well as assisting the claimant, this process will in some cases reduce the need for longer-term costs by providing timely intervention, and thus lessen the amount of the claim to the party held liable. In best circumstances interaction between the claimant's solicitor and services providing rehabilitation can prove beneficial to all concerned [11].

We turn now to longer term pensions for those unable to return to work.

Disability Pensions

Disability "pensions" as such may be provided by employers' superannuation schemes, private insurance schemes, or state provision.

Employers' superannuation schemes vary, but in the majority of cases the employee and employer both contribute to a fund from which the employee can draw, either at retirement on the grounds of age, or if they are unable to continue working due to disability or illness. The extent of the pension due will in some cases be linked to the salary of the employee at the point where they cease to be able to work, but in others will pay amounts linked to the size of the accrued fund. The former arrangement is becoming less common, as pension funds are challenged by increasing demands at a time of low investment income.

A typical arrangement would be that an employee who becomes sick will, for a time, receive full salary, following which there may be a period of reduced salary before salary ceases. If it becomes clear that return to work is permanently unlikely, the employee will seek retirement "on medical grounds". There will usually be medical evidence presented, perhaps gathered by an Occupational Medicine Physician, to determine whether this is an appropriate course to follow, before medical retirement is confirmed. It has been pointed out that "retirement on medical grounds" is in some cases a misnomer – individuals with similar levels of disability will not necessarily all opt for, or be awarded, medical retirement. Factors such as the age of the client, their financial circumstances, and their diagnosis, affect the decision, as does their personal motivation to return to work. The decision of the examining physician is likely to be influenced also in that for those who wish to return to work, there will probably be at least an initial examination of ways in which that may be enabled; but that is less likely in cases where no such desire is apparent. Clearly this depends on the extent of the disability; in many cases the decision may be obvious, but it is in the marginal cases that factors other than disability are relevant. Where the assessment is carried out by an Occupational Medicine Physician the practitioner will have to consider both the desires of the employee and the needs of the employer to reach a fair and correct assessment.

For many employers, the form of this assessment is not specified. Matters may be addressed more formally in certain occupations, e.g. the armed forces, or civilian air crew. Formal standards also may be used when jobs involve driving, especially public service or large freight vehicles. In some occupations, disability pensions may involve not just a monetary award, but also access to other benefits or services – the most obvious example is that of a pension due to injury during active military service.

For those who do not have such a scheme, some will have income protection insurance as a private scheme. This follows the standard model of an insurance scheme with regular premium payment, with, in return, provision of a pension by reason of permanent inability to work. Again, some form of medical assessment and certification is required to access this provision. Insurance companies have recognised that permanent absence from work, and consequent payment of the pension, may be avoided by vocational rehabilitation [11]. Thus some firms have appointed rehabilitation counsellors, or case managers, to work with those clients who have a potential claim to explore whether any alternative options are available. These case managers, after assessment, may decide to purchase retraining, treatment, or equipment from private suppliers. Although the principal aim is to reduce the potential claims, nevertheless it is clearly of advantage to the claimant to have the benefit of this assessment.

What of the state provision? To some extent this overlaps with the benefits payable to disabled people irrespective of their previous employment. Thus, Disabled Living Allowance incorporates components for mobility and self-care. This is paid in a series of tiers (three for the care component, two for mobility), meant to represent increasing severity of disability. Assessment for these is primarily by a self-report questionnaire but detailed medical information is sought in a proportion of cases, and a few clients are called for specific examination by medical staff working for the DWP. This has recently become much more standardised, with formal training being given to the examining doctors in disability assessment. Many are encouraged to obtain a specific diploma (the Diploma in Disability Assessment Medicine), which incorporates knowledge of the functional consequences of illness or injury, and familiarity with many standardised assessment tools. The intention of this more rigorous approach is to give confidence that decisions on entitlement to benefits are based on a consistent process: but there is no doubt that this has been perceived as attempting to force disabled people back to work by withdrawing, or reducing, their benefits.

DLA awards also act as a gatekeeper to certain other financial benefits. For example, payments from the Independent Living Fund – which exists to pay for sufficient personal assistance to allow very severely disabled people to continue living in their own homes or tenancies – are only available to those receiving the highest tier of DLA, representing the most severely disabled individuals.

In addition to DLA, disability or illness resulting from accidents at work, or occupational-associated illness, may result in payments under the Industrial Injuries Benefit Scheme. Here, disability – in reality, impairment – is assessed medically, and a "percentage disability" awarded on the basis of a Table of Maims. As in most systems using a Table of Maims, this ensures considerable consistency in awards for the impairments specified in the Table, but appreciable difficulties in estimating the disability of those not specified. Other benefits overlap with those described above. Certain prescribed occupational diseases, such as pneumoconiosis, occupational deafness, or vibration white finger, are also compensated by this benefit.

Thus disability pensions come from a variety of sources, which are assessed by differing techniques, some of more rigour than others, and which vary in the extent to which quantum of pension is related to severity of disability.

Responsibility for Vocational Rehabilitation

Responsibility for vocational rehabilitation primarily belongs to the State, although often commercial or non-profit making organizations are contracted to provide this. Several Government departments, however, are involved in this.

The point of contact for an individual requiring vocational rehabilitation after sickness or injury could be either a medical consultation, (usually with their family practitioner, but sometimes a hospital specialist), or the employment agencies, an arm of the Department of Work and Pensions (DWP). In either case, once a problem is recognised, cases may be referred to an agency providing vocational rehabilitation, but the more probable consequence for the majority will be an interview with the Disability Employment Advisor (DEA). These individuals are linked to Job Centres and Job Centre Plus whose primary users are those unemployed. These centres exist both for finding new employment opportunities, and to deal with benefits to support unemployed people.

Disability Employment Advisors will try to consider the options for the sick person. Do they need advice on job-seeking skills? Can they return to their previous occupation? Do they need to make adjustments to their pattern of work? Sometimes the DEA will liaise with prospective or previous employers.

The DEA has several options available to assist the client. If it is felt that further assessment is required, the client may be referred to other members of the Employment Disability Services, still an arm of the same Department. Assessments here could include psychology, or practical tests, partly aimed at identifying residual capacity, but also intended to decide on adaptations or assistance necessary to allow a return to work. This will inevitably entail liaison with employers, but where equipment needs to be purchased to maintain employments (e.g. a wheelchair, or perhaps equipment to allow computer access), the DWP may fund this through the "Access to Work" scheme. Access to Work benefits could also include transport to work, or the costs of a support worker. Although the Disability Discrimination Act (1995) lays a responsibility on employers of a certain size to make reasonable adjustments to enable the worker to continue employment, the DEA service may again be involved in facilitating this.

What if the assessment reveals that return to previous work, or the previous employer, is impracticable? If the client is deemed to be ready to return to suitable work, but that requires a different employer, the DWP staff will attempt to assist the client to find a suitable placement. Alternatively Work Preparation Schemes, or more prolonged vocational training may be recommended – this is likely to be purchased from a contracted independent agency, and in some cases may be residential. The agency will attempt to retrain the client for a different vocation where appropriate and in many cases provide counselling to assist in adaptation to different possibilities. Again, identification of goals and strengths is an important component of the work. Many will also assist in the eventual re-introduction to work, by providing support or possibly job coaching.

This describes the pattern for many of those who require vocational assistance. However, many small agencies exist to provide much more intensive assistance for particularly disadvantaged clients, e.g. those who have never worked, or been out of the labour market for some years. Other agencies may have particular interest in challenging diagnostic groups, such as acquired brain injury. Many of these problems are of course similar to those who have long-term unemployment or issues other than disability. Often the needs here may include pre-vocational issues, dealing perhaps with issues of confidence and social competence in some cases, or mental health issues in others. Clients with these sorts of difficulties may need assistance in job-seeking skills, such as writing applications and preparation for interviews, at least as much as specific adaptations for their impairment. Some of the work done in this area will not be funded by the DWP, but rather by grant-funding for particular charitable projects.

Some clients will continue to require supported employment, particularly those with complex needs. The WORKSTEP programme is available for this, and supports around 25000 people. Some later progress to open employment.

In recent years, there has been increased focus on those in Incapacity Benefit. Reviews of recipients of this benefit now take the form of a "work-focussed interview", aiming to establish reasons behind the continuation of incapacity and possibilities of re-employment. Although such interviews are not necessarily performed by officials with knowledge of disability, if issues relating to disability are identified, this may be a further source of referral to the Disability Employment Services. Recent Government initiatives intend to increase the approach of "job-focussed interviews", applying these more widely and at an earlier stage, before a pattern of long-term absence from work has been established. Pilot schemes are proposed whereby the first interview will be about eight weeks after the claim, and 4-5 regular reviews will follow. The aim is to keep the likelihood of return to work prominent in the minds of the client and those assisting him or her, and examine how and when to proceed with that. Participation in the interviews will be mandatory, but clients with very severe disabilities will be exempt unless they request an interview [3]. An action plan will be developed at the interview, but other activity will be voluntary.

There can be financial disincentives in returning to work. The schemes above, together with a Working Tax Credit, are expected to result in financial gains for those transferring to work from Incapacity Benefit in over 90% of cases. Job Grants for one-off expenses of starting employment, and continuation of some benefits until the first pay is received, should also ease clients' concerns over leaving benefit, together with guarantees that leaving a failed work trial will lead to re-instatement of previous benefits without a qualifying period [3, 10].

DWP also proposes other important initiatives in developing teams of advisers specifically trained to assist disabled people in seeking work by consolidating the skills of the DEA, benefits advisers, and New Deal Advisers. Welcome new thrusts include proposals, now being piloted, to establish short-term programmes combining work-focussed support (from DWP) and health focussed rehabilitation (from the NHS) – a move to remedy the dislocation of these agencies discussed in the introduction to this chapter.

Another major involvement in Vocational Rehabilitation comes from occupational Health Schemes. Rather than a Government Agency, these services are employed by, or contracted to, employers. Part of their rôle frequently will be review of employees of the company who have been absent from work often or for a certain period. These reviews may identify issues requiring further medical treatment or investigation – e.g. a worker awaiting imaging of an injury before treatment can be planned. Occupational Medicine practitioners will liaise with the employee's medical advisors in this instance, or they may initiate specialist referral (normally in consultation with the client's family medical practitioner) to deal with problems causing absence from work. Unfortunately, the National Health Service is not always organized in a way that allows rapid access to investigation or treatment for conditions which are not urgent on health (rather than vocational) grounds [11]. Access to private care for the employee, on the advice of the Occupational Health Service, may sometimes then be in the best interests of the employer.

The crucial importance of intervening early is increasingly recognized [11, 12]. The concept of "Work Instability" [13] may be important here in identifying those who require intervention to prevent them moving from employment to long-term sickness absence.

Employers' responsibilities are being stressed [2, 3, 14], as active sickness management plans have shown improvements in return to work. Health services are being challenged to consider questions of return to work early in treatment [15].

A further task for Occupational Health lies in assessing the requirements of the job in question and matching this with the employee's residual capacities. Detailed vocational capability testing and ergonomic assessments, are perhaps less widely available than is desirable; but some major companies have made arrangements to buy such assessments, from University Departments, for example. The Occupational Health practitioner, with knowledge of the employee's health and capacity, and the job's requirements, is then likely to be well placed to advise the employer on how to facilitate the employee's return to work, where this is possible.

Although this chapter has detailed processes which are available, nevertheless many, perhaps the majority, of those who become unable to work because of illness or accident do not undergo any serious attempt at Vocational Rehabilitation. This may well be because the practitioners dealing with the disability condition concentrate on treatment of that, without consideration of the consequences for employment. Since those most often responsible for certifying sickness absence are most frequently the family practitioners, there may be a conflict of interest between their desire to accede to the patient's request for sickness absence, and their function as certifying and, in a sense, legitimising this absence. Training schemes have now been put in place to address this problem, including a "web-based" approach.

Another acknowledgement of the necessity for early intervention is a series of Job retention pilots. Funded by the DWP and the Department of Health, these are essentially large scale research exercises into determining the most effective methods of helping people return to work quickly. Participants are randomised to receive workplace based interventions, health interventions, or a combination of these; there is also a control group. Results will not be available for some time, but anecdotal accounts of successes with these programmes are emerging. Participation in the schemes is voluntary, however, and recruitment has been slower than anticipated – perhaps a reflection of the low expectations amongst employees, employers, and health practitioners that assistance with return to work would be available.

Conclusion

Thus vocational rehabilitation is available through the initiatives of a number of agencies, and, at its best, can provide well managed effective programmes – albeit that there may be issues of the amount of service available. There is serious consideration of the ways that DWP, the NHS, and the independent sector can co-operate, to produce a better-linked process and challenge the sequential model of "treatment then work" so prevalent currently. Much has been done, but we started from a low base. Disabled people, employers, trade unions, and insurance companies have agreed that we need to research what works; and it is acknowledged that considerable training is needed if all the initiatives listed are to succeed. However, currently the vast majority of those absent from work on grounds of sickness have no contact with any vocational assistance. Perhaps, therefore, the greatest needs in vocational rehabilitation in the UK, however, lie in the education of health professionals, employees and employers, in the variety of forms of assistance that are now becoming available, and of the value of timely vocational rehabilitation – and the problems inherent in delaying vocational considerations for too long.

References

1. Grahame R (2002) The decline of rehabilitation srevices and its impact on disability benefits. J R Soc Med 95: 114-7
2. British Society of Rehabilitation Medicine (2003) Vocational rehabilitation – the way forward (2nd Edition): report of a working party (Chair: Frank AO). British Society of Rehabilitation Medicine. London
3. Department for Work and Pensions (2002) Pathways to work: helping people into employment. Department for Work and Pensions, London
4. Benefits Agency (1994) The medical assessment for Incapacity Benefit, Benefits Agency, London
5. Sawney P (2002) Current issues in fitness for work certification. Br J Gen Pract 52: 217-22
6. Cunningham J (2004) Can we cure the "sickie" culture of workers pretending to be ill? The Herald, 2 May 2004, 14. Newsquest (Herald and Times Ltd), Glasgow
7. Disler PB, Pallant JF (2001) Vocational rehabilitation: everybody gains if injured workers are helped back into work. Br Med J 323: 121-3
8. Benefits Agency (2000) Medical evidence for Statutory Sick Pay, Statutory Maternity Pay, and Social Security Incapacity Benefit purposes. A guide for registered medical practitioners. Benefits Agency, London
9. Allaire SH, Anderson JJ, Meenan RF (1996) Reducing work disability associated with rheumatoid arthritis: identification of additional risk factors and persons likely to benefit from intervention. Arthritis Care Res 9: 349-57
10. Department for Work and Pensions (2003) Pathways to work: helping people into employment – the Government's response and action plan. Department for Work and Pensions, London
11. Association of British Insurers, Trades Union Congress (2002) Getting back to work. A rehabilitation discussion paper. ABI/TUC, London
12. Frank AO, Sawney P (2003) Vocational rehabilitation. J R Soc Med 96: 522-4
13. Gilworth G, Chamberlain MA, Harvey A et al. (2003) Development of a work instability scale for rheumatoid arthritis. Arthritis Rheum 49: 349-54
14. Frank AO, Chamberlain MA (2001) Keeping our patients at work: implications for the management of those with rheumatoid arthritis and musculoskeletal conditions. Rheumatology 40: 1201-5

Vocational rehabilitation in Finland

H. Alaranta

Introduction

Rehabilitation of disabled persons and persons with impaired functional capacity is provided in Finland by a wide range of sectors such as workplaces/occupational health care, public health care, the Social Insurance Institution, earnings-related employment pension scheme, accident and traffic insurance, and labour administration [1, 2]. Cooperation between these systems on both local and national levels is strengthened by a separate piece of legislation on cooperation between rehabilitation legislation.

Workplaces/occupational health care

In the case of employed persons, the workplace is in a key position in the assessment of rehabilitation needs. The occupational health care system is often the first to see the employees in need of rehabilitation. The need is detected in conjunction with occupational health care services, such as workplace surveys, health examinations and absenteeism follow-ups. Surveys can also be initiated by occupational safety delegates, colleagues or superiors who see that an employee is finding it increasingly difficult to perform his duties.

The duty of occupational health care is to monitor the work performance of an employee who has become disabled on account of illness or some other impairment and, if necessary, to refer him/her for treatment or rehabilitation. That way the occupational health care sector can identify rehabilitation needs at an early phase.

Public health care

Early rehabilitation needs may be identified by child welfare counselling clinics or by school health care staffs. Guidance is provided for pupils in respect of diseases or other impairments restricting their performance. Secondary schools provide counselling to create the necessary capabilities required by the pupils´ individual study programmes or career plans. Schools and the public health care system work together to design education, training and rehabilitation plans for individual pupils. Student health care then revises these plans or designs new study and rehabilitation plans together with the student counsellors and teachers at the educational institution in question.

There are rehabilitation teams at health care centres whose main concern are the chronically sick and those suffering from sequelae of serious diseases or impairments. Customers requesting occupational rehabilitation surveys are referred to the vocational guidance services provided by employment offices. The process may also be initiated by drawing up a statement concerning vocational rehabilitation needs for the Social Insurance Institution or an insurance institution.

Social Insurance Institution

The duty of the Social Insurance Institution (SII) is to chart a person´s vocational rehabilitation needs and prospects. This must take place at the latest when a daily allowance has been paid for 60 days under the Sickness Insurance Act. The SII also assesses rehabilitations needs in conjunction with other social insurance benefits, such as reimbursement for medicine costs, disability allowance and unemployment benefits. The initiative can be taken by the person him/herself or cooperation parties such as public health care, social welfare or labour administration authorities. The need for a survey is assessed case by case by each local office of the SII.

In order to identify vocational rehabilitation needs and prospects, the SII arranges for rehabilitation examinations and work and training tryouts to be carried out by rehabilitation examination institutions and occupational clinics. A rehabilitation need assessment is an expert evaluation of rehabilitation prospects and of any need for more extensive examination.

The SII carries the cost of examinations, and the person´s subsistence is safeguarded with a rehabilitation allowance during the examination period.

Earnings-related employment pension scheme

Rehabilitation provided under the employment pension scheme is discretionary for all: the private sector, local authorities and the State. Therefore, the rehabilitation process is always based on the discretion of the pension institution in question.

In the employment pension scheme, vocational rehabilitation needs are identified in conjunction with pension applications or on the basis of an initiative taken by either the person involved or an outside party. When a person applies for a pension, it is usually fairly late with a view to starting a rehabilitation process, since the employee´s health and weak motivation set restrictions at this stage.

To get the rehabilitation process starting sufficiently early, the employee him/herself should ensure that the rehabilitation need is identified as soon as he/she finds that work performance is endangered by health problems. The need for rehabilitation can also be determined at the workplace, as was pointed out in the section on occupational health care.

Rehabilitation under the employment pension can begin when an employee´s health undergoes a long-term or permanent change weakening his/her work performance. The rehabilitation need can be assessed as soon as symptoms suggesting diminished work performance are detected. Not only health but also, factors such as burnout, stress, aging and "pension risk" must all be taken into account. If full identification of vocational rehabilitation needs and opportunities calls for a more detailed survey, a separate rehabilitation examination or a work or training try out period can be arranged by either the employment pension institutions or The Insurance Rehabilitation Association in conjunction with the rehabilitation process.

The employment pension institution in question carries the cost of the measures taken and sees to the customer´s subsistence security in the form of a rehabilitation allowance.

Accident and traffic insurance

Rehabilitation is provided on the basis of accident or traffic insurance when the need for rehabilitation is caused by an occupational accident entitling compensation, an occupational disease or traffic accident. Such rehabilitation is based on the principle of compensation and overrides other rehabilitation systems. As long as the terms laid down in the legislation on rehabilitation based on accident or traffic insurance are met, an injured patient has subjective right to rehabilitation.

If an impairment entitling a person to compensation causes long-term restriction on that person´s working capacity and opportunities for earning his living, the insurance institution is obliged to take immediate action on its own initiative to start the vocational rehabilitation process and to see to rehabilitation need surveys and the referral for rehabilitation. In assessing the need for a rehabilitation survey, attention must be paid to the nature of the impairment or disease, the restrictions it sets on working capacity and functional ability, loss of earnings, duration or threat of invalidity and handicap, as well as the age of the person concerned.

The initiative to start a vocational rehabilitation process can also be taken by the injured person, his/her employer, a health care unit, a manpower authority or some other party involved in evaluating the rehabilitation situation. The suggestion to start vocational rehabilitation is normally sent by the insurance institution to The Insurance Rehabilitation Association, which plans and implements rehabilitation programmes (Fig. 1). Insurance institutions must consider setting the assessment process in motion at the latest when the incapacity for work has lasted 120 days.

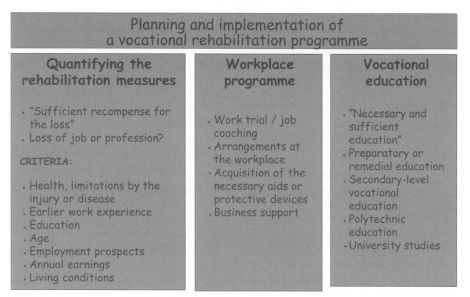

Fig. 1 – The Insurance Rehabilitation Association.

Where the identification of vocational rehabilitation needs and opportunities calls for more detailed surveys, separate rehabilitation examinations or work or training try out periods can be arranged by The Insurance Rehabilitation Association, with the insurance institutions carrying the cost of the measures and safeguarding the customer´s subsistence security in the form of a full-scale loss-of-earnings allowance.

Labour administration

Within the framework of the labour administration, either the customer or an involved official can take the initiative in identifying the rehabilitation need. The necessity to identify rehabilitation needs may emerge in connection with any type of employment services: the job placement service, vocational guidance, labour market training for adults and vocational information service and vocational rehabilitation services.

Vocational guidance has a central role. Its purpose is to use the interactive relationship between the customer and vocational guidance psychologist to help the individual customer to begin systematic, vocational planning and to carry out it. A person may need vocational guidance at any phase of his/her life, but in particular on completing his/her education and training, or when disease or some other impairment changes his/her life situation. The vocational guidance provided for disabled pupils takes place in close cooperation with the school´s health care staff and student counsellor.

Rehabilitation staff training

The rehabilitation staff consists of employees with a wide range of basic education, in the course of which each specializes in a certain sector of vocational rehabilitation or employment. The basic education must guarantee sufficient information on various forms of disability and their restrictive effects, as well as the support services available. Further training will be required as the service systems are elaborated.

The central principles in rehabilitation are cooperation and customer-orientation. Acquiring skills for these calls for work experience and cross-sectoral complementary training closely linked with the work in question. Cooperation means that the rehabilitation staff work with the customer to evaluate the situation, set mutually approved goals and take decisions together.

Complementary education should pay particular attention to the following skills:

– communication with the customer and other employees;
– the ability to solve problems in one´s own work and team;
– mastery of the group process and various teamwork models;
– interprofessional cooperation and negotiation skills;
– creation of a favourable and encouraging atmosphere;
– self-evaluation.

The need to include customers on equal terms in multiprofessional teams calls not only for cognitive training and skills on the part of professions but also for attitude training. Their training must therefore comprise long periods devoted to improving skills in which training events and independent study alternate.

It is particularly important to be able to understand the way other professions represented on work teams think and speak. Customer-oriented approaches require staff to see the customer´s entire life situation through his eyes. Training must provide the means to do this. Complementary training must further provide the skills required for working in multiprofessional teams and for genuinely customer-oriented work.

Complementary training has been provided by various organisations providing rehabilitation services and by universities and their further education centres. Training has enhanced the professional skills required in rehabilitation and clarified the theoretical foundation and framework of values involved.

Customer-oriented cooperation

Cooperation is often required between various authorities and rehabilitation parties in devising and implementing an individual rehabilitation programme. The legislation on rehabilitation creates the framework for local, regional and national cooperation. The cooperation organs of local authorities and of various rehabilitation organisations discuss principles related to the division of labour and cooperation and try to solve the problems of individual rehabilitation customers.

The most important form of cooperation in the view of the person undergoing rehabilitation and his/her entire rehabilitation process, however, takes place outside official teams in the normal interaction that all the rehabilitation workers experience in their daily work. The development of those cooperation and better customer-orientation call for new work models. In situations where the customer´s problems require simultaneous measures by a number of service systems, cross-sectoral cooperation networks should be established case by case, to establish a better tailored approach. This requires adoption of a new work culture in many organisations, since their basic purpose does not necessarily encourage cross-administrative action. The threshold to active participation in decisions concerning one´s own life should be as low as possible. The lower the threshold, the better the chances that the rehabilitation programme will succeed. Efficient customer-oriented cooperation requires clear rules of the game between the rehabilitation experts and commitment to the solutions agreed on.

Report on rehabilitation of the Council of State to the parliament

In the year of 2002 the Council of State handed in a report on rehabilitation to the parliament. Maintaining working capacity has been an important aim for rehabilitation policy. As employment pension legislation is revised the importance of the occupationally-oriented rehabilitation is emphasised. The occupationally-oriented rehabilitation of handicapped and disabled persons has been taken into account through improvements in the rights to rehabilitation allowance and work activity that support employment and by eliminating social security regulations that prevent employment.

Future challenges are to be found in maintaining the working capacity of the ageing workforce, maintaining the functional capacity of the older population, beginning rehabilitation at an early enough state, developing a multi-professional working group and in increased research on the effect of rehabilitation [3].

Today and tomorrow: Healthy at Work project

Healthy at Work is an extensive cooperation project, the objective of which is to promote such activities in the Finnish society that support employees to continue in the labour market and their ability to cope with their work by means of training and information.

The project provides information about rehabilitation within the statutory earnings-related persons scheme, the rehabilitation reform within in 2004 as well as general information about the advantages of continuing in working life.

The project Healthy at Work supports widely accepted efforts to raise the average retirement age by 2-3 years. A special object is also that the rehabilitation policies related to the reform of the statutory earnings-related pensions are put into practice at the workplaces. This presupposes improving cooperation and intensifying the distribution of responsibilities between the parties involved.

The project is backed by the Finnish Pension Alliance TELA and its members. Other central cooperation partners are the labour market organisations, the SII and the Finnish Institute of Occupational Health.

Rehabilitation within the statutory earnings related pension scheme

The rehabilitation which pension institutions in the statutory earnings-related pension schemes provide falls within the scope of vocational rehabilitation, and it applies to employees and self-employed persons who participate permanently in working life. The objective of the rehabilitation within the statutory earnings-related person scheme is that the insured person can remain in working life despite his or her illness.

Rehabilitation within the statutory earnings-related pension scheme is individual and discretionary. In practice, rehabilitation is based on the cooperation between the individual, the workplace, the occupational health care and the pension institution authorised to operate a statutory earnings-related pension scheme.

Rehabilitation legislation since the beginning of the year 2004

There have been changes in the vocational rehabilitation provided by the pension institutions authorised to operate a statutory earning-related pension scheme and the SII at the beginning of 2004.

The reform approved by the Parliament emphasises the primary nature of the vocational rehabilitation in respect to the disability pension. The objective is to support starting vocational rehabilitation so early that disability can be prevented or at least postponed.

With the reform, the insured person will receive the right to vocational rehabilitation

– if they are duly found to be under the threat of losing their work capacity and to have to retire on a disability pension;

– if this threat can be reduced by means of vocational rehabilitation;

– if rehabilitation contributes to reducing pension expenditure.

In future, the insured person can appeal against the rehabilitation decision stating that there is a threat of incapacity for work and whether this threat can be reduced by means of vocational rehabilitation. The actual rehabilitation measures are discretionary also in future.

The definition of the threat on incapacity for work will be the same in all the different acts on the earnings-related pension as well as in the Act on Rehabilitation Services according to which the SII provides rehabilitation. The rehabilitation allowance paid by the SII will be on a level with that provided by the statutory earnings-related pension scheme for all income brackets.

The rehabilitation reform will also increase the flexibility and incentive effect of rehabilitation within the statutory earnings-related pension scheme. According to the new provisions, the rehabilitated person will have the chance of drawing partial rehabilitation allowance.

Acknowledgement

The author is grateful to Rehabilitation Manager Juha Mikkola, Secretary General Heidi Paatero and Dr. Paavo Rissanen for sharing their valuable expertise in vocational rehabilitation.

References

1. Bergeskog A (2001) Labour market policies, strategies and statistics for people with disabilities. A cross-national comparison. IFAU - Office of Labour Market Policy Evaluation. Uppsala 2001: 13
2. Ministry of Social Affairs and Health (1997) From Disability to Ability. National programme of action for vocational rehabilitation and employment of disabled persons. Helsinki, Finland 1997: 5
3. Riipinen M, Hurri H, Alaranta H (1994) Evaluating the outcome of vocational rehabilitation. Scand J Rehab Med 26: 103-12

The French model of vocational rehabilitation
Existing legal plans of action for reimbursement for the deficiency
Plans of action enabling preparation for job retention

J.-M. André, C. Le Chapelain and J. Paysant

The right to work for everyone – and thus for disabled persons – is written into the French constitution. Therefore, the employment and placement of disabled persons forms an element of governmental policy [6, 15]. Complex regulations determine the various measures that aim to favour the guidance, training and professional integration of disabled persons from when they are recognised as "disabled workers"[1]. In these functions, an authority – the Technical Committee for Guidance and Professional Placement[2] – mainly adopts a decision-making role to allow disabled adults to benefit from plans of action, structures and established financial aid. Although the plan of action is available to everyone, the payment methods and, in particular, their financing vary depending on how the deficiency that caused the professional disability arose as a result of or caused by work, or whether it is a deficiency that arose in private life independently of professional activity.

General organisation of vocational rehabilitation in France

Deficiencies resulting from work (accident at work) or caused by work (occupational disease) are reimbursed in a compulsory manner and compensated for by and under monitoring of the state by means of the health insurance system. If they are caused by a third party (e.g. accident at work occurring *en route* caused by a third party and not the insured party), the health insurance company takes court action against the private insurance companies of those responsible.

---

1. "Any salaried employee who is the victim of an accident that results from or is caused by work is declared to be a victim of an accident at work. Any salaried employee who contracts a disease through his/her professional activity is declared to be affected by an occupational disease". Article L411-1 of the Social Security Code.
2. COTOREP.

Deficiencies contracted on the occasion of an affection that arises in the private area are covered by the health insurance system. The latter is frequently completed by mutual benefit societies and private insurances, in particular when the deficiency occurs on the occasion of an event involving third-party responsibility.

In the case of disease, payment is globally less beneficial for the insured party and depends on the contracts he/she was able to take out in a personal capacity.

In 2000, the number of disabled workers was estimated at 219,000[3], which represents an employment rate of 4.10; 223,000 were, incidentally, seeking work[4].

Numerous public and private organisations participate in vocational rehabilitation in a wide range of forms. Depending on the severity of the disability, the obligation to resort to work in a sheltered environment, the type of aid sought and the status, it may or may not be necessary to refer the case to COTOREP. Vocational rehabilitation can be initiated or guaranteed in hospital services and physical medicine and rehabilitation centres that use common (COMETE) or individual codified procedures, in ordinary training centres and in different job retention bodies. It can also be carried out in specific training structures aimed at disabled workers (vocational training centres) and involve work in sheltered environments and in sheltered jobs in an ordinary environment. The general organisation of the professional rehabilitation of disabled persons is represented schematically in Figure 1 [4, 9].

Structures responsible for organising vocational rehabilitation

Technical Committees for Guidance and Professional Placement

The Technical Committees for Guidance and Professional Placement (COTOREPs)[5] bring together all the individuals and institutions of a department with the aim of assessing the disability, suggesting guidance solutions and allocating financial aid. The consultation thereof constitutes an obligatory stage for every disabled adult wishing to benefit from measures aimed at facilitating his/her professional integration.

The committee is made up of[6] 3 departmental councillors, 4 persons of whom at least one is a representative of the National Employment Agency and one company physician, whilst the others are nominated because of their competence in health and social affairs. There is also a person put forward by the departmental service of the National Office of War Veterans and War Victims and a physician who advises Social Security organisations. Other members represent health insurance organisations and organisations that pay

---

3. Source: Ministry of Social Affairs, Labour and Solidarity.
4. Source: ANPE.
5. Created by the Guideline Law no. 75-534 of June 30, 1975.
6. Article D323-1 of the Labour Code.

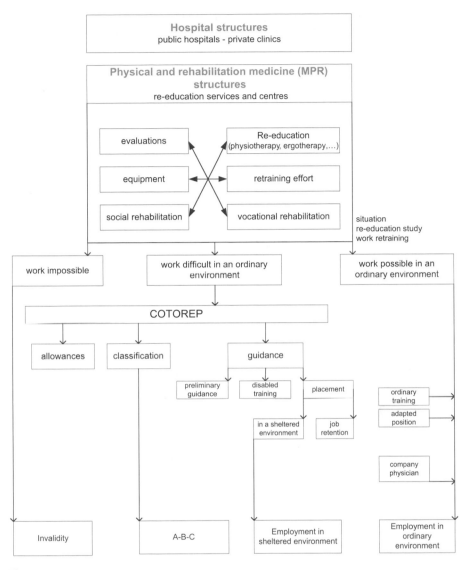

Fig. 1

family benefits, management organisations of vocational re-education centres, sheltered workshops and support centres for work, management organisations of accommodation centres for disabled persons, associations that represent disabled workers, employers' trade union organisations and the most representative salaried employees.

COTOREPs need to undertake a comprehensive overall examination of the situation of each disabled person who is presented to them. This consists of two specialised sections depending on the nature of the decision that needs to be made[7].

---

7. Article D323-3-8 of the Labour Code.

The first section gives a verdict mainly on the ability to work, the recognition of the status of the disabled worker and his/her classification as well as the guidance of the disabled worker. Recognition of the status of the disabled worker depends on the nature and severity of the disability, the qualification of the salaried disabled employee and his/her ability to hold down his/her previous job or any other job. The disability is assessed with regard to employment and not with regard to the medical condition. The disabled worker is guided either towards the ordinary working environment, towards the sheltered working environment, or towards training (apprenticeship, internship, re-education contract in the company). The section also has competence with regard to allocating the placement bonus (after a re-education internship or a professional training internship), the installation subsidiary in the case of pursuing an independent profession, the determination of rates of salary reduction (implemented by the employer on the salary of a disabled worker for whom productivity is reduced).

The second section determines the disability rate of the disabled person, the awarding of the disabled adult subsidy, the compensation allowance for third parties, the accommodation allowance, admission to a specialised establishment if the disability is incompatible with any professional activity and the awarding of the disability card and the disability badge.

Permanent secretary's offices ensure the welcome of and information for disabled persons, their family or representative, the preparation – in collaboration with the technical team – of the files to be submitted at meetings, and guarantee the necessary relationships with competent organisations.

Technical teams study the case submitted to the committee, gather the necessary opinions and present the synthesis of their work to the ruling committee. The disabled person – and if necessary his/her legal representative – is invited to the meeting where the committee examines the request.

A case can be submitted to COTOREP by the disabled person him/herself, his/her parents, his/her legal representatives, the people who are actually responsible, as well as various representatives of the institution that may take on the disabled person.

The decisions are well-founded and subject to periodic revision[8]. The decision needs to specify the period after which it will be revised – this period cannot exceed five years. The notification indicates how to submit for a legal settlement – either by means of submission for an out-of-court settlement before the competent authority or by means of submission to the court of the competent jurisdiction.

COTOREPs do not have any power to impose a decision upon employers with regard to a placement in the ordinary work environment. Its decisions, on the other hand, are imposed on reception establishments designed within the specialist area of which they are authorised to bear the title, namely on organisations that guarantee payments (social security and social aid) and on organisations responsible for paying the various allowances.

---

8. Article L323-11 of the Labour Code.

There are various ways of appealing against decisions that have been made: (i) before the technical Social Security litigation jurisdiction for decisions about establishments or a service combining re-education, placement and reception for disabled adults or with regard to the awarding of disability card allowances; (ii) before the Departmental Committee of Disabled Workers, Disabled Veterans and Those in Similar Categories for appeals relating to decisions on the guidance of a disabled person and the correct measures to assure his/her placement.

Departmental Committees for Special Education

The mission of the Departmental Committees for Special Education (CDES) is to evaluate and guide disabled children (physical, sensory and mental) and to award financial aid to their family (special education allowance (AES) and its complements as well as back-up and adaptation bursaries).

The CDES consists of 12 members, nominated by the "*Préfet*" and represents various departmental administrations and organisations: the ministry responsible for health represented by the Departmental Directorate of Social and Health Affairs (DDASS), the Ministry of National Education, social organisations, private and user organisations (parents of students, association of families of disabled students).

A case can be submitted to the CDES by the parents of the disabled child or by the child's guardians, the health insurance organisation, the payment service of the special allowance, the head of the educational establishment attended, the DDASS and various structures that may take responsibility for the child. The technical team studies the case submitted to the committee, gathers the necessary opinions and presents the synthesis of the work to the section responsible for making the decision. The family of the disabled child – and if necessary his/her legal representative – are invited to the meeting where the committee examines the request. The notification of the decision indicates how to submit for a legal settlement – either by means of submission for an out-of-court settlement before the competent authority or by means of submission to the court of the competent jurisdiction.

The decisions of the CDES apply to educational establishments (ordinary establishments and special educational establishments), payment organisations (national state health insurance office, office for family allowances) and children and their families.

Departmental Committees of Disabled Workers, Disabled Veterans and Those in Similar Categories

They provide their opinion on sector or enterprise settlement projects and rule on disputes regarding authorised salary reductions[9] and disputed COTOREP decisions. Their decisions may be the subject of an appeal to the State Council.

---

9. Article L323-6 of the Labour Code.

Regional Advisory Committees on the Employment and Placement of Disabled Workers

These committees[10], which are connected to the Regional Committee for Professional Training, for Social Promotion and for Employment, express an opinion on the adaptation at a regional level of the measures decided at a national level in favour of disabled persons. They evaluate the measures aiming to create and coordinate public and private initiatives for the creation of sheltered workshops, centres for re-education, rehabilitation, preliminary guidance and professional training. They give a verdict on the coordination of the various structures that are numbered and listed above, on the awareness policies that need to be implemented for heads of business, employers' unions and chambers of commerce and trade with a view to informing them of aid measures (in particular financial) that disabled workers can benefit from[11].

Advisory National Council of Disabled Persons (CNCPH)

It guarantees the participation of disabled persons in the drawing up and implementation of the national solidarity policy that affects them. It has a consulting role in any project, programme or study that is of interest to disabled persons, handles – on its own initiative – any question that relates to the policy concerning such persons and submits an annual report to the Minister of Social Affairs and National Solidarity on the implication of the policy that is of interest to disabled persons.

Higher Council for Professional and Social Placement of Disabled Persons

The mission of this council consists of: (i) promoting public and private initiatives regarding functional rehabilitation, professional re-education, rehabilitation and professional placements, organisation of sheltered work, teaching, education and adaptation to work for disabled adolescents; (ii) combining all the information elements regarding these problems and, in particular, employment possibilities in France and in the French overseas departments and territories (DOM-TOM); (iii) favouring the creation and functioning of research and experimental organisations for treatment and placement; (iv) taking on a consulting role towards public powers for all legislative and regulatory acts concerning disabled persons; (v) guaranteeing through all forms of media appropriate information and a favourable climate for professional placement.

---

10. Defined by article R323-84 of the Labour Code.
11. PLanned by article L323-9 of the Labour Code.

Recognition of the status of the disabled worker

Definition of the disabled worker

Any person is considered to be a "disabled worker whose possibilities of obtaining or maintaining employment have been actually reduced through an insufficiency or a reduction of his/her physical or mental capacities"[12]. With regard to the labour law, only the consequence and not the nature of the disability is decisive, i.e., it applies indiscriminately to physical, motor, sensory, psychological and mental disabilities of all origins.

Recognition and classification

All persons concerned can make a request for recognition of the status of the disabled worker by COTOREP[13]. Depending on the severity of the disability, the person is placed in one of the three following categories: 1) category A: slight and/or temporary disability, 2) category B: moderate and/or lasting disability, 3) category C: severe and definitive disability.

This classification is connected, in particular, to the obligation to hire and to the salary reduction in the case of reduced productivity. Recognition of the status of the disabled worker and the classification connected thereto cannot be legally imposed on the disabled person who remains free to take advantage thereof or not.

Professional guidance of disabled persons

Services and centres for physical medicine and rehabilitation

Although it is at an early stage, a job retention problem can be indicated on the occasion of a stay in a hospital service or a centre for physical medicine and rehabilitation on the initiative of a physician or social assistant. The physician can, with the patient's agreement, inform the company physician and the advisory physician of the Social Security of the hospitalisation and the predictable consequences of the disease or the accident at the origin of this hospitalisation. The patient is informed of the various existing vocational measures – even if, at this stage, the interested party is far removed from concerns of this kind – and certain steps are initiated with the patient.

---

12. Article L323-10 of the Labour Code.
13. Article L323-11 of the Labour Code.

Professional department of services and centres for physical medicine and rehabilitation

Certain centres have a vocational department. *The indication for a stay is given in the face of the clear existence of a problem of resuming work.* Payment, irrespective of a decision by COTOREP, has several aims, namely pursuing re-education treatment (kinesitherapy, ergotherapy, etc), intensifying the level of physical training effort of by means of re-education programmes that last several weeks (these are particularly well developed in patients with spine diseases, i.e. common chronic low back pain), automating re-education exercises in everyday life then in work situations, retraining with effort and at work either in the work position previously held or in a close or similar position. It also allows the analysis and evaluation of professional aptitudes and competences through different practical situations as well as the establishment of contact with the company physician and the employer, and placement in a business internship either with the former employer or with another employer. If necessary, it sets up a vocational placement project, which requires dynamic job-seeking techniques, psychotechnical tests and an educational refresher course. The establishment of a new vocational project is only possible if the interested party is aware of the fact that he/she will not be able to return to his/her previous job and if all solutions aiming at retaining his/her job within his/her company have been looked into. Job-seeking aid by means of contacts, in particular with ANPE, are advantageous in integration and placement.

Preliminary guidance centres

Based on the COTOREP decision, preliminary guidance centres welcome people who have been recognised as disabled workers whose vocational guidance is posing difficulties that cannot be resolved by the committee's technical team. With an interdepartmental or regional vocation, they may be attached to establishments of functional or

Table I – Levels of aptitude.

Level III	Staff employed in jobs normally requiring training for a superior vocational training certificate or a diploma from a technology institute or the end of the first academic cycle in higher education.
Level IV	Staff employed in supervisory work or with a qualification of a level that is equivalent to the technical baccalaureate or the technician's baccalaureate or a vocational training certificate.
Level V	Staff employed in jobs normally requiring a level of training equivalent to that of the technical school certificate (BEP) or a vocational training certificate (CAP) or – by assimilation – the professional training certificate (CFP), first degree.
Level V bis	Staff employed in work presupposing a short training period of a maximum duration of one year leading to a professional education certificate or to any other certificate of the same kind.

vocational rehabilitation or of vocational re-education. In this case, they are managed autonomously.

This preliminary guidance is carried out during an internship lasting no longer than 12 weeks and that is adjusted to the needs of the interested parties. During this period, the disabled worker draws up a professional project and selects various jobs. He/she is placed in a work situation for each job, is informed of the professional perspectives offered by these jobs and draws up his/her professional project in relation thereto with the services of the National Employment Agency and the companies. At the end of the internship, the centre prepares a detailed report on the desires and intellectual and physical adaptation capacities of the person, which are observed during the internship. The committee expresses an opinion on subsequent guidance based on this report.

Professional integration of disabled persons

Obligation to hire disabled persons

The obligation to hire requires the employment of a number of disabled persons, which is schematically proportional to the size of the company or, failing that, the conclusion of subcontracting contracts with the sheltered sector, a collective agreement providing a programme in favour of disabled workers, or the contribution to the development fund for the professional integration of disabled persons.

Employment of disabled workers [11, 14]

Any employer employing at least 20 salaried employees is subject to the obligation to hire disabled workers or workers in similar categories. This obligation affects employers irrespective of whether they are in the private or public sector. Companies consisting of at least 20 salaried employees, either at the time of their creation or because of an increase in their workforce, are required to employ – either in a full-time or a part-time capacity – disabled workers in a proportion of 6% of the total number of salaried employees; they need to conform to the obligation to hire within three years[14].

The number of disabled workers is calculated according to a calculation taking into account the severity of the disability (category B: 1.5, category C: 2.5), the victims of accidents at work or occupational disease (1.5 if the degree of permanent incapacity lies between 66 and 85%, and 2.5 if it lies above this percentage), the work contract (increase for holders of a work contract of indeterminate duration), depending on the age (increase for a disabled worker aged under 25 or over 50), training, previous placement (sheltered workshop, support centre for work or medical-professional institute).

---

14. Article L323-41 of the Labour Code.

Beneficiaries of the obligation to hire[15] include (i) workers recognised as disabled by COTOREP, (ii) victims of accidents at work or occupational diseases who have sustained a permanent incapacity of at least 10% and are entitled to a pension from the general Social Security system or from any other obligatory social protection system, (iii) holders of an invalidity pension from the general Social Security system or from any other obligatory social protection system or through the provisions that regulate public agents providing that this invalidity reduces their capacity to work or earn money by at least 2/3.

Subcontracting contracts with the sheltered sector

Companies can, in part, settle their obligation to hire by setting up supply, sub-contracting or service contracts either with sheltered workshops, outwork distribution centres or support centres for aid. The conclusion of a contract of this kind is equivalent to employing a certain number of beneficiaries of the obligation to hire.

Application of an agreement planning a programme in favour of disabled workers

A sector, company or establishment agreement on the implementation of an annual programme in favour of disabled workers allows companies and establishments to make plans in the context of various actions for the benefit of disabled workers: an employment plan in the ordinary work environment; an integration and training plan; an adaptation plan for technological changes; a retention plan in the company in the case of redundancy.

Payment of an annual contribution to the development fund for the vocational integration of disabled persons

The amount of the annual contribution is fixed at 300 to 500 times the minimum wage depending on the number of salaried employees in the company. All employers[16] are affected[17], namely the state and – if they have more than 20 salaried employees – public establishments of the state, territorial communities and their public establishments other than public, industrial and commercial establishments[18].

Annual declaration

Any employer in the private sector or employing at least 20 salaried employees needs, every year, to submit to the administration, a declaration relating to the positions

---

15. In accordance with article L323-3 of the Labour Code.
16. Article L-323-1 of the Labour Code.
17. Article L-323-2 of the Labour Code.
18. Article L323-1 of the Labour Code.

occupied by disabled workers, accompanied by a justification of one of the legal exemption possibilities from the obligation to hire. A company that does not adhere to its obligation to hire, either by not employing the required number of disabled workers or by not justifying the application of the legal exemption possibilities, must pay a penalty (increase of 25% for every position that is not filled).

Integration into the ordinary work environment [7, 8]

Aids for job retention or professional integration

Job placement and follow-up teams (EPSRs) support disabled persons through all the stages of their reintegration process with the aim of facilitating their access to a stable professional and social life, whilst taking into account their wishes and aptitudes. Their role essentially aims for the professional integration of disabled persons. To this effect, EPSRs – like the ANPE – have a double mission, namely on the one hand towards recognised disabled workers by helping them to overcome personal and social difficulties that may form obstacles for them and, on the other hand, towards companies. EPSRs are compulsorily made up of a social services assistant who guarantees psychological and social support for the disabled worker and a specialised ANPE employment officer or a person with an equivalent qualification nominated for this position by the aforementioned agency.

The *development fund for the professional integration of disabled persons*[19] [5, 10] has the mission of increasing the funds dedicated to the integration into the ordinary environment of disabled workers and persons in similar categories. Employers[20] can settle their obligation to hire by paying an annual contribution for each of the beneficiaries they should have employed. The fund is managed by a private legal association that is administered by representatives of salaried employees, of employers, of disabled persons and of qualified personalities.

The *National Development Fund for the Professional Integration of Disabled Persons* (AGEFIPH) has developed an intervention programme containing 20 measures, which are completed by a three-year programme. It also ensures, by guaranteeing resources for disabled workers, to complement the remuneration of persons employed in an ordinary work environment when their salary is subject to a reduction following a COTOREP decision.

Integration plans for disabled workers (PDITH) were established to favour integration into an ordinary environment through the development of various lines of action (job seeking, course and training, information for and raising awareness in companies, job retention within the company).

---

19. Created by the law of July 10, 1987 (law on the professional integration of disabled persons).
20. Mentioned in article L323-1.

The *National Employment Agency* (ANPE) has a privileged role at various levels in the field of guidance and placement of persons recognised as disabled workers. It is situated among COTOREPs and liases with the job placement and follow-up teams of other organisations. The ANPE participates in the functioning of COTOREPs by contributing to the work of the technical team, to plenary meetings and to the implementation of decisions.

Preventive measures for job retention

The *verdict of invalidity in terms of Social Security* is given by the advisory physician of the state health insurance office when the person paying social security contributions has lost at least two thirds of his/her capacity for work or earnings because of an accident or a disease of a non-occupational origin.[21] This verdict can only be given by the advisory physician when the state of health of the insured party has stabilised or when his/her healthcare payment rights lapse. There are three categories of invalidity classification. The person who is declared to be an invalid according to Social Security benefits from work legislation provisions relating to the obligation to hire disabled workers or workers in similar categories.

The *company physician's verdict on fitness.* When a work contract is concluded, the salaried employee is subject to regular medical examinations, which evaluate his/her state of health in relation to holding down his/her job. Thus, the salaried employee regularly meets with the company physician when he/she is hired and then on the occasion of periodic appointments[22] or especially arranged appointments and when work is resumed again after an occupational disease or an accident at work requiring time off work of at least eight days, a disease or a non-industrial accident requiring time off work of at least 21 days and in the case of repeated absences. The role of the company physician towards the employer is to provide information on any changes in the health of workers in the company. On the occasion of the medical examination, the company physician checks whether the salaried employee has not contracted a condition that is dangerous to other workers and whether he/she is medically fit for the position that the head of the establishment plans to entrust him/her with.

If the company physician expresses reservations about the fitness of the salaried employee to take up his/her position, a procedure is initiated with the aim of providing the salaried employee with a professional placement within the company. After at least 15 days have elapsed, the company physician again examines the salaried employee and it is only on the occasion of this second visit that he can express a verdict of unfitness.

Preparation for job retention [2]

Medical appointment initiated by the salaried employee: the salaried employee can benefit from a medical examination with a view to – together with his/her company physician –

---

21. According to article L341-1 of the Social Security Code .
22. Article R241-49 of the Labour Code.

assuring her/himself of his/her fitness for the post[23]. This procedure, which is initiated by the salaried employee, has the advantage of being voluntary and not necessitating any preliminary procedures. A verdict on fitness is not compulsory following this appointment.

Medical appointment before resuming work: when any salaried employee stops working as a consequence of an accident or a disease, the salaried employee, the attending physician or the Social Security advisory physician can request that the company physician carries out a medical examination in preparation for the resumption of professional activity.[24] The aim of this visit is to set up a prognosis of the worker's fitness for when he/she resumes his/her position. It allows the consequences of restricted fitness for work to be anticipated and appropriate solutions to be thought of before the procedure of professional placement is initiated because of medical unfitness for the position.

Suggestions made to the employer by the company physician: in the context of fulfilling the work contract, when the company physician submits an opinion on the work fitness of a salaried employee, he encloses written conclusions for the employer. These conclusions contain indications on the fitness of the salaried employee for performing such and such a task and formulate the conditions in which the salaried employee's employment could continue in the company, in particular by means of the implementation of a change to or transformation of his/her position. The employer is obliged to consider these suggestions when fulfilling his professional placement obligation in favour of the salaried employee who has been recognised as unfit for his/her position.

The *liaison form*[25] is a means of support that the Social Security advisory physician can use to enter into a relationship with the company physician with a view to planning the return to the company of the salaried employee who has sustained an accident at work or occupational disease. It forms part of Social Security issues. The Social Security advisory physician is obliged, with the agreement of the person paying social security contributions, to inform the company physician about the state of his/her medical condition, while the company physician has to provide – within 15 days – a prognosis of the salaried employee's fitness for his/her position. Nonetheless, it remains little used in practice.

The *AGEFIPH job retention measure*[26] consists of funding[27] destined to facilitate concerted job retention action.

The *competence balance sheet*[28] allows the evaluation of experience and analysis of the possibilities and professional motivations of the salaried employee. Any salaried employee with five years professional experience (consecutive or not), of which 12 months have been in the current company can benefit – either on his/her own initiative or on that of his/her employer with his/her agreement. This needs to be compiled by

---

23. Article R241-24, paragraph 3 of the Labour Code.
24. Article R241-51, paragraph 5 of the Labour Code.
25. Article R434-4 of the Social Security Code.
26. Measure no. 3.
27. Subsidy of 30,000 French francs, subsequently completed by a sum of 20,000 French francs (2003 values).
28. Article L900-2 of the Labour Code.

an independent organisation of the company or by a professional training centre. Its contents are confidential. Only the salaried professional finds out about them.

The *professional balance sheet* is available to any salaried employee benefiting from the law of July 10, 1987. As someone paying social security contributions, the salaried employee can benefit from payments and from a balance sheet aiming to evaluate the deficiency, the consequences thereof and his/her functional, professional and educational aptitudes.

Working time management

Therapeutic part-time work allows vocational activity to be resumed in a progressive manner even if one's state of health is not yet stabilised to a degree where resuming work would favour recovery. Daily benefits can be maintained wholly or in part by the health insurance organisation. Therapeutic part-time work is a way of facilitating the return of the salaried employee to the company during the treatment period and progressively paves the way for resuming full-time professional activity. When this period of time has elapsed, either (i) the salaried employee has not recovered and is not yet able to resume his/her work under the initial conditions. In this case, therapeutic part-time work can be pursued if the state of health has improved; or (ii) the situation of the insured party has stabilised or been consolidated by the Social Security advisory physician. The latter then needs to analyse whether the person can resume his/her work contract under the previous conditions or whether another solution needs to be initiated (invalidity, professional placement, training, etc.).

Progressive early retirement allows the salaried employee with difficulties to retire progressively under favourable conditions. *The salaried employee definitively ends his/her professional activity after a progressive reduction of his/her working hours.* This has the benefit of not being too disadvantageous in monetary terms.

Work post management

Management of the work post and its environment requires collaboration between the employer, the salaried employee, the company physician, the works council and the Hygiene, Safety and Working Conditions Committee (CHSCT). The cost of managing the work post, including the advice of an ergonomist on workplace accessibility, may be financed by AGEFIPH.

Compensation for loss of worker's productivity

The authorisation granted to the employer to reduce part of the salary of one of the company's workers whose productivity is diminished is a decision that is made by the departmental management of work and professional training. The employer pays the worker his/her whole salary and then recovers the part that corresponds to income maintenance from the AGEFIPH to an upper limit of 130% of the minimum wage.

Integration of disabled persons into a sheltered work environment

Disabled persons for whom placement in the normal work environment proves to be impossible may be admitted to a sheltered workshop, either in an outwork distribution centre or a Support Centre for Work[29].

Institutions in the field of sheltered work

Sheltered workshops and outwork distribution centres are made up of economic production units that enable disabled workers to carry out a professional activity as salaried employees in conditions that have been adapted to their possibilities. These establishments need to favour their promotion and access to employment in an ordinary work environment[30]. They can only hire workers whose work capacity is at least equal to one third of the normal work capacity[31]. It is possible to hire disabled persons whose work capacity does not reach this minimum, but which may do so by the end of the trial period; this period may last six months at most. Depending on their production requirements, sheltered workshops may hire able-bodied employees within a limit of 20% of their workforce. They function like any company that is subject to the vagaries of the market, either by guaranteeing their own production or by entering into subcontracting contracts, and are obliged to guarantee a balance through their own means. They may, however, receive running cost subsidies through the enforcement conventions that have been agreed with the state, the department, communities and Social Security organisations.

Support Centres for Work (CATs), which were created in 1954, offer "disabled adolescents and adults, who are temporarily or permanently unable to work in ordinary companies or in a sheltered workshop or for an outwork distribution centre, or unable to carry out an independent professional activity, possibilities of various activities of a professional nature, medical-social and educational support as well as a living environment that favours their personal development and their social integration"[32]. In legal terms, CATs are medical-social institutions with the mission of production and support. Admission is subject to three conditions: (i) to be older than 20 years of age (dispensation possible from 16 years of age through a CDES decision); (ii) to have a work capacity of less than a third of normal work capacity (this capacity may be higher if medical, educational, social or psychological support is necessary); (iii) to obtain a favourable decision from COTOREP. This decision is provisional for a duration of six months and can be renewed once. At the end of this period, COTOREP rules on the definitive guidance of the disabled person. CATs function on the basis of a daily price that may be paid by social aid.

---

29. Article 167 of the Family and Social Aid Code.
30. Article R323-60 of the Labour Code.
31. Articles L323-30 and D323-25-1 of the Labour Code.
32. Law 75-534 of June 30, 1975, article 30.

Status and remuneration in establishments
in the sheltered work environment

In *sheltered workshops or outwork distribution centres*, disabled workers are considered to be salaried employees in legal terms. However, the employers, i.e. the management organisations of sheltered workshops or of outwork distribution centres, do not have the usual management powers. Thus, at the end of the trial period, decisions on hiring are the responsibility of COTOREP and not of the establishment and are based on a report set up by the Labour Inspector and after consultation with the person who is responsible for the sheltered structure. The minimum salary is equivalent to the minimum wage and is based on the same percentage as that of the productivity of the interested party in relation to normal productivity without being less than 35% of the minimum wage. The amount of income maintenance is fixed at 90% of the minimum wage. The statuses are identical to those of any salaried employee.

In *Support Centres for Work*, disabled persons do not have the status of salaried employees because they are not linked to the CAT by a work contract. The remuneration received depends on the productivity of the interested party and cannot be less than 5% of the minimum wage. Income maintenance is fixed at 70% of the minimum wage.

Sheltered work for disabled persons
in the ordinary environment

Subcontracting contracts allow the establishment of relationships between the ordinary work environment and establishments in the sheltered environment. Sheltered work establishments enjoy considerable additional appeal as subcontractors of companies in the ordinary environment with prices that are often lower than market prices, a low rate of accidents at work, marginal absenteeism and partial exemption from the obligation to hire.

The disabled worker employed in a sheltered workshop can be *provisionally made available to another employer*[33] but remains under the responsibility of the authority of the sheltered workshop, or may be *authorised to carry out his/her professional activity outside* the latter. The external activity must be of a professional nature. The person providing work may be a physical or moral body (individual, company, local community). Disabled workers must be able to continue to benefit from their usual medical, educational and social treatment. The disabled worker involved is not party to the contract established between CAT and the provider of work, which is a contract of a maximum duration of one year, which may be subject to renewal. He/she continues to number among the workforce of the people accommodated by CAT and remains protected in the same way as any other salaried employee with regard to insurance for accidents at work.

---

33. Article L125-3 of the Labour Code.

Vocational training of disabled persons

Any disabled adult who has left compulsory education can benefit from rehabilitation, re-education and vocational training[34].

Apprenticeship and training [13]

The goal of an apprenticeship is to provide a vocational qualification resulting in a technical education diploma. It is available to everyone and, thus, also to disabled persons. Arrangements[35] are possible for young disabled workers who have been guided by COTOREP and who sign an apprenticeship contract[36]. The duration of the apprenticeship can vary between one and three years. It may be prolonged in the case of failing the examination, dispensation on the start date of the apprenticeship or suspension of the contract for reasons not pertaining to the will of the apprentice. Remuneration, which is determined in relation to working hours, is fixed as a percentage of the minimum wage. It depends on the age of the apprentice and on the length of the apprenticeship contract.

Aids may encourage apprenticeships, namely an apprenticeship bonus and an integration bonus that are paid to the employer[37] and a fixed subsidy for the disabled apprentice[38].

Vocational training of disabled persons

This represents one of the key elements of professional integration. Disabled persons may have access to "ordinary" vocational training plans of action or to specialised structures.

The "ordinary" training plan of action

The disabled person can access the ordinary training plan of action, either within the context of his/her work contract, in the context of all training policies or in the context of various block-release integration contracts.

Within the context of his/her work contract, the disabled person has access to all the plans of action relating to continued vocational training.

Continued training within the company: any employer is obliged to organise and finance training for his employees. The object of this obligation is to enable salaried employees to adapt to the evolution of technologies and work conditions and to favour his/her social promotion[39].

---

34. Article L323-15 of the Labour Code.
35. Article 119-5 of the Labour Code.
36. Article L115-1 of the Labour Code.
37. For the conclusion of a contract of indeterminate duration or a contract of determinate duration of at least 12 months at the end of the apprenticeship contract.
38. Fixed subsidy of 1 524,49 paid by AGEFIPH (in 2003).
39. Article N901-1 of the Labour Code.

Individual leave for training (CIF) is an authorised absence granted by the employer to the salaried employee so that the latter can pursue training independently of his/her participation in internships included in the company's training plan. Any salaried employee may request a CIF if he/she has been a salaried employee for 24 months, whether consecutively or not (36 months for companies with fewer than 10 salaried employees), of which 12 months have been in the current company.

Block-release integration contracts are offered by centres of the Association for Vocational Training of Adults (AFPA) and institutional community or professional business training centres to guarantee accelerated vocational training of the *employee*[40]. Supervised by the Ministry of Labour, they are part of the plan of action for the rehabilitation, re-education and professional training of disabled workers.

Specialised vocational training centres

Disabled adult training relies on three main types of specialised training centres that pursue a double objective of "re-education" and "rehabilitation", which presupposes that the disability arose after initial professional experience. These are centres of re-education-rehabilitation and of vocational training that were created by the state, by a public group or by a public establishment such as the National Office of War Veterans (ONAC), state-approved private centres of re-education and vocational rehabilitation, such as the centres created by Social Security, and back-to-work training centres, managed by a group or a company subject to a ministerial agreement.

Professional re-education schools of the National Office of War Veterans[41] were initially destined for servicemen of the two last wars and have progressively opened their doors to other groups. Currently, 90% of interns are persons who sustained an accident at work and who belong to various social insurance programmes[42]. Basic training lasts 21 months and is spread over two school years with eight to twelve weeks spent on an internship in a company. It may be preceded by preliminary training of three to six months destined to refresh general knowledge. Diplomas are awarded upon completion of these forms of training (vocational training certificate (CAP) and technical school certificate (BEP)), which are issued by the Ministry of National Education.

Private centres of vocational re-education, whether profit-oriented or not, are subject to the double protection of the ministry responsible for Social Security and the ministry responsible for labour and employment. They provide a wide spectrum of training ranging from level V bis (preparation within one year for the certificate of primary studies: CEP) to level III (preparation for the higher technical certificate: BTS). A vocational training certificate issued by the Ministry of Labour is awarded at the end of the training provided. Admission depends on age (less than 45 years) and psychotechnical level.

---

40. By the decree of November 9, 1946.
41. According to the law of January 2, 1918.
42. In 1995, ONAC managed ten schools and offered 40 training sections, divided into four large teaching categories: industrial, commercial, production and agricultural.

Financial reimbursement of the costs of the internship and remuneration stem, in part from national solidarity, i.e. the state, and may be completed by AGEFIPH financing[43].

The aim of corporate *Back-to-Work Training Centres* is to allow salaried employees who had to interrupt their professional activity following disease or accident to resume work and – after a brief period of time – to resume his/her previous position or – if this fails – to have direct access to another position. Any establishment (or group of establishments with the same professional activity) with more than 5000 salaried employees must guarantee – following a medical opinion – retraining for work and vocational re-education for ill and injured persons belonging to the group or the establishment or group of establishments[44].

The aim of the *Back-to-Work Contract*[45] (CRE) is to get people back to work who – because of their disability – have become unable to carry out their function or who will only be able to do so after a new adaptation. It provides essentially practical vocational training either in a new job or in the carrying out of the former job. The CRE is only used to an extremely low degree although it makes it possible to provide training in an ordinary environment at a low cost, simplifies vocational reintegration and often leads to employment.

Remuneration

Unemployed disabled workers who are undertaking a training internship authorised by the state or a region and who carried out a salaried activity for six months in a twelve-month period or for twelve months in a 24-month period receive monthly remuneration[46] equal to their former salary, adjusted by a revaluation coefficient[47]. Unemployed disabled workers who do not fulfil these conditions as well as young disabled individuals who are seeking a first job receive fixed remuneration[48] when they pursue a training internship that is authorised by the state or a region.

A *placement bonus*[49] can be paid to the disabled worker at the end of a re-education, rehabilitation or vocational training internship if he/she fulfils several conditions, in particular having been admitted to a retraining, rehabilitation or vocational training internship, of having pursued this internship in full under conditions considered to be satisfactory by the director of the centre or the employer[50].

---

43. Measure no. 11.
44. Article L323-17 of the Labour Code.
45. Article L432-9 of the Social Security Code.
46. Decree of April 15, 1988.
47. Within the limits of a minimum of 4225.50 French francs and a maximum of 12676.50 French francs (2003 value).
48. Fixed at 3803 French francs in 2003.
49. Article L323-16 of the Labour Code.
50. The amount is fixed as a sum between € 76.22 and € 152.45 (2003 value).

Financial aid for the employment of disabled persons

Financial aids that favour the employment of disabled persons in a company comprise: apprenticeship bonuses, aids for managing work situations, salary reductions, AGEFIPH aids, financial aids and exemptions from paying social security contributions for hiring and aids for machine constructors.

Apprenticeship bonuses

Heads of companies who train disabled apprentices may obtain[51] a bonus destined to compensate for the additional expenses or the "lack of earnings" that may result therefrom.

Aids for managing work situations

The state may grant financial aid to establishments, organisations or employers who are subject to the obligation to hire disabled workers for the adaptation of workplaces and the additional supervision costs to facilitate the employment or resumption of work in an ordinary environment. These aids may apply to the adaptation of machines or tools, work post management (individual equipment necessary for the disabled worker to occupy his/her position), access to the workplace, the evolution of work posts thanks to new technologies. The cost of technical assistance provided by an external ergonomist may also be taken into account.

They also allow compensation for additional supervision costs to cover salary expenses, social security contributions and, generally, all expenses directly linked to the employment of staff guaranteeing the specific supervision of disabled workers.

Salary reductions

The salary of a disabled person cannot be lower that that resulting from the application of the provisions of the collective labour agreement that applies in the company. However, when the professional productivity of the disabled worker is manifestly diminished, reductions in salary can be authorised under certain conditions. The percentage of the reduction is fixed by COTOREP, either when it places the disabled worker in category B or C, or on request of the parties to the work contract. Reductions are limited and, in category B, cannot exceed 10% of the salary normally allocated to an

---

51. Article L119-5 of the Labour Code.

able-bodied worker carrying out the same task and, in category C, cannot exceed 20% of the salary evaluated as above. Classification in category A does not authorise any salary reduction.

AGEFIPH aids

The allocated aids do not replace those of the state or the territorial communities, but complete them and are allocated after checking the appropriateness and examining the costs Companies and employers in the private sector, irrespective of their legal form, public companies, organisations and establishments that are subject to private law may benefit therefrom. The AGEFIPH intervention programme comprises different measures in favour of access for and retention in employment of disabled persons. It consists of information on and awareness of the law of 1987, diagnostic analysis and advice on the issue of employing disabled persons in the company, an evaluation and guidance balance sheet, training, apprenticeship aids, integration support and follow-up, management of work situations, accessibility of workplaces, secondment to companies of people working in a sheltered environment, bringing the sheltered environment closer to the ordinary environment, job retention, integration bonuses, support for integration in the ordinary environment and aid for innovations. It may be possible to combine these different forms of aid. The file requesting intervention must be submitted to the regional AGEFIPH delegation and each subsidised action is the subject of a meeting.

Other work incentive aids

The aim of *vocational integration contracts* is to plan for a duration of three years the integration policy for disabled workers. These contracts are concluded between the state and the employers. They appear to have become obsolete.

"Light employment" covers particular jobs in the ordinary production sector, which are part-time and destined for disabled workers who cannot be employed in a normal or full-time rhythm because or their physical or mental condition. They are destined for workers suffering from a severe physical or mental disability who, in principle, require work in a sheltered work environment, but cannot work there because there are no establishments of this kind close to where they live or because their condition or family situation does not allow this.

Tele-work is interactive long-distance work that utilises all means of telecommunications as well as possibly telematics and information technology. It is particularly adapted to certain disabled persons and covers eight main employment groups: secretarial work, accounting, information service, commercial action, management, file management, communication and studies.

Machine constructors who make adjustments to their machines to enable disabled persons to use them, can obtain financial aid from the state.

Financial resources and protection for victims of an accident at work or suffering from an occupational disease

Independent resources following an accident at work or occupational disease

Disabled adult subsidy (AAH)

This subsidy aims to guarantee minimum resources to severely disabled individuals and is paid like a family benefit. It is paid to French nationals, European Union nationals and to persons with residence permits and residing in France in the case of permanent incapacity of at least equal to 80% or between 50 and 80% with a recognised impossibility[52] of obtaining employment because of the disability. Beneficiaries need to be older than 20 years of age and younger than 60 years of age and their resources may not exceed the fixed limit for the calendar year preceding the one in which the law starts to apply[53]. The decision to pay this allowance is taken by COTOREP for the duration of at least one year and at most five years. The monthly AAH amount is equal to one twelfth of the overall total allowance paid to old salaried workers.

Compensation allowance

Irrespective of the preceding subsidy, the compensation allowance is destined to compensate for the costs that arise through having to rely on a third person for essential acts of everyday life and/or the supplementary costs that arise through carrying out a professional activity. It is paid to people between 16 and 60 years of age when the incapacity is at least 80% according to the same means tests as is used for the AAH. It varies from 40% to 80% depending on the nature and the permanence of necessary aid and depending on the level of supplementary costs. It comes on top of the AAH and any old-age or invalidity benefit.

Accommodation allowance

This is destined to reduce rent for accommodation to a level that is compatible with means.

---

52. COTOREP.
53. In 2003, the means limit was € 6999.68 for a single person, € 13399.35 for a household and a supplementary € 3349.84 for each dependent child.

Health, maternity and old-age insurance

Disabled persons benefit from health insurance and maternity [3] benefits if (i) they carry out a professional activity and are covered by their activity's system; (ii) they benefit from the disabled subsidy (disabled adult subsidy or AAH) and are covered by the general social security system; (iii) they have the rights of those paying social security contributions; (iv) they benefit from universal healthcare coverage (CMU)[54] and from old-age insurance under common law.

Particular resources following an accident at work or occupational disease

Benefits in kind [1]

The insured party does not need to pay for any treatment. The health insurance companies transfer the allowances (payment by a third-party system) to the practitioners, pharmacists, medical assistants, service providers and to the care establishments[55]. Apart from reimbursing medical, surgical and pharmaceutical costs, these benefits in kind[56] comprise the supply, repair and renewal of prosthetic and orthopaedic devices, the repair or replacement of devices that have become useless because of the accident, transport costs and the reimbursement of costs necessary for treatment. The period of professional re-education is taken into account for calculating old-age pension rights[57].

Cash benefits

Compensation for temporary incapacity

The insured party receives daily compensation starting from the first day of work being stopped as a consequence of the accident at work for the whole period of time he/she is unable to work (including the period of functional re-education and vocational rehabilitation)[58]. This period of inability to work ends with complete recovery, either with consolidation of the injury – this corresponds to recovery without sequellae – or with the stabilisation of the medical state – with or without sequellae – or with death. Daily compensation can be maintained totally or in part if work is resumed if this resumption of work is of a nature that will favour recovery or consolidation of the injury, or can be paid once more after consolidation in the case of regression or worsening.

---

54. Any person who does not carry out a professional activity and does not benefit from any social reimbursement through any other situation can benefit from the CMU if he/she is resident in a town or in a French overseas department (DOM).
55. Article L432-1.
56. Article L431-1 of the Social Security Code.
57. Article L432-6.
58. Article 431-1.

Daily compensation is calculated and is equal to a proportion of the daily salary. It is set at 80% of the latter from the 29th day after work is stopped as a consequence of the accident[59]. The total amount of compensation may not exceed the normal salary of workers in the same professional category or, if it is higher, the salary on which the daily compensation calculation was based.

Compensation for permanent incapacity

In the case of permanent incapacity, the victim of an accident at work benefits from compensation in the form of capital calculated using the rate of incapacity of the victim and determined by a scale that is fixed by decree (official scale for accidents at work). This rate depends on the nature of the disability, the general condition, age, physical and mental faculties of the victim, his/her aptitudes and professional qualification.

Work protection measures

The work contract is suspended for the whole time that work is stopped and during the waiting period and period of any rehabilitation, re-education or professional training internship. The employer cannot terminate the working contract except in the case of serious misconduct on the part of the salaried employee or because of an external factor making it impossible to maintain it. Priority is guaranteed in terms of access to professional training actions. When work is taken up again, a study of placement possibilities needs to be carried out between the employer, the salaried employee and the company physician. This study must be backed up with regard to the common-law obligation. In the case of redundancy, compensation is doubled. Incidentally, the victim of an accident at work profits from provisions relating to the obligation to hire disabled workers or those in a similar category in the ordinary work environment.

Conclusion [12]

In December 2001, the active disabled population in France numbered 840,000 individuals in work and 218,000 individuals seeking work. This population of job seekers differs from the general job-seeking population in three main characteristics: older, predominantly male and under-qualified. In addition to the medical problems and functional consequences thereof, this population is confronted by a situation of social disability. In response to the problems of this population, the plans of action and structures of vocational rehabilitation in France are weighty and complex. This comprises the complexity of the COTOREPs, the length of time required to access the plans of action for specific forms of training, the uneven spread of training centres around France, the relative rarity of sheltered work structures such as sheltered workshops. There is a clear imbalance between "administrative" and medical-social reimbursement, which is predominant, but

---

59. Article R-433-4.

often occurs late in the rehabilitation process, and "health" and medical reimbursement, which is less developed and even non-existent in some areas and which should occur at an earlier stage. Where it exists, this "health" reimbursement is sometimes oriented towards certain pathologies (for example, common lombalgia) and is not generalised. In response to this imbalance, the "COMETE" structures were put into place a few years ago. Their aim is to reintegrate disabled persons vocationally at an early stage of their re-education and they support vocational rehabilitation departments of the services and centres of physical medicine and rehabilitation.

Nonetheless, despite this state of affairs, new perspectives are opening up. On the occasion of his election in 2002, the President of the French Republic put forward as a national priority taking care of disabled persons. The guideline law of 1975 is in the process of being revised and consists of 75 propositions, some of which express a true desire to deal with obstacles in the way of vocational integration (for example: the current impossibility of drawing salary and allowance at the same time). One of these propositions aims to redefine existing allowances around integral disability compensation. Finally, COTOREP and CDES should truly become places where people listen to and evaluate the needs of individuals so that they can work out a life plan with them.

References

1. Rogier A (Association Handiface).Handicap: éléments médico-légaux (clinique, évaluation, expertise). Paris: ESKA, p 571
2. GIRHP, Groupe de réflexion sur le maintien dans l'emploi. Le maintien dans l'emploi en question. Paris: ENSP, p 223
3. Rogier A. Dommage corporel: éléments médico-légaux à l'usage du juriste et du médecin. Paris: ESKA, p 342
4. Triomphe A (1995). Les personnes handicapées en France. Données Sociales. Paris: INSERM-CTNERHI, p 303
5. Blanc A (1998) La loi de 1987: ambition et résultats d'une action collective. In: Solidarité MdlEedl, editor. L'intégration des personnes handicapées: quelques éléments de bilan. Paris: La documentation française, p 115-27
6. Chaix M (1998) La politique de l'emploi des personnes handicapées. In: Solidarité MdlEedl, editor. L'intégration des personnes handicapées: quelques éléments de bilan. Paris: La documentation française, p 93-101
7. Mollinier A (1998) L'emploi des travailleurs handicapés: le point de vue d'un praticien. In: Solidarité MdlEedl, editor. L'intégration des personnes handicapées: quelques éléments de bilan. Paris: La documentation française, p 133-5
8. Podesta Le Poittevin G (1998) L'intégration professionnelle des personnes handicapées: notes sur les réflexions du Conseil de l'Europe. In: Solidarité MdlEedl, editor. L'intégration des personnes handicapées: quelques éléments de bilan. Paris: La documentation française, p 151-5
9. Ravaud J-F, Held J-P (1998) Handicap et travail. In: Held J-P, Dizien O, editors. Traité de Médecine de Médecine Physique et de Réadaptation. Paris: Flammarion, p 812-8

10. Ségura J-L (1998) Bilan général et chiffré de la loi du 10 Juillet 1987. In: Solidarité MdlEedl, editor. L'intégration des personnes handicapées: quelques éléments de bilan. Paris: La documentation française, p 103-13

11. L'obligation d'emploi des travailleurs handicapés (1999) Trav. Sécurité 581: 20-31

12. Velche D (2000) L'emploi des personnes handicapées: accompagner la transition vers un nouveau modèle ? Handicap 88: 43-69

13. The company and disabled persons. Liaisons sociales 2001, October

14. Professional integration of disabled persons into an ordinary environment. Report of the Economic and Social Council. Paris

15. www.handicap.gouv.fr

Vocational rehabilitation and participation in working life: the German model

H.M. Schian

The paradigm shift – introduction

The introduction of Social Security Code IX (SSC = SGB – Sozialgesetzbuch) on 01.07.2001 represented a milestone in vocational rehabilitation, in particular, and in the participation of human beings in working life. It saw the start of a paradigm shift in policies for the disabled in Germany. This "Draft legislation to promote the training and employment of the severely disabled" is a further development that will become effective after passing the arbitration commission. The following path is being pursued: from the welfare and passive care given to the disabled (also to people threatened by disability) through to participation and active self-determination. This represents a change in role for all involved: providers are in the role of customer-oriented service providers while the people concerned assume the active role of self-determined service claimants. In order to achieve this goal, SSC IX has summarized the regulations that apply uniformly to several social security sectors and their bodies. In addition, supplementary regulations were created.

Overview of important facts created by Social Security Code IX

Creation of a uniform concept of disability that is measured on the basis of a condition typical of a person's age without any functional health problems. This means: if physical function, mental ability or emotional health are extremely likely to deviate from this "typical condition" for longer than six months and – participation in life in society – is affected. For the first time, people threatened by disablement are included.

Particular aspects:

– prevention has priority;
– priority of benefits for the purpose of participation;

– coordination of benefits, combined effect of the services of the seven rehabilitation agencies, obligation of rehabilitation agencies to cooperate, formation of joint cross-agency service points to advise, inform and accompany those concerned, priority given to the promotion of self-help, principles designed to assure quality in rehabilitation.

In principle, legislators have followed the concept of the International Classification of Functioning, Disability and Health, WHO 2001. The paradigm is the participation model, the active participation and active involvement of those concerned to attain this goal. In order to achieve this, the right of beneficiaries to request and to choose was introduced and combined with the possibility of receiving a personal budget in order to handle their own path to rehabilitation by themselves. The possibilities open to organizations for the disabled are clearly reinforced.

Important key aspects with reference to vocational rehabilitation and integration to facilitate participation in working life – an overview

Sign language is compulsory in the field of assistance and advice for the hearing-impaired.

Accompanying benefits to achieve participation in working life. They are not listed here individually.

Due consideration is given to the special requirements of the problems encountered by disabled women and children.

Due consideration was given to more recent findings on the participation of people with mental problems.

The gradual resumption of work based on time and content is legally binding for all rehabilitation agencies. The coordination instruments between agencies, those concerned, general practitioners, work doctors and companies are regulated.

Working assistance for people with particularly pronounced disablement in working life is increased.

Fundamentals for job-site integration management

Integration teams can be formed in companies or integration services can operate for smaller companies as external service providers. The integration agreements, which can be compiled in agreement between the tariff partner and/or employer and employee representation as well as union workplace representatives for the severely disabled in companies with the enlistment of the help of experts in occupational rehabilitation form an important element.

Another possibility is the conclusion of company agreements within a company that integrate integration agreements.

What is of particular importance, however, is that job-site integration management is based on integration, a method that also clearly follows preventive targets. Put simply:

Exclusion from working life must be prevented with all available means, integration into working life "as a one-stop system" must be promoted with all available means.

Overview of benefits for the participation of disabled people with due regard for the seven rehabilitation agencies

Figure 1 shows the seven rehabilitation agencies that are now covered by Social Security Code IX. The table in Figure 2 shows the "Benefits for the participation of the disabled" as an overview. The second column (Fig. 2) contains the benefits for participation in working life, which are of special significance for vocational rehabilitation in Germany.

Social Security Code IX spells out the benefits and thus spreads a cooperative and organisational net over the seven rehabilitation agencies. Their individual benefit rights are described in the relevant social security codes and are only reproduced here in the form of an overview. With regard to Figures 3, 4, it will be clear to the reader that the coordinating statutory intention of Social Security Code IX with its participatory paradigm shift was absolutely imperative.

Overview of a summarizing, simplified description of the services of the seven agencies (q.v. Figs. 1, 2 in this connection)

Health insurance: (SSC V) the treatment of the sick and the integration of the disabled, the payment of sickness benefits, no matter whether this is a private accident, an acute or chronic sickness. Using the instrument of gradual reintegration, health insurance has a direct effect on the goal of participation in working life.

In cases of sickness and accidents (if these are not clearly caused by work such as occupational diseases and accidents at work), compulsory health insurance is responsible for outpatient and inpatient treatment irrespective of cause. (Under certain circumstances, income, etc. private health insurance can be an alternative).

From the first day of working incapacity caused by illness, the employer pays for six weeks, what is more or less a wage benefit, (wage continuation, compensation payment). The responsibility of the statutory medical insurance begins from the seventh week on; it pays sickness benefits (for 78 weeks). If working incapacity threatens or takes place, the pension insurance takes over with medical and/or vocational rehabilitation and the corresponding financial coverage (transitional payments).

Statutory Health Insurance	Statutory Pension Insurance	Federal Employment Office	Statutory Accident Insurance	Carriers of social Compensation for Disadvantages caused by Disease	Social Assistance	Public Youth Welfare
Local health insurance	State insurance carriers	State labor offices	Industrial professional associations	State maintenance offices	Interregional social assistance carriers	Interregional public youth welfare carriers
Compagny based health insurance	Federal railway insurance	Employment offices	Associations of marine professions	Maintenance offices	Local social assistance agencies	Local public youth welfare agencies
Guild health-insurance	Seamen's pension insurance		Agricultural professional associations	Main welfare offices*		
Seamen's health insurance	Federal insurance carrier for employers		Community accident insurance associations	Welfare offices		
Supplementary health insurance	Federal miner's insurance		Executive offices of the accident insurance of the federal government, the states and the communities			
Federal miner's insurance	Agricultural pension insurance		Firemen's accident insurance agencies	*simultaneously, these are also responsible according to the Severely Disabled Persons Act		
Agricultural-health insurance						

Fig. 1 – Carriers of rehabilitation.

Medical measures	Vocational rehabilitation	Measures for integration in school age pre-school age, measures for social integration, others measures	Supplementary measures
Especially: – Medical and dental treatment – Medication and bandages – Remedies including physiotherapy, kinetotherapy, speech therapy and occupational therapy – Prostheses, orthopaedical aids and other aids – Work tolerance tests and work therapy, also in hospitals, rehabilitation facilities	Especially: – Assistance in maintaining or getting a job – Measures for finding a job, work tolerance tests and preparation for the job – Vocational adaptation, education, further training and retraining – Other assistance for furtherance of the economic activity or occupation in the general labour market or in a workshop for disabled persons	Especially assistance: – In developing the mental and physical abilities before the child gets to school age – For an appropriate education in school including the necessary preparation – For disabled persons, that can only be trained in practical work, in order to enable them to participate in society – In carrying out an appropriate occupation, as far as measures for vocational promotion are impossible – In making communication possible or easier – In maintaining, improving, restoring the physical and mental flexibility and the emotional equilibrance – For making it easier or possible to keep the household – To improve housing accommodation – In organizing leisure time and in other kinds of participation in social and cultural life	Especially: – Transitional payment, sickness benefits, injury benefit, special sickness benefit for war disabled people – Other assistance in life-supply – Contributions to the statutory health-, accident- and pension insurance and to the federal labour office – Paying the costs that are associated with measures of vocational promotion – Financing travel expenditures – Rehabilitation-sports in groups under medical surveillance – Housekeeping assistants

Fig. 2 – Rehabilitative measures.

(Healthcare insurance: care benefits and introduction, coordination and provision of participatory benefits, care services, healthcare payments, etc. – it is not included in SSC IX, but naturally has a supplementary effect).

Pension insurance: (PI-SSC VI) On the one hand, pensions due to a reduction in earning capacity, on the other hand, the integration of the disabled, particularly into gainful employment:

In principle, it can be assumed that – if the prerequisites for claims are fulfilled and reduction in earning capacity is imminent or present – the statutory pension insurance is responsible for medical or occupational rehabilitation. For the purpose of speeding up the introduction of medical rehabilitation procedures, one of the special examples of inpatient rehabilitation is what is known as the follow-up healing process. This is made possible by a direct transition from inpatient hospital treatment to inpatient rehabilitation establishment. If an application for vocational rehabilitation is approved, the range of benefits provided by pension insurance also includes financial cover for the person concerned as well as almost all flanking measures.

Depending on the situation of the individual case, all (seven) rehabilitation agencies can be involved in *medical rehabilitation*. They do so irrespective of the cause (q.v. previously mentioned exceptions, however).

Statutory accident insurance: (SSC VII) A peculiarity as here, consequentially caused, compensation by means of financial payment is combined with all the "one-stop" benefits for the integration of the disabled into working life. The other task is occupational and health protection as well as prevention.

In the case of an occupational disease or accident, full responsibility for all benefits rests with the statutory accident insurance. The involvement of the latter is more or less only over when healthcare, medical and vocational rehabilitation have resulted in integration into gainful employment. In addition, the statutory accident insurance pays – in accordance with certain rules – compensation that is income-related, i.e., it also pays the pension resulting from disability or sickness if working capacity can no longer be attained. The degree of reduction regarding working capacity as interpreted by accident insurance on the general labour market serves for the percentile assessment of compensation obligation and not the reduction in earning capacity as interpreted by the statutory pension insurance.

Federal Labour Agency: (SSC III – Promotion of labour) Procurement of training and further training places, finding work for the disabled in gainful employment by means of placement service. For this purpose, there are links with the business world and with individual employers. In the case of imminent or actual unemployment, the federal Labour Agency pays unemployment benefits and assistance, intercedes and bears exclusively qualifying shares in occupational rehabilitation among a wide range of different specialist institutions for qualifying occupational rehabilitation.

Law of social compensation in the case of health impairment: Special assistance in individual cases, including occupational promotion as well as pension payments. These are subsidiary benefits, which – dependent on the situation of each individual case – can encompass all the benefits required including medical and vocational rehabilitation.

Help for young people: Help in education and integration, in particular for mentally disabled children and young people.

Simplified schematic description of the path following illness or accident from acute treatment through to integration

This path can best be followed using Illustrations 3 and 4 below. The stages given there correspond to the overviews in sections 3, 4 and 5 and are described in detail in section 7.

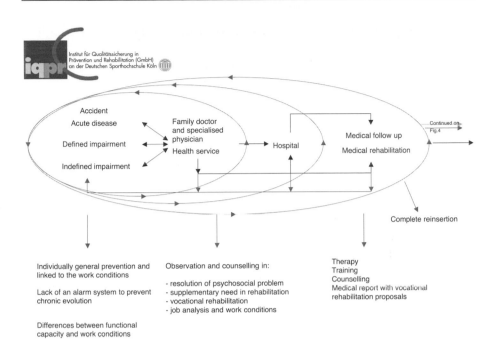

Fig. 3 – Graphic simplified and schematic representation of the path from the treatment of the actue phase to the reinsertion after a disease or an accident.

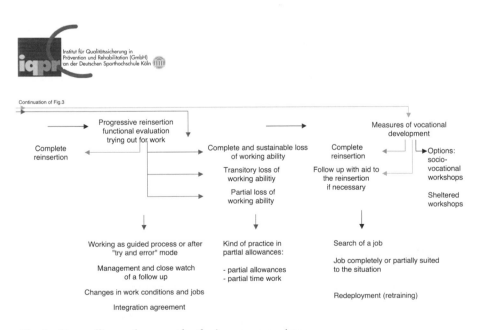

Fig. 4 – Counselling and support by the insurance carriers.
Particular models: institutional services.
Specialised services in reinsertion after the new law on disability.

Current state of affairs created by SSC IX

The overviews given in the beginning of this chapter and illustrations 1 to 4 are individually described below and arranged in accordance with SSC IX.

Introduction

There is not one single independent social benefit fund which holds responsibility for participation-oriented benefits as a whole or even individual benefit categories; instead they are part of the miscellaneous tasks of a number of benefit funds which, in the context of participation-oriented benefits, are referred to as *rehabilitation funds*. According to section 6 of Book 9 of the Social Code:

– *medical rehabilitation benefits* are provided by the health insurance, pension insurance and occupational accident insurance funds as well as by the funds providing compensation benefits in the event of damage to health;

– *benefits aimed at participation in working life* are provided by the Federal Employment Service, the pension and occupational accident insurance funds as well as by the funds providing compensation benefits in the event of damage to health,

– *benefits aimed at participation in community life* are provided by the occupational accident insurance funds and by the funds providing compensation benefits in the event of damage to health.

Because of their comprehensive range of responsibilities, the funds responsible for public youth welfare and social assistance step in as subsidiary funds in the case of all benefits aimed at participation where the required benefits cannot be obtained from funds responsible in the first place because the respective eligibility requirements are not met in individual cases. On the whole, participation-oriented benefits are provided by seven categories of rehabilitation funds:

Benefit aimed at	Occup. accident ins.	Social compensation	Health insurance	Pension insurance	Fed. employment service	Youth welfare	Social assistance
Medical rehabilitation	X	X	X	X		X	X
Participation in working life	X	X		X	X	X	X
Participation in community life	X	X				X	X

The question as to which benefits aimed at participation are provided by which rehabilitation fund and under which conditions depends on the benefit laws applying to the individual rehabilitation funds (section 7, clause 2, of Book 9 of the Social Code); this takes account of the fact that the system consists of various branches. Thus pension insurance benefits may only be granted to persons who are covered by that scheme, and social assistance benefits only to those who meet the requirements of that scheme; the relevant regulations are laid down in the respective Books of the Social Code and in other laws on benefits. In contrast, regulations *on the nature and objectives of participation-oriented* benefits which can be similar for various social benefit areas are to be found only in one place – in Book 9 of the Social Code – which is also meant to illustrate that the common objective – a participation of disabled persons and persons who are in danger of becoming disabled in the life of society to the largest possible extent – is generally pursued in the same way by all rehabilitation funds that are responsible in individual cases. Due to the consolidation of regulations which apply uniformly to several social benefit areas, Book 9 of the Social Code is similarly effective across the board as the regulations of Books 1, 4 and 10 of the Social Code already were before. Because of the particularities of a system which consists of various branches, these uniform regulations can only apply if the benefit legislation applicable to the individual rehabilitation funds does not provide otherwise; in the context of the drafting of Book 9 of the Social Code, however, many special regulations of individual benefit laws were repealed, replaced by references to Book 9 of the Social Code or adjusted in terms of their contents.

Section 11 of Book 9 of the Social Code provides that in so far as it is necessary in individual cases, the responsible rehabilitation fund examines at the time when medical rehabilitation benefits are initiated, while they are provided and after their completion whether the earning capacity of a person with disabilities or in danger of becoming disabled may be preserved, improved or restored by means of suitable benefits aimed at participation in working life. If it becomes evident during the provision of medical rehabilitation benefits that it may be difficult for a person to keep his present job, the question whether benefits aimed at participation in working life are necessary is clarified without delay in consultation with the person concerned and the responsible rehabilitation fund.

In addition to the benefits aimed at participation in working life that are granted if the requirements are fulfilled, severely disabled persons may also receive special benefits and other assistance under Part 2 of Book 9 of the Social Code to attain this objective; further details are given in nos. 92 to 107. These benefits are financed from the compensatory levy which employers have to pay if they fail to meet their obligation to employ severely disabled persons. The benefits of the statutory long-term care insurance whose funds do not belong to the rehabilitation funds are described separately.

Benefits aimed at participation in working life

Vocational training cannot guarantee permanent participation in working life; it is nevertheless indispensable, since disabled persons can only survive competition in working life with non-disabled persons if they have the best possible vocational qualifications. It is therefore a primary task of educational and social policy together, also and particularly in case of problems on the labour market, to provide *comprehensive training opportunities for disabled persons* in order to give them the greatest possible degree of equality of opportunity when competing with non-disabled persons for permanent employment.

According to section 33 of Book 9 of the Social Code, *benefits aimed at participation in working life* should include all forms of benefits necessary to sustain, enhance, generate or restore the earning power of disabled persons or persons in danger of becoming disabled in accordance with their capability, thereby assuring their permanent participation in working life, if possible. The selection of benefits aimed at participation in working life must take sufficient account of the aptitude, inclinations and earlier occupation of the disabled person as well as of the situation on and development of the labour market. It is ensured that disabled women enjoy equal opportunities in working life.

Other benefits aimed at participation in working life, in addition to those mentioned under no. 67-73, are, in particular:

– assistance to keep or obtain employment, including counselling and placement services, training measures and mobility aids;

– preparation for employment, including basic training necessary due to the disability;

– vocational adaptation and further training, also if benefits include a school-leaving diploma required for participation in the measures;

– vocational training, also if benefits include, for less than half of the time, school-type training;

– bridging allowances in compliance with section 57 of Book 3 of the Social Code, to be provided by the rehabilitation funds according to section 6(1), no. 2-5;

– other forms of assistance to promote participation in working life in order to allow disabled persons to obtain and keep appropriate employment or self-employment.

There is, partially, a *legal right* to the benefits required in each individual case for participation in working life; partially, benefits are subject to dutiful discretion.

In numerous cases, benefits *such as technical equipment for the workplace*, aids for the disability-specific adaptation or for the acquisition of a *motor vehicle* – the details are regulated by the Motor Vehicle Assistance Regulation –, *training subsidies* and *integration assistance* to employers are sufficient to achieve the goal of rehabilitation. However, vocational training measures form the core of benefits aimed at participation in working life.

The primary objective of vocational training for disabled persons is training in an *officially recognised training occupation* under section 25 of the Vocational Training Act or section 25 of the Handicrafts Regulation Act. This is to take place, whenever possible, in a company or administration along with non-disabled persons; at the same time, this training is supplemented in accordance with the legislation of the Länder by attendance at a vocational school (dual training). On-the-job training is often made possible by providing training subsidies to employers.

The special circumstances of disabled persons are taken into account, where appropriate, for training in an officially recognised training occupation. This possibility is granted by section 48(1) of the Vocational Training Act and section 42b(1) of the Handicrafts Regulation Act. Recommendations adopted by the Central Committee of the Federal Vocational Training Institute contain information as to how the special concerns of disabled persons may be taken into account in intermediate, final and qualifying examinations. For instance, individual training units may be dispensed with where these are of secondary importance as far as subsequent employment is concerned. If there is a need to modify the standard required in examinations due to the candidate's disability, this fact will be recorded on the certificate.

For young people who cannot be trained in officially recognised training occupations, despite extra assistance and the possibility of derogating from training regulations, because of the nature or severity of their disability, section 48b of the Vocational Training Act and section 42d of the Handicrafts Regulation Act give the competent regional authorities the possibility of creating *regulations on training outside officially recognised training occupations* to take account of the special circumstances of disabled persons. The special training courses are intended to lead to a final qualification which can be used to seek employment in the labour market and guarantees access to officially recognised training occupations. According to Federal Employment Service statistics, the number of young disabled persons participating in these special training courses was 21,372 in December 2002. A large number of these special courses were in the metalworking trades, followed by housekeeping and the building and allied trades. To obtain some degree of uniformity in these training courses, the Federal Vocational Training Institute drafted, as part of the recommendations put forward by its Central Committee in 1978, standardised forms of nationwide training courses in the form of model recommendations, the regional implementation of which is subject to the decisions of the relevant chambers and the other "competent bodies" under the Vocational Training Act and the Handicrafts Regulation Act.

The aforementioned principles governing the vocational training of disabled persons also apply to the *further training of adults* rendered necessary because of a disability; it is possible for adults, however, to be retrained in other professions than the officially recognised training occupations. Section 37 of Book 9 of the Social Code provides that under normal circumstances the *duration* of payment of vocational further training benefits should not exceed two years.

Where appropriate conditions exist, both disabled and non-disabled persons should receive training in *companies and administrations*; the same applies to further training of disabled adults or adults who are in danger of becoming disabled. Experience shows that such training offers particularly good opportunities for lasting participation in working life since it enables the trainees to grow accustomed to the conditions and demands of everyday working life, and trainees are normally taken directly into employment afterwards. If the company and the vocational school are willing and able to provide training while taking adequate account of disabilities, priority is also given to this kind of training for disabled persons. At the end of December 2002, 147,254 disabled persons assisted by the Federal Employment Service in the context of participation in working life were taking part in work preparation or vocational support measures, 45,719 of them in the new Länder. Of these persons, 59,651 completed vocational training courses and 33,917 further training courses, 24,356 took part in support courses and 18,049 in measures carried out in the context of the admission procedures and in the vocational training sections of workshops for disabled persons.

Where training measures carried out within companies make it necessary, because of the nature or severity of the disability or in order for participation to be successful, to accommodate the persons away from their own or parental home, expenses for *board and lodging* are covered (section 33(7), no. 1, of Book 9 of the Social Code).

Where it is required by the nature or severity of the disability or in order to guarantee successful participation, vocational training measures are implemented in special *centres for vocational rehabilitation* (section 35 of Book 9 of the Social Code). These centres for the initial training of young disabled persons (50 vocational training centres with around 13,000 places) and for the retraining of disabled adults (27 vocational retraining centres with around 15,000 places) are equipped with the necessary specialist (medical, psychological, educational and social) services. In the case of these measures, the rehabilitation fund responsible accepts all expenses related to the benefit, including board and lodging. The training programmes are to take account of the inclinations and abilities of persons undergoing rehabilitation and be geared to the progressing demands of the labour market and adapt these training programmes to developments in technology. The fact that the work done by vocational training and retraining centres is successful is, for example, shown by the *good placement results* of those who complete the courses at these centres: according to surveys carried out among former trainees one year after the payment of benefits has ended, they amount to roughly 70 per cent (covering a wide range of different professions). The success of participation in working life is due not least to the fact that participants in these benefit measures are continually introduced to modern technologies such as numerical control machines, computer-controlled drawing systems, modern data processing equipment and microelectronics and, therefore, have greater opportunities than others for employment in modern industries. For the future, however, increasing placement difficulties must be expected so that more follow-up care will be necessary for those having completed courses in rehabilitation centres.

In addition to the vocational retraining and vocational training centres, particular importance is assigned to the *centres for medical and occupational rehabilitation* (18 with 3,915 places) where, in the case of certain (e.g. neurological) illnesses, initial steps of vocational assistance (e.g. assessment of aptitude for work and work testing, benefits for further training) are already initiated while benefits for medical rehabilitation are being paid. These centres bridge the gap between purely medical-based centres for acute treatment and primary care on the one hand and the occupational rehabilitation centres on the other, which provide training and further training.

When paying benefits aimed at participation in working life, the rehabilitation fund responsible usually provides *cash benefits* (training allowance for initial training, *bridging allowance* to assure subsistence), provided that the eligibility criteria of that particular fund are satisfied, and also pays social security contributions (section 44(1), no. 2, of Book 9 of the Social Code). The bridging allowance usually amounts to 68 per cent of previous regular earnings (80 per cent of previous earnings, but no more than the full amount of previous net earnings), rising to 75 per cent if the beneficiary has at least one child within the meaning of section 32(1), (3) to (5) of the Income Tax Act or if the spouse with whom the disabled person shares a home is unable to obtain gainful employment due to taking care of the beneficiary or because this spouse is in need of care also and is not entitled to benefits from the long-term care insurance. In addition to this, other *supplementary benefits and benefits to guarantee subsistence* are possible such as:

– rehabilitation sports or functional training if prescribed by a doctor (section 44(1), no. 3, of Book 9 of the Social Code),

– travelling expenses (section 53 of Book 9 of the Social Code),

– domestic help or help at work (section 54(1), (2) and (4) of Book 9 of the Social Code), and

– costs linked with child care (section 54(3) of Book 9 of the Social Code).

For a *course of study* at a university, college or similar educational establishment, *disabled persons* can normally only be given assistance according to the Federal Education Assistance Act; in many instances, however, there is also a need for intervention by social assistance, which also classifies this type of training as vocational training for disabled persons (section 13 of the Integration Assistance Regulation).

Special forms of assistance are often required to facilitate participation in working life – for example, immediately after successful completion of some form of vocational training. To facilitate the *taking up of employment*, the relevant stipulations in section 33 of Book 9 of the Social Code provide for benefits to the disabled persons themselves or their employers. Forms of assistance available to the persons concerned include:

– the coverage of costs linked with course fees, examination fees, expenses for study aids, working clothes and working equipment;

– motor vehicle assistance according to the Motor Vehicle Assistance Regulation;

– compensation of unavoidable loss of income arising for the severely disabled person or a person accompanying the disabled person due to travelling to and from training measures and job interviews;

– costs for work assistance which the disabled person may need in order to find a job;

– costs for aids which may be necessary due to the type or severity of the disability in order to exercise an occupation, participate in benefits aimed at participation in working life or increase the safety of the disabled person travelling to and from the workplace and at the workplace itself, unless the employer has an obligation in this respect or such benefits can be granted as medical benefits;

– costs for technical aids necessary to exercise an occupation due to the type or severity of the disability, and

– reasonable costs for procuring, equipping and maintaining a home fit for disabled persons.

Of the *funds responsible for benefits aimed at participation in working life*, the Federal Employment Service is almost exclusively responsible for the initial participation of disabled persons in working life and in many cases bears the responsibility for restoring participation in the event of disabilities occurring at a later stage. The accident insurance and social compensation funds, on the basis of their obligations, have a clearly defined group of persons to assist. Pension insurance provides discretionary benefits aimed at participation in working life especially where the earning capacity of an insured person, after 15 years of paying contributions, is substantially threatened due to a potential disability, where a pension on account of reduced earning capacity is paid, or would have to be paid without these benefits, or where such benefits are to be provided directly after benefits for medical rehabilitation granted by the pension insurance funds.

Because of the comprehensive nature of benefits aimed at participation in working life from other funds, *social assistance* benefits are relevant only in individual cases. However, these benefits are of great importance for workshops for disabled persons (see also nos. 108-112). To assist disabled persons in obtaining a type of work which is suited to their disability, assistance is also given as part of integration assistance to support work at home. In all other instances, the general regulations on working at home (Homework Act) apply to disabled persons.

For the whole area of benefits aimed at participation in working life, the Federal Employment Service also has the special task, over and above its function as one of the funds responsible for rehabilitation, of producing, upon request of another rehabilitation fund, a report on the need for, the type and the scope of benefits, while taking into account their effectiveness with regard to prospects in the labour market (section 38 of Book 9 of the Social Code).

Special forms of assistance for participation of severely disabled persons in working life

To improve the opportunities of *severely disabled persons* in working life, special forms of assistance are available, in addition to the benefits aimed at participation in working life, which can also be claimed by severely disabled persons under Part 2 of Book 9 of the Social Code. In order to secure employment for the disabled persons covered by this legislation and at the same time improve the individual conditions, this Act provides for the following, in particular:

– the duty of public and private employers to fill 5 per cent of the positions with severely disabled persons or pay a compensatory levy for unfilled compulsory places (sections 71 et seq. of Book 9 of the Social Code);

– special responsibilities of employers toward severely disabled employees (sections 81 et seq. of Book 9 of the Social Code);

– a special protection against unlawful dismissal for severely disabled employees following expiry of a six-month period (sections 85 et seq. of Book 9 of the Social Code);

– protection of the interests of severely disabled persons at work by the representatives for severely disabled persons (sections 93 et seq. of Book 9 of the Social Code), and

– supplementary benefits granted by the Federal Employment Service and the integration offices to severely disabled persons to facilitate their participation in working life (sections 101 et seq. of Book 9 of the Social Code).

On the basis of the "*Points of reference* for those issuing medical reports" published by the Federal Ministry of Health and Social Security, the compensation office *determines* which persons are to be classified as severely disabled. The severity of the limitation is expressed as a "degree of disability" in increments of ten degrees between 10 and 100. The fact that this determination is made on a general basis and not in relation to a particular job means that severely disabled persons are also and particularly protected in jobs where their disability has little effect. Severely disabled persons may receive a *pass* upon application, which verifies the degree of disability ascertained and makes it easier to exercise certain rights and obtain compensation for disadvantage. If disabled persons having a degree of disability of less than 50 but of at least 30 are unable, because of their disability, to find or retain suitable employment, they are accorded *equal status with severely disabled persons* by the employment office upon application.

Part 2 of Book 9 of the Social Code obliges all employers to examine whether persons with severe disabilities or persons of equal status could be employed when *vacancies are to be filled*. The same Act also provides for work to be adapted to accommodate the disability by:

– equipping workplaces with the requisite technical equipment;
– designing and maintaining the working environment, furnishings, machinery and appliances with the aim of allowing the highest possible number of severely disabled persons to be employed;
– employing severely disabled persons in such a way that they are able to fully develop and use their knowledge and skills, and
– promoting occupational advancement and facilitating participation in on-going vocational further training.

The special regulations and principles for filling civil service and judicial posts are also to be formulated in such a way that the engagement and employment of severely disabled persons is promoted and there is an appropriate percentage of severely disabled persons amongst civil servants and judges.

The *employment obligation* is of particular importance for securing the participation of severely disabled persons in the labour and training places market. Employers with a workforce of 20 or more are obliged to ensure that at least 5 per cent of their workforce is made up of severely disabled persons. This obligation applies not only to private, but also to public employers. In calculating compulsory places, the employment office may take into account more than one, at most three, compulsory places for one severely disabled person if participation of that person in working life is particularly difficult.

Fulfilling the employment obligation is not always easy if no suitable severely disabled candidate is available when a vacancy arises; yet solutions can often be found with good will and by drawing upon all available forms of assistance. Nevertheless, many employers obliged to employ severely disabled persons are still not willing to meet their obligation and pay the compensatory levy.

Of the 151,595 employers who were subject to the employment obligation in 2001, 30,900 (around 20 per cent) had fulfilled their obligation or were above the obligatory number. However, 80 per cent of all employers failed to meet their obligations or did not meet them in full. In 2001 the employment rate amounted to 3.8 per cent in Germany.

The *compensatory levy* payable by employers monthly per unfilled compulsory place amounts to:

– € 105 in the case of an annual average employment quota of 3 per cent up to less than 5 per cent;

– € 180 in the case of an annual average employment quota of 2 up to less than 3 per cent;

– € 260 in the case of an annual average employment quota of less than 2 per cent.

The revenue from the compensatory levy may only be used for participation purposes of severely disabled persons; the details are embodied in the Severely Disabled Persons Compensatory Levy Regulation.

The revenue from the compensatory levy – around DM 1,013 million in 2001 – is used primarily for the engagement and employment of severely disabled persons, which means that the greater part of it is returned to employers. A 55 per cent share goes to the integration offices of the Länder (which used to be called "main welfare offices") where it is used for benefits to boost the supply of jobs and training places for severely disabled persons, benefits towards supplementary assistance in working life and other measures for the participation of severely disabled persons. Forty-five per cent of the revenue is invested in the *Compensation Fund* set up by the Federal Ministry of Health and Social Security to promote nation-wide benefits aimed at participation of severely disabled persons in working life. The Compensation Fund allocates to the Federal Employment Service the resources necessary for the special promotion of the recruitment and employment of severely disabled persons. In addition, it promotes nation-wide projects for participation of severely disabled persons in working life.

Special Promotion for severely disabled persons with particular difficulties

Special promotion of engagement and employment of severely disabled persons concerns those severely disabled persons who, as a result of their disability, old age or other reasons, have particular difficulties on the labour or training places market. This includes those severely disabled persons who require a special assistant or other exceptional expenses to enable them to work, whose employment will permanently cause exceptional expenses for the employer due to their disability, whose performance is obviously reduced considerably on a permanent basis due to their disability, or whose degree of disability caused solely by a mental or psychological disability or pathological fits reaches a level of 50, or who due to the type and severity of their disability do not have a vocational training diploma as defined under the Vocational Training Act, as well as severely disabled persons aged 50 and over (section 72(2) of Book 9 of the Social Code). Where employers who fulfil or are not subject to the employment obligation engage severely disabled persons from the above groups, they may be entitled in accordance with section 222a of Book 3 of the Social Code to receive wage cost subsidies from the Federal Employment Service of up to 70 per cent of the wage paid to the severely disabled person for up to three years, and in the case of older severely disabled persons, for up to eight years.

Supplementary assistance in working life is implemented by the integration offices or – on their behalf – by the local welfare offices in close co-operation with the Federal Employment Service. The intention is to ensure that the social status of severely disabled persons does not decline, that they are employed in jobs in which they are able to fully use and develop their skills and knowledge, and that they are enabled to assert themselves at work and in competition with non-disabled persons.

In addition to the financial assistance provided by the integration offices, in particular for a disability-suited equipment of training places and workplaces and to compensate for extreme difficulties resulting from the employment of particularly severely disabled persons, the other forms of assistance they offer also play an important role. The *counselling* of severely disabled persons, mainly at work, and *company visits* are of particular significance. The integration offices may also involve independent funds in the provision of psychological and social care as part of their supplementary assistance programme in working life; such care is important not only for psychologically disabled persons but for all severely disabled persons and persons of equal status (in the latter instance, the need for this type of care will depend upon the circumstances in each individual case).

On the basis of experience and findings gained in model projects, and by involving other existing services, local *specialist services for integration* were set up all over the country. These services are to support employment offices, the other rehabilitation funds and integration offices in fulfilling their tasks, especially when it comes to counselling severely disabled persons before taking a job, when looking for a job, in application procedures, after they have taken a job, and to assisting them in gaining mental and social stability; moreover, they can provide information, advice and support to companies and administrations. In addition to focusing on severely disabled persons who are unemployed or in danger of becoming unemployed, the activities of the specialist services will also concentrate on the transition of severely disabled persons from workshops for disabled persons to employment in the general labour market, and from school to employment under the conditions of the general labour market, if the persons concerned could otherwise only be employed in a workshop for disabled persons.

Further special promotion

A further important instrument for securing and preserving jobs for severely disabled persons is the *special protection against dismissal*; this commences six months after the start of employment. The employer's obligation to obtain the approval of the integration office *before* giving notice of dismissal is intended primarily to examine all forms of assistance which might secure continuing employment and to weigh the interests of both parties; should these measures serve to show that the continued employment of the severely disabled person is unreasonable, given the circumstances of the individual case, the dismissal is approved. This is what happens in the majority of proceedings initiated; consequently, this protection against dismissal is not an obstacle to recruitment – a view which is still held by many employers despite increased information.

The special interests of severely disabled persons are looked after by works and staff councils in companies and administrations. Where more than five members of permanent staff are severely disabled, a spokesperson as a *representative for severely disabled persons* is to be elected. The main task of this representative is to monitor adherence to all provisions in favour of disabled persons and to support these persons by providing advice and assistance. The representatives of severely disabled persons are able, on the basis of their specialist knowledge and experience of procedures in companies and administrations, to make a valuable contribution to improving participation of severely disabled persons in working life.

Employers should normally ensure that these representatives are consulted when determining whether vacant jobs or training places might be suitable for severely disabled persons, particularly those who are registered with the employment service as unemployed or seeking employment.

The representatives are entitled to be fully informed and to be heard. If a measure has been determined without their involvement, its implementation or execution must be suspended until the representatives have been involved.

They must be included in all monthly discussions between the employer and the works or staff councils, since these may deal with matters affecting severely disabled persons.

They must maintain constant contact with the local employment office and with the integration office and cooperate closely with these authorities (section 99, clause 2, of Book 9 of the Social Code).

Details of the election of representatives are set out in the Severely Disabled Persons' Election Regulations.

According to section 104 of Book 9 of the Social Code, the Federal Employment Service is responsible for the provision of vocational guidance and the placement of severely disabled persons into training and employment; it is also responsible for counselling employers in cases where severely disabled persons may be recruited to fill vacant jobs or training places. Special *counselling and placement centres* have been set up at the employment offices for the employment promotion and vocational assistance of disabled persons.

The compensation for disadvantages experienced by severely disabled persons includes entitlement to a paid *supplementary leave* of regularly five days per year (section 125 of Book 9 of the Social Code). Severely disabled persons must also be exempted on their own request from working *overtime* (section 124 of Book 9 of the Social Code).

Workshops for disabled persons

For disabled persons who, because of the nature or severity of their disability and in spite of every assistance, are not or not yet able to participate (again) in the general labour market, workshops for disabled persons offer suitable vocational training and employment while paying wages that are commensurate with the disabled persons' performance (section 136 of Book 9 of the Social Code). According to this provision, the workshops are open to all those disabled persons, irrespective of the nature and severity of their disability, who are capable of doing a minimum amount of economically useful work, at the latest after having participated in measures in the vocational training section; the workshops must make it possible for the disabled employees to develop, enhance or recover their skills, abilities and earning capacity and, in so doing, further develop their personality. The technical requirements to be met by workshops for disabled persons and the approval procedure are set down in the Workshop Regulation. In the year 2001, around 186,000 disabled persons were employed in 669 approved workshops.

The workshops for disabled persons are also meant for persons who, because of their disability, require special personnel to provide care and individual assistance for them and who, therefore, receive care and assistance in special support groups. Disabled persons who do not or have yet to meet the requirements for employment in a workshop for disabled persons may be admitted to institutions affiliated to the workshop.

To prepare for employment in the workshop, benefits are awarded in accordance with section 40 of Book 9 of the Social Code for up to 3 months to promote participation in measures in the *entry procedure* offered by approved workshops for disabled persons, and in the *vocational training section*, benefits are awarded for up to 2 years, with the vast majority of them being granted through the Federal Employment Service. It is the task of the workshops to assist disabled persons in such a way that by the time they have completed the vocational training measures, they are in a position to deliver a minimum amount of economically useful work; beyond this primary aim, the workshops' task is to assist and encourage each individual in such a way that he attains his full potential. To fulfil these tasks, workshops for disabled persons must offer the widest possible range of vocational training and actual work opportunities.

Assistance in *the work section* is generally one of the functions of integration assistance for disabled persons, in accordance with section 40(1), no. 7, and section 41 of the Federal Social Assistance Act in conjunction with section 41 of Book 9 of the Social Code; according to section 100 of the Federal Social Assistance Act, the bodies responsible are the social assistance funds, which in 2001 raised around 3,100 million EUR for this purpose. *Wages* for disabled persons working in the workshops amount to an average of € 125 per month. In addition, those working in workshops and earning up to € 325 receive an employment promotion allowance of € 26 per month. The involvement of disabled employees in workshops for disabled persons is governed by the Regulation on the Involvement of Disabled Persons in Workshops.

The disabled persons who are employed in the work section of the workshops normally have a *legal status* similar to that of employees. They are compulsorily insured with sickness insurance, long-term care insurance, pension insurance and occupational accident insurance funds. After a period of employment of least 20 years they receive a pension on account of totally reduced earning capacity from the statutory pension insurance.

Vocational rehabilitation: the Greek model

X. Michail, K. Stathi and M. Tzara

The Greek social security system

Concept of social security [1]

The Greek social security system is a rather complex model of social protection that is promoted through the application of three different techniques: social insurance for persons within the labour market, social assistance for needy uninsured persons and a national health scheme for all persons living in the Greek territory. As far as its administrative structure is concerned, the social insurance system is regulated and supervised by the Ministry of Labour and Social Insurance, while health care and welfare policies are monitored by the Ministry of Health and Social Assistance.

The social insurance system is the cornerstone of the domestic social security model. Its function, as has been developed since the 1950s, aims at covering social risks of workers and employees through the provision of cash benefits and services, which address problems related to the reduction or loss of income gained through employment. The system is based on three insurance pillars:

– the first pillar corresponds to the public schemes of compulsory main and supplementary insurance, which function through legal entities supervised by different ministries;

– the second and the third pillar have not yet been developed equally with the first pillar. Recently, the government adopted legislative measures to introduce occupational funds with the aim to extend the protection of insured persons and to strengthen the adequacy of insurance benefits; these funds will form the second pillar in Greece.

The Greek health care system today can be characterised as a mixed system: the health care branches of the various social insurance funds co-exist with the national health care system *(E.S.Y. - ethniko systima ygeias)*. The national health system was established by law in 1983, designed to guarantee free health care for all residents of Greece. Although from a legal point of view the national health system constitutes the cornerstone of health care protection, this harmonizing concept suffered serious drawbacks due to the parallel functioning of the health care branches of the various social insurance schemes. Policy makers have been seriously discussing since 1996 the possibility to integrate the health care branches of the various social insurances schemes into the general framework of the national health care system.

The national health system covers the entire Greek population, without any special entitlement condition, regardless of professional category or region. Health care services are also provided to European Union and non-EU citizens on the basis of multilateral or bilateral agreements.

Within the ESY context, primary health care services are provided through rural health centres and provincial surgeries in rural areas, the outpatient departments of regional and district hospitals, the polyclinics of the social insurance institutions and specialist in urban areas. Secondary care is provided by public hospitals, private-for-profit hospitals and clinics or hospitals owned by social insurance funds.

The social assistance system forms the final safety net for needy persons without sufficient means. It is based on categorical minimum income schemes, which cover specific welfare target groups, such as the elderly, the disabled, the single parent families and the children in need. These schemes were introduced in the 1960s and developed during the 1980s.

The categorical social assistance schemes normally require the Greek nationality and permanent residence in Greece in order to qualify for the cash benefits and social services. However, E.U. citizens are equally covered as welfare benefits fall into the definition of social advantages, to which the principle of equal treatment is applied according to the provisions of E.C. Regulation 1612/68.

The current system provides cash benefits, benefits in kind and personal social services through decentralized legal bodies supervised by the Ministry of Health and Social Assistance. Social services are also provided through local communities and a network of voluntary bodies and NGOs actively involved in the framework of policies for children, refugees and persons with special needs. Their role is influential as far as domiciliary services and services for socially excluded persons is concerned.

Since, the introduction of the so-called "prefectural self-government" in 1993, regional public law bodies assumed responsibility for certain activities in the social welfare area. In each prefecture there is a social welfare department, which bears responsibility for the implementation of welfare programmes in the region; this department administers cash benefits financed by the ministry of health and social assistance and promotes personal social services financed both by the ministry and the prefecture concerned.

A national social care scheme was introduced in 1998. This scheme decentralizes personal social services and develops new forms of open care that tend to prevail over the out of date institutional care.

Personal social services include institutional and domiciliary care. Institutional-type services are mainly provided by centres for disabled and elderly persons. Open care services are provided by rehabilitation centres for disabled and the Centres for the Protection of the Elderly (KAPI). These centres function on a local level aiming at preventing biological, psychological and social problems of the elderly; coordinating the cooperation of competent institutions and the public sector in dealing with the problems of the elderly and researching relevant matters. Their services include entertainment (excursions, summer camps, further education); instructions for medical and pharmaceutical care; social work; physiotherapy; occupational therapy and home help.

Apart from direct cash allowances and personal social services, benefits for needy persons in Greece include favourable tax treatment and tax credits. Relevant benefits were introduced through the design of the first National Action Plan on Social Inclusion (submitted in July 2001 to the European Commission), aiming, among others, at the coverage of poor persons in rural areas (they receive a lump-sum allowance equal to 293 euros per year, under the condition that their annual family income does not exceed 2,200 euros and the tax treatment of households with children under 16 (they receive marginal tax credits, under the condition that their annual income does not exceed 2,990 euros).

The statutes and the administrative acts [2, 3, 4]

In the Greek context, the term statute must be understood as referring to acts that stem from the plenum of the Parliament or departments thereof, as well as the legislative texts issued by the government or, under certain conditions, by the President of the Republic. Statutes dealing with pension issues are discussed by the plenum on a proposal by competent ministries, followed by an opinion of the Chamber of the State.

The main social insurance legislation is to be found in the acts that regulate main and supplementary schemes as well as in the new provisions on the modernisation of the system adopted during the 1990s and finalised by the issue of the Law No 3029 / 2002. There is no codification of the existing legal norms. Nevertheless, the Ministry of Labour and Social Insurance will soon promote a codification process with the view to simplify administrative procedures and to strengthen the access of citizens to social insurance funds.

The large number of the first tier social insurance schemes and the pluriformity of supplementary funds and mutual aid societies are responsible for the fact that social security law has been laid down in hundreds of legislative texts. A degree of harmonisation is urgently required and indeed efforts to this effect are currently being undertaken, namely the introduction of general statutes in 1992, 1998, 1999 and 2002 that deal with the unification of affiliation rules as well as entitlement conditions to receive benefits between different first tier schemes. Already at this stage the legislative framework of the social insurance institute (IKA: idryma koinonikon asphaliseon) scheme serves as a model for the other social insurance schemes. IKA is the largest Social Security Organization in Greece. It covers 5,530,000 workers and employees and provides 830,000 pensioners with retirement pension.

Through the right insurance scheme, an employee is entitled to an entire range of benefits from both IKA and other Organizations, such as OAED 32 (the State Employment Services of Greece), Ergatiki Katikia (equivalent to Council Housing Services) and Ergatiki Estia (labourer's Union).

The administrative organisation
of social insurance in Greece [4, 5, 6]

Social insurance policies in Greece were developed in a piece-meal way through the establishment of main and supplementary funds for different socio-professional categories. There is no single universal scheme for all active persons but different schemes according to the occupation of the relevant persons concerned.

In 2002 there were as many as 170 social insurance institutions, each of them being more or less different from the others. The majority are supervised by the Ministry of Labour and Social Insurance; four other Ministries are involved in the monitoring of socio-professional based schemes (Ministry of Labour and Social Insurance, Ministry of Defense, Ministry of Economy and Finance, Ministry of Marine, Ministry of Agriculture, hellenic parliament, insurance agencies, mutual aid societies).

The plurality of the existing schemes and the function of relevant insurance funds should be attributed to the adoption of socio-professional principles for the cover of persons active in the domestic labour market, as identified in the following table.

Social Insurance Funds according to employment criteria.

Number of funds supervised by the Ministry of Labour and Social Insurance	Socio-professional categories
22	Employees and workers under private law
10	Employees in the banking sector
12	Persons employed in public utilities
6	Self-employed people
11	Independent professionals
6	People employed in the press
1	Farmers
17	Civil servants

The role of OAED in Greek society [3]

The task of OAED is completed by:

– the acquisition or/and improvement of the vocational skills of manpower through training and its support with employment programmes, so that it will correspond to the continuously changing conditions of the Labour Market and

– the Social Security Benefits and Allowances granted to the social groups that have already been mentioned. The Organization contributes with the best way possible to the protection of the citizen's right for employment and social welfare given by the Constitution, contributing to the co-existence of development and social cohesion by taking responsibility for finding the proper work placement for each unemployed person and by delivering Social Security Services to the various groups of the population.

OAED is a member of CEDEFOR and participates in a 15-member Organizations Network named EVTA (European Vocational Training Association).

OAED, in order to meet the differentiated needs of Labour Force, is going to have its role and activities, structures, systems and functions redefined according to a master plan which is going to be elaborated. Accordingly, its strategy and transition towards a new model have to be decided.

Employed persons' insurance schemes

Personal scope of application [6, 7]

There is no general social insurance system covering all active persons in the case of the occurrence of any of the traditional social risks. Each first tier fund applies its own affiliation conditions. A common general characteristic is that, in order to be affiliated to a scheme, a person must be engaged in employment. It depends upon the character of the specific employment (sometimes also upon the region) to which social insurance institution a person belongs.

Manual workers and private employees are affiliated to the IKA. The affiliation conditions for the IKA apply for the whole nation; if a person satisfies the affiliation conditions, he is insured with the IKA wherever he works in Greece (or sometimes even outside the country). A worker is affiliated to the IKA scheme unless he is covered by another insurance scheme for employees. Such special social insurance schemes exist, for example, for employees in the banking sector and for employees of state companies.

Types of insurance forms [6, 7, 8]

The domestic social insurance schemes for employees and manual workers distinguish between different types of insurance periods.

The most usual form of a permanent legal relation between an insured person and the relevant fund is the *compulsory social insurance period*. Only the state or legal persons under public law can be institutions of compulsory insurance. Other forms of social insurance are the formal insurance and the voluntary insurance.

Formal insurance refers to the period in which a person contributes to a social insurance scheme, for a reasonable time and in good faith, without actually fulfilling all the legal conditions to affiliate to the concerned institution. Although the legal conditions were not met, the social insurance institution, which accepted the contributions under those circumstances must accept the contributor as a member.

Voluntary insurance takes three different forms. In the strict sense of the term, voluntary insurance is mainly created for Greek nationals living abroad. A second form is the voluntary continuation of a interrupted compulsory insurance period. The third form is the additional voluntary insurance for which a special branch has been established within the IKA. In order to qualify for the second form of voluntary insurance the person who was insured with IKA should request on termination of his employment to continue the insurance relation in the pension, sickness and auxiliary insurances; the voluntary insurance period can however not be taken into account for the completion of the 10,500 working days required for entitlement to a full old-age pension.

Risks and Benefits [6, 7, 8]

The legal regulation of risks, eligibility conditions and benefits for those insured with the IKA scheme is different according to the period during which the person in question is/was affiliated to IKA. As the conditions for entitlement for social insurance benefits under IKA were changed in 1992 for the future, it will be important to make the distinction between persons who first joined IKA after 31-12-1992 and those already insured before 1-1-1993.

Old age

Old age forms the main insurance risk in the light of funds used to guarantee the payment of pensions and the number of pensioners in Greece. The main benefits here (contributory pensions) are supplemented by auxiliary contributory pensions and means-tested non contributory supplements, while there are minimum amounts of pensions that correspond to mixed social pensions.

Incapacity for work

Incapacity for work is regulated within the Greek social security system according to its effects on the insured people. In respect of social insurance schemes a distinction is made between sickness insurance and invalidity insurance.

As far as the IKA scheme is concerned, the sickness insurance branch covers medical care and the loss of income as a result of sickness and maternity. Invalidity is covered through the pensions branch; the benefits which are payable due to permanent incapacity to work often bear strong similarities to old age pensions.

The cover of sickness

The insured person unable to work due to illness, is entitled to sickness benefits which include cash allowances and benefits in kind.

In order to be entitled to a sickness allowance, a person must satisfy the following conditions:

– he/she must be incapable for work and abstain from work;
– he/she must have established a contribution record of at least 100 working days in the year before the sickness or in the first 12 of the previous 15 months (in respect of incapacity for work due to industrial accident or occupational disease there are no contribution conditions;
– he must not be a pensioner.

In principle, sickness benefit provides 70% of the estimated income of the insurance class to which the claimant belonged the last 30 days of the previous year. A sickness benefit is payable from the fourth day of incapacity (3 waiting days) over a period of maximally 6 months. However, if the claimant has established a contribution record of 300, respectively 1,500 working days in the two, respectively five last years preceeding the sickness, the maximum duration is 1 year, respectively 2 years. It must also be noted that during the first month of sickness the employer is obliged to additional payments, as a supplement on top of sickness benefit; so the last wage level remains intact.

Benefits in kind include medical and health care treatment provided on the first day of the disease. IKA employs salaried doctors who provide primary medical care and dental services; IKA also contracts out private doctors for primary care services reimbursed on a fee for service basis. IKA members receive free treatment in public hospitals of the national health system or contracted private clinics. The insured people are also entitled to free consultations from a local IKA practitioner (both general practitioners and specialists).

Furthermore, the costs of medicine on prescription of an IKA doctor, are covered by the IKA subject to a personal change of 25% of the costs of the product. A personal charge is not demanded if the patient is being treated in a recognized hospital, in cases of pregnancy, when the patient is suffering a chronical disease or in cases when medicine is prescribed in respect of an occupational disease or industrial injury. Tuberculosis patients only pay a personal contribution of 10% of the costs.

Employees in higher earnings classes and their dependents may have a right to treatment in hospital accommodation of a higher grade than the one to which persons from lower earnings classes may be entitled. However, such a right is subject to extra working days requirements.

The cover of invalidity

Invalidity benefits are payable after the right to sickness benefit has expired. The insured person is regarded to be invalid when a medical committee assesses a serious illness or physical or mental disability resulting in a radical reduction of the earning capacity. The person concerned should therefore not be able to earn more than 50% of the normal average earnings of a worker in the own profession and this for at least one semester.

The amount of the pension depends on the degree of invalidity:

– an invalidity rate of 80% or more opens a right to a full pension;

– an invalidity of 66,6% at least (but not 80%) gives entitlement to 3/4th of the full pension rate, unless the insured person has established a contribution record of at least 6,000 days or 20 years; in the latter case he receives a full-rate pension;

– an invalidity rate of at least 50% (but not 66.6%) entitles to half of the full rate pension, unless the insured person shows a contribution record of at least 6,000 days or 20 years; in the latter case he receives 3/4 of the full-rate pension.

The basic amount of the pension is increased by specific supplements for a dependent spouse and/or dependent children. The spouse supplement is however only awarded to persons insured with IKA before 1993; this monthly benefit amounts to one and a half daily wage of an unskilled worker (22.35 euros in 2002).

Special supplements are provided to persons with increased needs due to invalidity:

– Paraplegics and tetraplegics who have established a contribution record of at least 1,000 days are entitled to a special monthly allowance equal to 20 times the minimum daily wage of an unskilled worker (20 × 22.35 euros in 2002).

– Persons with an invalidity degree of 100%, who are in need of constant care by a third person, are entitled to a monthly allowance equal to 50% of the basic pension rate.

The minimum levels of invalidity pension are the same as those for old age pension; also the method of calculation is the same as for old age pension (mutatis mutandis).

Industrial accidents and occupational diseases

Industrial accidents and occupational diseases are covered through the provision of sickness benefits, invalidity and survivors' pensions.

Sickness benefits (cash allowances and benefits in kind) are provided during a period of six months, without any contribution requirements.

Invalidity pensions are also paid without any contribution requirements. Here, the normal invalidity pension is payable, albeit that for persons insured with IKA already before 1993, the minimum benefit level is 60% of the estimated income in the relevant earnings class. The minimum rate for persons insured since 1993 is equal to the amount of an old age pension paid after the establishment of a contribution record of 15 years.

Survivors' pensions are paid in case of death of the insured person.

Unemployment

Social insurance coverage due to unemployment is restricted to persons affiliated to the IKA scheme. Eligible persons receive cash benefits and integration services from OAED (the manpower employment organization), a legal body of public law supervised by the Ministry of Labour and Social Insurance, acting as the responsible agency for integration and passive employment measures within the Greek social policy context.

The main benefit is the ordinary unemployment benefit. In order to become entitled to this benefit under OAED and IKA and the insured person must satisfy the following conditions:

– to be capable for work;
– to be involuntarily unemployed;
– to be registered with the labour exchange;
– to establish a contribution record of 125 working days during a period of 14 months preceding the two months prior to the commencement of unemployment (in cases of first claims, proof must be given of at least 80 working days in each of the three years prior to the commencement of unemployment).

Benefit is paid after a waiting period of six days. The period during which the unemployment benefit is being paid depends upon the contribution record the applicant established during the 14 months before becoming unemployed.

Unemployed persons, who take part in vocational training programmes, enabling them to acquire working experience are covered by IKA for risk of sickness (only for benefits in kind) and for employment injuries. Beneficiaries who receive ordinary unemployment benefits may also receive a training allowance during their participation in vocational training programmes. Nevertheless, unemployment benefits are not paid whether the rate of the training allowance exceeds their daily amount.

As far as active employment measures are concerned, traditional vocational training and job-placement schemes are supplemented by innovative measures developed during the Greek National Action Plans for Employment (NAPs for 1998, 1999, 2000, 2001 and 2002). In fact, amongst the various initiatives planned within the framework of the NAPs, over 50 programmes designed to promote employment and vocational training for the unemployed were set up involving some 140,000 unemployed people with a view to taking up employment and to acquiring vocational training.

Special subsidies have been planned for businesses which recruit older unemployed people or the long-term unemployed. They will be obliged to complete 1,500 days of insurance cover or five additional years of work in order to be entitled to a pension totaling 4,500 days of insurance cover. The subsidy period may not exceed a total of 60 months and may not be less than 18 days per month.

Moreover, in accordance with recent regulations, unemployed people of any age (the young unemployed up to 29 years of age, unemployed people between the ages of 29 and 55 and the long-term unemployed over 55) are entitled to receive free medical care (benefits in kind).

The financing of social insurance

The funds required to cover the cost of social insurance branches in the Greek system are obtained in different ways according to the distinction between the statutory first pillar and the occupational second pillar. First pillar schemes are financed according to a tripartite model in case of private employees (employers contributions, employees contributions and state subsidies) and a bipartite model in case of self-employed, independent professionals, farmers and civil servants (insured persons contributions, state subsidies).

Occupational schemes are financed by employers and employees contributions.

	Employees	Employers	State
Basic pension	6.67%	13.33%	10%
Sickness	2.55%	5.10%	3.80%
Supplementary pension	3%	3%	–

Government funds

The State itself also contributes towards the financing of the social insurance schemes by means of periodical (mostly annual) subsidies to the social insurance institutions. Thus the shortages of the IKA or other statutory schemes are annually made up out of general taxation. In the last years the state subsidies have gradually increased. The State finances most of the expenditure of the social insurance schemes for civil servants and farmers.

Tables

GREECE: Health Care [1, 2, 4, 9]
Applicable statutory basis

Applicable statutory basis	Law of 14 June 1951 Law No 1902 / 92 last modified by Law No 2676/99 of 5 January 1999

Basic principles

Basic principles	Compulsory social insurance scheme for employees and assimilated groups

Field of application

1. Beneficiaries	Employees and persons assimilated thereto Pensioners Unemployed
2. Exemptions from the compulsory insurance	No exemptions
3. Voluntarily insured	No voluntarily insurance
4. Eligible dependants	Dependant members of the insured family

Conditions

1. Qualifying period	50 days of work subject to contribution over the preceding year, or in the 12 first months of the 15 months preceding the illness
2. Duration of benefits	Unlimited

GREECE: Long-term Care [1, 2, 4, 9, 10]
Applicable statutory basis

Applicable statutory basis	Old age and invalidity No special legislation. The Law 1140/1981 (revised version) JO 68A/20-3-81, provides for some benefits

Basic principles

Basic principles	Old age and invalidity: insurance scheme Guaranteeing sufficient resources: social welfare scheme

Risk covered

Definition	Old age and invalidity: Pensioners and persons affiliated to social insurance institutions, suffering from paraplegia/tetraplegia and absolute disability if the person is in permanent need of supervision, care and support provided by a third party Guaranteeing sufficient resources: Elderly persons in need of care

Field of application

Field of application	Old age and invalidity: Persons affiliated to social insurance institutions Guaranteeing sufficient resources: Permanent residents

Conditions

1. Age	No age limit
2. Qualifying period	Old age and invalidity: 4,050 days of insurance Guaranteeing sufficient resources: no qualifying period

GREECE: Sickness - Cash benefits [4, 7, 9, 11]

Applicable statutory basis

Applicable statutory basis	Law of 14th June 1951, modified

Basic principles

Basic principles	Compulsory social insurance scheme for employees with contribution-related benefits

Field of application

1. Beneficiaries	Employees and persons assimilated
2. Membership ceiling	No membership ceiling
3. Exemptions from the compulsory insurance	No exemptions

Conditions

1. Proof of incapacity for work	Incapacity for work certified by the Institute's doctor
2. Qualifying period	100 days of work subject to contributions during the previous year or the 12 first months of the 15 preceding the illness (duration of benefit: 182 days)
	300 days subject to contributions during the 2 years, or 27 months of the 30 preceding the illness (duration of benefit: 360 days)
	1,500 days of insurance during the last 5 years preceding the incapacity for work due to the same illness (duration of benefit: 720 days)

GREECE: Employment injuries and occupational diseases [7, 8, 10, 11]

Applicable statutory basis

Applicable statutory basis	No particular insurance exists, the risk being covered under sickness, invalidity and survivors by specific regulations

Basic principles

Basic principles	No particular insurance. The risk are covered by insurance systems for sickness, invalidity and survivors

Field of application

1. Beneficiaries	Employees and persons assimilated
2. Exemptions from the compulsory insurance	No exemptions
3. Voluntarily insured	No voluntary insurance

Risks covered

1. Employment injuries	Accident injury occurred because of and during employment
2. Travel between home and work	Covered
3. Occupational diseases	List of occupational diseases

Conditions

1. Employment injuries	1 day of insurance
	Time limit for declaration: 5 days following the accident
2. Occupational diseases	The list of occupational diseases fixes minimum affiliation periods

GREECE: Invalidity [8, 10, 11]
Applicable statutory basis

Applicable statutory basis	Law 1846 / 51 of 14th June 1951, last amelioration on 24th December 1997 with the publication of Law No 2556/97

Basic principles

Basic principles	Compulsory social insurance scheme for employees with contribution-related benefits

Field of application

Field of application	Employees

Exemptions from compulsory insurance

Exemptions from compulsory insurance	No exemptions

Risks covered

Definition	A person is considered to be suffering from severe invalidity when, as a result of illness or physical or mental disability which appeared or worsened after affiliation, he or she cannot earn more than a fifth of the normal earnings of a worker in the same category or training during at least 1 year
	However, those who can no longer earn more than 1/3 of the normal earnings obtain 75% of the benefit and those who can no longer earn more than 1/2 obtain 50% of the pension

Conditions

1. Minimum level of incapacity for work	50%
2. Period for which cover is given	From the date when invalidity is deemed to exist.
	• Periodically (after 1 or 2 years depending on circumstances) the insured persons are reassessed by the health committees
3. Minimum period of affiliation for entitlement	Persons insured before 31-12-1992:
	4.500 working days during the whole active life required or period of contributions depending on age:
	21 years: 300 days
	22 years: 420 days
	23 years: 540 days
	24 years: 660 days
	53 years: 4.140 days
	54 years: 4.200 days
	If none of these conditions are fulfilled, 1.500 working days are required, 600 of those in the 5 years preceding the invalidity
3. Minimum period of affiliation for entitlement	Persons insured before 31-12-1992:
	In case of employment injury and occupational disease: no minimum period of membership. If injury is due to an accident taking place out of the workplace, 2.225 or 750 working days (of which 300 in the last 5 years preceding the invalidity) are required

Persons insured since 1-1-1993:
working days: 4,500 working days or 15 years of insurance, 1,500 working days (600 within the 5 years preceding the invalidity) or 5 years of insurance contribution period (depending on age):
Up to the age of 21 years: 300 days (or 1 year of insurance)
This time increases progressively up to 1,500 contribution days, if for each year beyond the age of 21, an average of 120 days (or 5 years of insurance) can be added
Employment injury and occupational disease: full eligibility starts if one day insured
Injury due to an accident not occurred at the place of work: eligibility as soon as 50% of the conditions for invalidity as result of normal disease are fulfilled

Vocational Orientation [3, 11]

The Vocational Orientation is an institution with an educational (pedagogical) nature implemented by OAED, that refers to the employable manpower. The Directorate of Vocational Orientation is the Service of the Organization which is consisted by four Departments and is responsible for carrying out this task.

Apart from the Directorate of Vocational Orientation, there are the Local Services of the Organization that deliver Vocational Orientation services.

The role of the Directorate of VO is to define the strategies of implementation and to coordinate the local VO Services. In addition to this, it provides the VO Services with necessary technical means for the delivery of VO and secures the quality of the services offered.

Local VO Services have not yet been expanded to all Regions of the country. There were three kinds of Services, where a person may get help with the VO.

VO and Information Services are the most advanced VO Units. Such Services exist in Athens, Thessaloniki and Heraklio.

The VO Offices at regional level. The staff of these services are specialised and consist of psychologists, VO councilors and VO supervisors.

The Employment Services where VO is offered in local level, as well as in the new Employment Promotion Centres (delivering Vocational and Training Orientation plus job-seeking techniques).

Hellenic Society
for Supported Employment (HELASE) [4, 11]

Supported Employment for individuals with disabilities places, trains and maintains them with ongoing psycho-educational support in the open work market.

HELASE was founded in 1997 as a private, non-profit, social benefit organization. The goals of the Association are:

– to organize, plan and develop work options for the disabled in service centres, organizations and job finding agencies for people with disabilities.

– to inform, educate and make the public more aware of Supported Employment and so create new opportunities in the open work market.

– to represent Greece in European Union of Supported Employment (EUSE) as an active participating member.

For the accomplishment of these goals HELASE aims to put in place the following improvements throughout Greece:

– conduct collaborative programs with various service provider agencies for the disabled in order to develop, enhance and upgrade their services in job finding, training and employing people with disabilities;

– provide continuing education for staff working with the disabled;

– collaborate with various organizations (universities, public and private services and European agencies) for the development of education and research programs which will help promote and establish the practice of Supported Employment;

– compiling and publishing relative information, advertisements and use of media for the promotion of Supported Employment.

Because Supported Employment means:

– enhancing quality of life for people with disabilities;
– development of self-esteem and self-confidence;
– opportunity in the world of actual employment;
– equal participation in social activity and everyday life - social inclusion.

People with disabilities [4, 10, 11]

For people with disabilities the interventions aim mainly at timely prevention, diagnosis and rehabilitation as well as their integration and support within the family and social environment and their integration in the labour market. These aims are achieved either by means of ensuring working posts or through alternative forms of employment (sheltered work - social cooperatives).

An effort is also being made to convert closed care institutions into modern rehabilitation structures and at the same time steps are taken in order to de-institutionalize people treated in these institutions.

Centres of Education, Social Support and Training for Persons with Disabilities (KEKYKAMEA) [12]

The Centres of Education, Social Support and Training for Persons with Disabilities (KEKYKAMEA), according to the Law No 2646 / 1998, article 13, paragraph 1b, are bodies belonging to the National Organization of Social Care.

The KEKYKAMEA aim at:

Timely diagnosis with the provision of advice and support in response to the biological, sociological and psychological needs of people with disabilities and of their families.

The provision of services and the development of programs for the social support of people with disabilities as well as the more complete and equal social integration in various areas of daily life (employment, independent leaving, sports, etc.).

The professional training of people with disabilities, their functional rehabilitation and the support for their integration in all forms of our society.

The provision of reliable information and briefing to the people with disabilities and to their families concerning issues related with disability.

Raising the awareness of the local society and briefing it on issues concerning people with disabilities.

Addressing and guiding people with disabilities to specialised services on a local or regional level.

The development of methods and techniques that will help in dealing with issues concerning people with disabilities.

The development of policies and programs for these.

The KEKYKAMEA are staffed by specialised personnel: psychologists, special psychiatrists for children, educators of special education, speech therapists, nurses, physiotherapists, occupational therapists, social workers, health visitors, experts in the professional orientation, etc.

In some areas where the people with disabilities are far from the KEKYKAMEA there will be guesthouses of hospitality for people with disabilities so that these people can profit from all the services offered by the KEKYKAMEA and so that the maximum number of people with disabilities can be professionally trained.

References

1. Robolis S, Romanias G, Margios B (2001) An Actuarial Study for the Greek Social Insurance System. Labour Institude, Athens
2. Kremalis K (1996) (ed) Case Law on Social Security Issues. AN Sakkoulas Publishing Athens
3. http://www.oaed.gr
4. http://www.ggka.gr/english/asfalistikoinen2.htm

5. Sissouras A, Amitsis G (1999) The Social Safety Net and its Implementing Mechanisms in the Greek Social Protection System, p 537-566 in Th. Sakellaropoulos (ed) The reform of the Social State, KRITIKI Publishing, Athens
6. Stergiou A (1994) The Constitutional Guarantee of Social Insurance. A.N. SAKKOULAS Publishing Thessaloniki
7. Stergiou A (1999) The Regulation of Disability in the IKA Legislation. A.N. SAKKOULAS Publishing Thessaloniki
8. Report 2002 of Ministry of Labour and Social Security - General Secretariat of Social Security: "The Greek Social Security System", Athens
9. Amitsis G (2002) Current Policies and Reform Plans for the Greek Benefits Framework. Benefits and Compensation International 31(7): 12-9
10. http://www.disability.gr
11. http://europa.eu.int/comm/employment_social/missoc2001/el_part2_en.htm
12. http://www.ypyp.gr

Vocational rehabilitation: the Italian model

N. Pappone, C. Dal Pozzo and F. Franchignoni

In Italy the legal source for protection of people with disabilities lies, first of all, in Constitutional principles. Article 2 introduces the duty of political, economical and social solidarity, and Article 3 states the need for the removal of social and economic barriers limiting freedom and equality among citizens. Moreover, Article 38 specifies types of intervention towards citizens incapable of work and without means of living and workers with reduced or abolished work capacity.

Citizens incapable of work and "disabled" people have the right to a means of living and social assistance. They also have the right to education and vocational training [1]. These rights are guaranteed by the National Health System (NHS) and Social Security System.

The Italian NHS – rehabilitation services

In 1998 the Italian Minister of Health defined guidelines for the organisation of rehabilitation services as until then rehabilitation had been delivered in a non-structured fashion across the country (i.e. treatments were performed in varying modes, times and contexts for similar conditions) (Act 7th May 1998).

Therefore guidelines for medical rehabilitation were drawn up promoting a network of structures included in the NHS. The guidelines were designed to preserve the autonomy of the Italian Regions and leave them free to devise their own programs within a framework of national regulations. Among others, the guidelines stress the importance of appropriate individual rehabilitation projects and programs (in order to optimise the effectiveness of the interventions), and the need for assessment of the residual capacity of the disabled (more than of the severity of damage) and for a proper occupational and social settlement of people with disabilities.

An efficient network among different clinical departments and units was established, the main goal of which was to "take charge of the rehabilitation patient", aiming at ensuring the best level of autonomy and quality of life. The network is also intended to provide systems for continuous quality improvement and program evaluation, and progressively identify the best treatment protocols and practice standards. The procedures to follow start from the early stages of the disease, pointing out the links between emergency (either surgical or medical) departments and rehabilitation units.

The guidelines of the Ministry of Health take into account both "intensive" and "extensive" rehabilitation programs. The "intensive" activities deal with significant disabilities (particularly those due to severe brain damage and spinal cord injury) that require major medical care and rehabilitation treatment in terms of complexity and duration of intervention, while "extensive" rehabilitation activities (mainly delivered in day care, outpatient services, long-term care facilities, nursing homes, home services, etc.) are directed at the treatment of transient and/or minor disabilities, or of stabilised functional conditions and require a lower intensity of therapeutic commitment. Some NHS structures for rehabilitation interventions include laboratories for the assessment of the residual functional capacities, and units for occupational therapy and vocational training. These structures are identified as tools for both medical and social rehabilitation aimed at (re-)allocating the disabled to work whenever possible; they strictly collaborate with the Work Integration Services (see below). In particular, according to the new ICF classification, the procedures to analyse the residual capacity of disabled people consist of a comprehensive vocational evaluation, assessing the whole person (on the basis of biological, vocational, and technical-professional characteristics) and the environment, and including abilities, skills, interests, physical capacities and other crucial factors affecting vocational potential. Physiatrists (supported by the rehabilitation team) play a pivotal role in this kind of assessment and intervention.

The Italian Social Security System

The Social Security System in Italy is divided into two parts: one is based on public assistance for citizens incapable of work (i.e. who never entered the labour market or suffers from acquired disability); the other, for working citizens, deals with social insurance respectively against: a) common illnesses; b) industrial injuries and occupational diseases. Special categories are civil servants and military forces, which will not be specifically examined here.

This approach reflects the above mentioned Constitutional principles and the complex history of Social Security System development in Italy. However, a debate has been going on for years about the opportunity of merging different policies on disability and offering disabled persons a global approach to managing their needs. The Table summarises the economic and non economic benefits of our national Social Security System.

Table – Economic and non economic benefits of the Italian Social Security System.

Legal nature of disability	Disabled People who did not pay a set contribution or never entered the labour market (civil invalidity)	People who become disabled during working life (common illnesses)	People who become disabled during working life (industrial injuries and occupational diseases)
Board	Ministry of Economy and Finance	INPS	INAIL
Cash benefits (short term benefits)	Not applicable	Sick pay	Temporary employment-injury benefits
Cash benefits (long term benefits)	Monthly allowance for unemployment periods (>74% loss of work capacity)	Ordinary invalidity allowance (>2/3 loss of work capacity)	Indemnity (lump-sum) (6-15% reduction of psychophysical integrity) Monthly benefit (>16% reduction of psychophysical integrity)
	Inability pension (100% loss of work capacity)	Inability pension (complete loss of work capacity)	
Work (re-) integration	Law 68/1999 (2) Quota system (>45%) loss of work capacity)	–	Law 68/1999 and 38/2000 (2,3) Quota system (>34% loss of work capacity)

Social assistance: non contributory benefits

The Ministry of Economy and Finance administers non-contributory benefits to those people who were born with disabilities or never entered the labour market or did not pay the set contribution because of an acquired disability. Subjects below 18 years with persistent disabilities have the right to an indemnity if they attend school. Subjects over 65 years receive health and social welfare assistance. Subjects between 18 and 65 years (working age) with a reduced work capacity of over 33% qualify for Civil Invalidity, of over 45% have right to "compulsory" employment (quota system) [2, 3], of over 74% receive a monthly allowance when not employed. In the case of complete loss of work capacity they receive a monthly pension. At any age the incapacity to walk or to perform basic activities of daily living entitles the subject to an extra indemnity.

Insurance against common illnesses: contributory benefits

INPS (National Institute for Social Security) administers, besides short term sick pay, the invalidity allowance and inability pension for people that become disabled during working life due to "common illnesses". The term of reference for the invalidity allowance is a more than two-thirds reduction of work capacity according to education and work experience. The requirement for the inability pension is the loss of all-work capacity. These benefits represent a sort of early retirement [4, 5].

Insurance against industrial injuries and occupational diseases: contributory benefits

INAIL (National Institute against Industrial Injuries and Occupational Diseases) administers benefits granted to workers that become disabled due to an industrial injury or an occupational disease.

The legal framework is complex. The former legislation (TU n. 1124/1965) was based on the assessment of impairments causing reduction of work capacity (invalidity), so-called "barèma". The worker with an invalidity between over 10 and 100% was entitled to receive a proportional monthly allowance. This law is still operating for some benefits (i.e., long term allowance for continuing assistance for special categories of disabled workers, and as a basis for qualifying return to work in the *quota system* according to law 68/1999 [2] when invalidity is over 34%) but the core of the system is the statutory order 38/2000 [3]. The novelty of this small revolution is the introduction into an insurance system of the principles of the liability. The term of reference is no longer the incapacity for work but the reduction of psychophysical integrity of the individual assessed via a legal *baréma*. This implies that the value of an individual lies not only in the capacity to produce income but in all aspects of personal life (e.g. in the previous law scars were irrelevant; today they must be assessed). The economic benefits are a daily compensation for total temporary disability (as in the past); a lump sum for injury to psychophysical integrity resulting in a 6-15% invalidity and a monthly annuity for invalidity over 16%.

The other major change brought about by law 38/2000 is the global approach to the subject: not only is economic protection taken into account but all other relevant aspects of social security, ranging from prevention to rehabilitation and return to work. In the field of industrial injuries and occupational diseases it is common experience that small impairments are easily compensated and return to work is relatively simple, particularly in semi-skilled jobs, but - as the level of impairment grows - finding a job or returning to work may be critical without intensive vocational rehabilitation programs and specific support for work integration (see below).

Role of the National Institute against Industrial Injuries and Occupational Diseases (INAIL)

INAIL is an integral part of the National Social Security System. As part of its main goals it pursues the reduction of accidents at work (prevention), the insurance of workers involved in risky activities and the re-integration into the labour market and in the social life of work accident or occupational disease victims. In the past the Institute's aim was to protect only a few categories of workers (such as factory employees and farmers), but more recently many other categories have been included (e.g., clerical jobs, housewives and sporting professionals). Moreover it is involved in the assessment of many other potentially disabling conditions since the decree N° 179/88 of the Constitutional Court extended the protection to any other disease that could be proved to have been caused by a working activity.

In recent years INAIL has had a growing interest in the areas of prevention, rehabilitation and research into all occupational diseases ("new and old").

One could say that protection of workers is becoming a fully encompassing protection system aimed at re-integration in social and working life.

At present, clinical rehabilitation is provided by the National Health System (through the local health authorities) and INAIL acts only to control and co-ordinate treatments for its clients.

However, the Institute is committed to carrying out several initiatives in the field of rehabilitation.

A major commitment of INAIL is in the supply of prosthesis and assistance to people with work-related amputations, as well as the supply of all technological aids to increase the activities and participation of its clients in social and working life.

The INAIL Prosthesis Centre at Vigorso di Budrio (BO) is an avant-garde research institute at the forefront in both the production and research of prosthetics. The centre implements customised prostheses and ortheses, as well as holding rehabilitation and training courses aimed at a more effective use of these prostheses, which are a fundamental step along the individual path towards autonomy.

In the framework of rehabilitation INAIL has promoted several projects. In the field of New Technologies, the Institute has implemented a call centre and a web portal for the disabled called "*SuperAbled*". This provides an integrated information and counselling service on issues such as architectural barriers, autonomy and mobility, rules and regulations, rehabilitation, technological means and prostheses, travel, sport and leisure.

In the field of return to work, INAIL gives a contribution to remove architectural barriers at the workplace, at home and in public places.

With regard to work re-integration, a multidisciplinary team in each INAIL Unit carries out an individual rehabilitation project for those clients qualifying for the "quota system" (Law 68/99 see above). The method is matching the residual abilities with the requirements of the workplace offered in the areas of residence. The individual rehabilitation projects are vocational rehabilitation projects contracted to dedicated institutions or associations and subordinated to a real job offer.

Italian policies for raising the employment level of people with disabilities

All countries of the European Union have cash benefits for people with disabilities and special policies to promote work integration. But, as in many other countries, a large number of Italian disabled people (regardless of aetiology) have remained on benefits rather than been actively helped to return to work through special rehabilitation programs. In fact, rehabilitation - which should precede the economic phase of social protection - is not recognised in Italy as a pre-condition for a cash benefit. At present, in our country (as more generally in Europe) people with disabilities have a rate of employment at least 20-30% lower than that of the general population [4, 5].

For these reasons, enhancing the employment level of people with disability is an Italian as well as European goal, as reported in the European Community Household Panel (1994), the European Employment Strategy, the 1998 Member States' National Action Plans and many other official documents.

The strategy is to open the following fronts to tackle the unemployment rate of disabled people:

Upgrading disabled people's skills: improving education (mainstream); facilitating transition from school to work (vocational training and counselling). Disabled people are involved in the mainstream education with a support teacher if needed. Vocational training is actively interfaced with the open labour market, within a continuing education strategy, rather than limited to a pre-employment phase.

Creating suitable jobs for people with disabilities: facilitating self-employment; sustaining sheltered and supported employment; encouraging social cooperatives. Social cooperatives, as non-profit organisations, are especially tailored to promote the work integration of people with disabilities, have lower working costs and greater facility to obtain work opportunities from public institutions.

Adjusting work organisation to the needs of individuals with disabilities: building a safer workplace (risk maps); harnessing new specific technologies. The framework on handicap law 104/92 foresees Regional interventions aiming to introduce technical equipment in the workplace of people with disabilities. At regional level the law 46/80 gives the NHS Units responsibility to take such action.

Building an equal opportunity environment (e.g. through non-discrimination provisions, quota system, and persuasion measures), and enhancing the employability of people with disabilities, moving from passive to active measures such as retraining, rehabilitation, and work integration services.

The quota system (although regarded as one of the most significant anti-discrimination measures) has been revealed as insufficient to solve the problem of raising the employment level of people with disabilities in Italy [2, 3]. As shown in Table, disabled people who never entered the labour market with invalidity > 45% are entitled to enrol in job centres (from 18 to 55 years) according to the law 68/1999; for people with work-related invalidity the minimum level is set at 34%. Those people whose level of invalidity is 74% or higher receive a monthly allowance for periods of unemployment. Low employment growth and lack of enforcement of the previous law on compulsory employment (Law 482/1968) has transformed the monthly allowance into a permanent income replacement for many people with disabilities.

Data from the Ministry of Labour in 1995 showed that 158,416 disabled people entitled to a benefit according to the Law 482/1968 were employed (43%) versus 207,150 on the waiting list (57%).

In the meantime, at regional and local level, new procedures and active policies have been tested to facilitate an exchange between disabled job seekers and businesses.

Work Integration Services (WISs) are special Guidance and Placement Services within the Social Services of the NHS Units. They represent the interface between disabled job seekers and local businesses. Typical tasks of WISs are: 1) to help the disabled person to assess his/her potential and personal motivation and training needs; 2) to understand the local labour market and increase awareness on the issue of work integration for disabled people; 3) to build a work integration project orientated to individual training needs, adjustments of the workplace, choice of right tasks and support for relational problems; 4) to counsel companies on legislation and management of work integration.

In general, regional laws assign NHS Units' specific functions to mediate between people with disabilities and the labour market based on the assumption that leaving them out of the productive context is not only economically expensive but – more importantly – socially incorrect. As disabled people have different needs and capacities, WISs develop flexible projects according to the individual's characteristics and behaviours. The projects can include orientation (to assess in real work contexts the potential and attitudes of the person with regard to independence, socialisation and learning in view of a possible work integration), training (to promote development of personality, enhancement of psychological, psychomotor and social functions, and learning of work skills), and other kinds of support to promote specific job skills and obtain and maintain a job. The instrument to carry out these projects is often that of a temporary engagement or "stage" in real work situations. As an example, in the Veneto Region (4.5 million inhabitants), WISs users were 1,140 in 1991 and 2,805 in 1997 (69% physically disabled, 25% mentally disabled, 5% addicts and 1% others). In 1997, 1,607 stages were promoted in the Region in public employment (367), industry (323), social co-operatives (302), handcraft industries (251), trade (141), agriculture (46), and others (177): 56% of stages were for training, 28% a mediation for employment, and 16% for work orientation. With regard to the subsequent employment, industry employed the highest number of subjects, followed by social co-operatives, trade, handcraft, public employment, and others. Almost 70% of work contracts were made in private companies. Public employment is keener to help in orientation and training projects rather than in employment.

For severely disabled people a social integration program within real occupational contexts is a valuable alternative to sheltered workshops. It is not related to the quota system and does not lead to an employment. However, severely disabled subjects who would not be successfully integrated as workers in the labour market may benefit from spending their time in real work contexts to practice their skills and to consolidate their level of independence.

WISs work in co-operation with job centres, local offices of the Ministry of Labour created to promote work integration for all unemployed citizens regardless of disability. Job centres are contacted by enterprises with vacancies, and directly or via the mediation of WISs may promote work integration. Job Centres have also been given responsibility to receive subscriptions of those disabled people who are entitled to benefit of the quota system, and to allocate them.

In conclusion, WISs promote co-ordination among forces involved in active work politics, creating a so-called Guidance Group for employment of people with disabilities: this includes local authorities, the national social security system, NHS units, training centres, job centres, trade unions, user associations, and enterprises.

References

1. Law no. 104 (February 5, 1992) on assistance, social integration and rights of people with handicap.
2. Law no. 68 (March 12, 1999) on norms on the right of job for people with disabilities.
3. Statutory order no. 38 (February 23, 2000) on employment injuries and occupational diseases.
4. Missoc – Mutual Information System on Social Protection in the EU Member States and EEA (web site: http://europa.eu.int/comm/employment_social/missoc2001/index_it_en.htm).
5. Blöndal S, Scarpetta S. Early retirement in OECD countries: the role of social security systems. Organisation for Economic Co-operation and Development (OECD) Economic Studies No. 29, 1997/II.

Vocational rehabilitation: the Irish model

A. McNamara and B. Miller

Introduction

For the majority of people, work is central to their lives and to the way they think of themselves. Disability may create a major disadvantage impacting upon quality of life at all levels. The disability may arise from congenital conditions or it may be caused by injury or disease. If serious incapacity arises from the disability, it may prove very difficult for an individual to enter or re-enter the world-of-work and to carry out the normal and expected duties of the work environment in a chosen career or profession. It is the case that the longer a person who is disabled from injury and is absent from the work environment, the longer and harder it is likely to be before they can satisfactorily re-enter fully into the employed environment.

The Irish model of vocational rehabilitation has changed fundamentally since 2000 following the Report of the Commission on the Status of People with Disabilities – A Strategy for Equality (1996). From 1967 to 2000 the National Rehabilitation Board (NRB), which reported to the Department of Health and Children, had statutory responsibility for advising and guiding vocational rehabilitation for people with disabilities. NRB had a staff of professional vocational rehabilitation advisors throughout the country NRB also a psychology and medical department. Their role included arranging training and placement of people with disabilities in employment and this was part of the continuum of linking rehabilitation from health through to employment.

NRB was dissolved by the government in 2000 and responsibility for employment and vocational training policies for people with disabilities was transferred to the Department of Enterprise, Trade and Employment. The relevant vocational responsibilities and services then became mainstreamed into other state bodies. This resulted in the direct link between medical rehabilitation and vocational rehabilitation services being severed. Responsibility for the rehabilitative life skills training and sheltered work for people with disabilities remained with the Department of Health and Children.

Research shows that vocational rehabilitation plays an essential role in the process of enabling a return to work [1]. The research also shows that employers have a pivotal role to play in the provision of employment opportunities for people with disabilities. It further shows that Vocational Rehabilitation professionals may be able to improve the employment outcomes of people with disabilities by assisting employers to recognize the potential of employees with certain types of disabilities to perform the essential functions in specific jobs.

This article highlights the current measures of support provided by the State to people with disabilities to enter and remain in employment, and to improve their overall quality of life. Future research into the assessment of the effectiveness of these supports will determine whether the changes to the policies derived mainly from the work of the Commission will require further adjustments or fundamental change going forward.

Policy Context

Report of the Commission on the Status of People with Disabilities - A Strategy for Equality, which was published in 1996, is the key policy framework document that sets out the overall approach to disability policy in Ireland.

The Commission engaged in the most widespread consultation with people with disabilities and their families ever undertaken in Ireland. The membership of the Commission was made up of over 60% people with disabilities and their families.

Three fundamental principles underpinned the recommendations of the Commission:

– enabling Independence and Choice;
– equality;
– maximising Participation.

A key recommendation of the Commission [2] was the mainstreaming of services for people with disabilities. Mainstreaming means the delivery of services for people with disabilities by the public bodies that provide the services for the general population.

Following the adoption of the mainstreaming policy by the Government, all existing government policies and services were examined and realigned to comply with this principle. This review had immediate and widespread implications for the model of Vocational Rehabilitation in Ireland.

The Department of Health and Children had responsibility for matters relating to the vocational training and rehabilitation of people with a disability. Following the mainstreaming policy this was seen as outdated and reflected the medical model of disability rather than the social and rights model of disability, which is now the currently accepted model.

The Department of Enterprise Trade and Employment now has responsibility for employment and vocational training policies for people with disabilities and this is now dealt with as part of general labour market policy.

A primary goal of the Department of Enterprise Trade and Employment is to achieve improved integration of people with disabilities into the open labour market in a way that maximizes their potential and contributes to economic growth and social cohesion.

The implication of this policy decision by Government was the dissolution of the National Rehabilitation Board. This Board, which reported to the Department of Health and Children, was responsible, among other things, for the Vocational Rehabilitation of people with disabilities. This function transferred to two government departments mentioned above.

Responsibility for the Rehabilitative Life Skills Training and Sheltered Work for people with disabilities remained with the Department of Health and Children. Overall the Department of Health and Children is responsible for the provision of the full range of health and social services from acute hospital services to continuing care in the community.

Vocational rehabilitation in Ireland – a model in transition

The Model of Vocational Rehabilitation in Ireland is best understood within this context of the mainstreaming policy and the adoption of the social and rights based model of disability.

It may be described as a model in transition. As we have seen programmes and supports previously provided by the Department of Health and Children are now being provided by the Department of Enterprise Trade and Employment.

The implementation of the mainstreaming policy has led to increased fragmentation of services to people with either an acquired or congenital disability as they engage with vocational rehabilitation. With several government departments now taking a more active involvement in the provision of services to people with disabilities there is a tendency for each department to keep within its own boundaries. Linkages and pathways between health and employment programmes and education programmes are diffused and confused.

There is a marked absence of a Case Manager Role that provides a link between the various strands of programmes. Prior to the dissolution of the National Rehabilitation Board the Vocational Service of the Board provided a case manager role for individuals undergoing vocational rehabilitation.

Of particular concern is the pathway from medical rehabilitation to the appropriate vocational rehabilitation. Although provision of programmes to support individuals has stayed at a constant level if not increased, the practical supports such as the case manager role, to engage individuals with these programmes are now more fragmented and where available is linked to sets of programmes provided by individual departments rather than between programmes.

A recent report by the National Disability Authority (NDA) summed this up when it concluded a review of training and employment services for people with a disability by stating:

"Though there have been some improvements in the mainstreaming of service provision to people with disabilities this has been at the expense of greater fragmentation of responsibility for policy development and service delivery. There is no evidence that mainstream service training providers are increasing their intake of people with disabilities". [3]

Prevalence of disability in Ireland

In the Quarterly National Household Survey [4] held in the second quarter of 2002 the figures showed that 10% of adults of working age have a longstanding disability or health problem.

Over 10% (271,000) of all persons aged 15 to 64 indicated that they had a longstanding health problem or disability. The prevalence of disability and health problems varied by age group, with a quarter (84,400) of all persons in the 55 to 64 age group suffering from a longstanding health problem or disability. This compares to less that 5% (30,600) of persons in the 15 to 24 year age group.

Just over 40% (108,600) of all persons aged 15 to 64 with a disability or health problem indicated that they were in employment which compares to an overall rate of 65% for the total population in the same category. Of the 108,600 in employment, over three quarters were in full time employment. The majority of those in employment were employees (87,600) with just over 20,000 falling into the self employed and assisting relative categories.

The most common reported disabilities/long standing health problems were chest or breathing problems (41,500) followed by heart, blood pressure or circulation problems (39,200) and back of neck problems (37,800).

Approximately 15% (40,500) of all persons with a disability/longstanding health problem have had their condition since birth. Just under one third (84,900) have had their condition for ten years or more.

Assistance was provided to 8,900 (8.2%) of the 108,600 persons in employment who reported a longstanding health problem or disability. Just over 3,000 worked in sheltered or supported employment. Almost 22,000 persons with a disability or longstanding health problem not in employment stated that they would require assistance in order to work.

Legislative context

The legislative context in Ireland has changed in the last six years with equality and anti-discrimination legislation providing a strong framework to support the equality agenda pursued by people with disabilities.

Employment Equality Act 1998

This act outlaws discrimination both direct and indirect in employment on nine grounds including disability.

The Equal Status Act 2000

This act prohibits the discrimination across nine grounds including disability in the provision of goods and services. The act requires providers of services to make reasonable accommodation to meet the needs of people with disabilities. In 2002, 44 individuals with a disability made claims under the Employment Equality Act and 50 under the Equal Status Act, this represents 14% and 5% of the claims.

Proposed Disabilities Bill

A new Disabilities Bill is currently being drafted. This Bill is intended to provide for an independent assessment of needs for all people with disabilities. As yet the exact details and provisions of this Bill are not in the public domain. Those representing the Disability Groups have lobbied for an independent assessment of need supported by a rights based delivery system.

A key issue for many people with disabilities, which they hope will be addressed in the new Bill, is the separate and disparate access to fragmented services many of which undertake or request a separate assessment of need. The intention is that the new Disabilities Bill will provide a comprehensive assessment that will be applicable across services and programmes.

National agreements and social partnerships

Since 1987 there have been five national agreements negotiated with the social partners and the government. The social partners are made up of employers, trade unions, farmers and community voluntary sector representatives. These agreements are the overarching agenda of government and the social partners. They are seen as a powerful way to address issues and to reach consensus with the social partners.

The success of the Irish economy in the 1990s was attributed in part to the social partnership approach to wage increases and economic development. Each successive agreement has seen increasing commitments to improving and addressing the issues of people with disabilities in Ireland. Many of these commitments include improved access to employment, new schemes for accessing employment, reviews of sheltered work, exploring the issue of a cost of disability payment, strategies for rehabilitation and reviews of services to people with disabilities.

Medical rehabilitation

Responsibility for medical rehabilitation rests with the Department of Health and Children. Individuals who have completed a period of medical rehabilitation are referred on to the appropriate government agency. The main difficulty here is that there is, however, no single assessment gateway or route to retraining. The local area health boards provide a Guidance Service to Rehabilitative Training and Sheltered Work. Foras Aiseanna Saothair (FAS) the state Training and Employment Services agency provides a gateway through its employment services for all of its services.

There is a marked absence of bridging programmes and supports for individuals to move between programmes.

Rehabilitative training

Rehabilitative training focuses on the development of an individuals core personal capacities such as life skills, social skills. Some area health boards provide the training themselves or make provision with voluntary agencies. Rehabilitative training courses are delivered in a range of locations from training centres, home based programmes and community based programmes. Health Boards have Occupational Guidance Officers who are the first point of contact for the individual seeking retraining and rehabilitation. Following assessment the Occupational Guidance Officer refers the individual to the appropriate training programme that meets the needs of the individual.

In total there are 2,557 Rehabilitative Training Places provided throughout the country by the area health boards. Many of the Rehabilitative Training Programmes are provided by Voluntary Bodies that provide a range of other services such as residential services, sheltered work and day care programmes.

The Department of Health and Children has responsibility for the development, funding and administration of rehabilitative training and sheltered work. These policies are operationalised by local Health Boards (ten in total but soon to be reduced to four as part of a wide ranging health services reform programme currently the focus of the government's attention).

Sheltered work

The traditional model of sheltered work is defined as work which people with disabilities undertook in a sheltered setting. However, following concerns expressed about the position of individuals in sheltered work, a re-definition of sheltered work is in the process of taking place. A new code of practice on sheltered work is awaiting approval by the Minister for Health and Children. A number of existing sheltered workshops will more than likely be reclassified as employment. A report commissioned by the Department of Health and Children in 1997 estimated that approximately 8000 individuals with a disability were in sheltered work in over 215 centres throughout the country.

Labour market services for people with disabilities

Employment and training are important routes for people with disabilities to achieve economic and social independence.

To this aim, the Department of Enterprise Trade and Employment has taken a three-pronged focus:

- provide employment skills to people with disabilities;
- promote the employment of people with disabilities to employers;
- provide employment supports to employers and people with disabilities.

In practice, the mainstreaming of vocational training and employment services, meant that FAS – the state agency responsible for the provision of training to the workforce needed to provide services to people with disabilities in an integrated way offering them more choice and options then were previously available. This means that FAS needed to ensure that people with disabilities have the same right of access to labour market services as their non-disabled peers. To this aim, FAS:

– worked towards increasing the capacity of services already available through FAS, such as FAS mainline service provision, Local Employment Services (LES), Job Clubs and Community Training Workshops (CTWs), Community Employment (CE), etc.;

– designed and developed new grants for employers such as the Disability Awareness Training Support Scheme (DATSS) and the Employee Retention Grant, as well as new employment initiatives such as Supported Employment;

– promoted services and programmes for people with disabilities to potential users and employers;

– assisted in the formulation and development of policies and strategies for the provision of labour market services for people with disabilities by working closely with government departments, and other major stakeholders, including a National Advisory Committee on Disability, to identify emerging issues and gaps in service provision.

FAS National Advisory Committee: This Committee, consisting of members who represent organisations of and for people with disabilities, relevant government departments, FAS, ADM and the social partners, aims to assist and advise FAS on matters relating to the development and provision of services and programmes for people with disabilities. Its inaugural meeting took place in June 2002 and it meets four times a year.

Vocational training

Vocational training is one of the primary routes available to people towards realising their full occupational potential. Therefore, it is important that people with disabilities have access to the widest possible vocational training provision whether that be provided by specialist training providers or mainline FAS centres.

FÁS provides a large range of training courses of an industrial and commercial nature, for unemployed and redundant workers, those wishing to update their skills or change their career and for school leavers. These courses are designed to equip participants with specific skills which will enhance their prospects in securing employment through training, and include:

– FÁS Training Centres;
– Community Training Workshops;
– Traineeships;
– External Training Courses.

FÁS also offers Interactive Training courses at its FÁS NetCollege.

To increase participation of disabled people within these courses a number of interventions are available, namely:

– the provision of assistive technology in its broadest sense, such as braille text, JAWs and close circuit televisions (CCTVs);
– the use of training support assistants and sign language interpreters; and
– assistance towards additional transport costs.

Additionally, because some people with disabilities may require:

– additional training duration;
– adapted equipment;
– enhanced programme content;
– reduced trainer to trainee ratios, and/or;
– staff, specially qualified in training people with disabilities, FÁS currently contracts with approximately 20 specialist training agencies to provide this type of training - Specialist Training Providers (STPs).

These Specialist Training Providers, for example National Training and Development Institute (NTDI), provide Introductory and Specific Skills training to approximately 2,500 people with disabilities in 60 centres throughout Ireland. They are required to meet minimum standards in relation to the design and delivery of training programmes and all these programmes lead to nationally recognised certification. Therefore, employers may be assured that if they employ a person with a disability, who has completed one of these vocational training programmes, they are employing a person with certified skills.

Initiative to facilitate the employment of people with disabilities

Many people with disabilities, having overcome significant barriers in normal day-to-day activities, are often highly motivated, flexible and loyal, and will bring these strengths to the workplace. Studies of organisations that employ people with disabilities have readily identified these positive qualities. Discussions with employers, who have employed people with disabilities, reveal other benefits such as enhanced customer relations. These factors, coupled with the obligations on employers to comply with recent employment equality legislation, make failure to attract people with disabilities an unnecessary waste of human resource.

Employment Support Scheme

Whereby financial support is offered to employers who employ people with disabilities whose work productivity levels are between 50% to 80% of normal work performance. There are currently 460 people with disabilities on this Scheme, and the average weekly subsidy is €66 per week.

Workplace Equipment/Adaptation Grant

Whereby employers who have to adapt their workplace or equipment for an employee with a disability, may apply for a grant of up to € 7,000 towards the cost.

Job Interview Interpreter Grant

Available to people with a hearing or speech impairment, who are attending job interviews.

Personal Reader Grant

Available to people who are blind or visually impaired and may need assistance with job related reading.

All private sector employers are eligible for funding under these Grants, provided they are:

– about to employ a person with a disability;
– continuing to employ a worker who has become disabled;
– if the person is self employed, with a disability.

FÁS also took over responsibility for the Pilot Employment Programme (PEP), whose aim is to grant assist commercially viable enterprises, of which 50% of the employees are disabled people.

From the onset, given the complexity of the tasks ahead of us, FAS realised that provision of existing services and programmes alone would not provide equality of access. Many people with disabilities may be able to access the labour force with supports and/or by overcoming barriers of attitude among the workforce. To broaden the labour market options for people with disabilities, and to address these issues, a number of new initiatives are currently being developed and implemented by FAS. These are:

Supported Employment

Launched in 2000, this Programme is an open labour market initiative that works towards the placement and support of people with different types and varying degrees of disability, who genuinely need the initial support of a Job Coach to obtain and maintain employment. Under this initiative:

– contracts were awarded to consortiums, consisting of organisations of and for people with disabilities;
– Job Coaches provide the employee with a disability with the necessary support and coaching in the workplace, and the employer and co-workers, in facilitating the integration of the employee with a disability into the workplace;
– nine hundred plus (900+) people with disabilities obtained employment in the open labour market as a result of this initiative by June 2002.

An evaluation to provide an assessment of the operation and impact of the national pilot for Supported Employment has been completed. The evaluation will identify areas which may be built upon to ensure that the Programme achieves maximum effectiveness in meeting its objectives, and recommendations will be used to further develop the Programme from the end of 2002, when the current round of funding will be completed.

Disability Awareness Training Support Scheme

One of the key factors in assisting the integration of people with disabilities into the workforce is to overcome mistaken perceptions of people with disabilities and their capacity to work. To increase awareness, and overcome these perceptions, this grant is available to employers to cover the cost of disability awareness training for their organisation's staff and personnel. This grant has been available since January 2002.

Employee Retention Grant Scheme

The purpose of this grant is to assist employers to retain employees that acquire a disability that jeopardizes their employability. The aim of the grant is to identify the supports and accommodations necessary to retain employees in their current job, or to re-train them for another position in the organisation. To date this grant has been endorsed by industry and unions alike, e.g. Irish Business and Employers Confederation (IBEC), Irish Small and Medium Enterprises (ISME), Small firms Association (SFA), Health and Safety authority (HAS) and Irish Congress of Trade Unions (ICTU), and the National Advisory Committee on Disability.

This is a two-stage grant. Stage I provides funding to the employer so that he or she may hire in an external specialist to develop a "retention strategy". Stage II provides funding for the implementation of the "retention strategy", including, where required, re-training, use of job coaches, and/or an external co-ordinator to oversee and manage its implementation. This grant has been available since October 2002.

Irish Income Maintenance System

Underpinning and a key element in the vocational rehabilitation of individuals with acquired or congenital disabilities is the Income Maintenance System. Over the last ten years and arising from the high unemployment in Ireland in the 1980s the Department of Social and Family Affairs developed a range of innovative supports to assist the long term unemployed regain entry to the workforce.

The income maintenance payments available under the Irish social welfare system consist of social insurance benefits, social assistance payments and universal schemes, all of which are administered by the Department of Social and Family Affairs.

Social insurance benefits

Are payable to people who experience one of a range of internationally-recognised contingencies, such as illness, unemployment, old age, maternity, etc. Entitlement to these benefits is based on prescribed social insurance contribution conditions.

Social assistance payments

Which broadly complement the range of social insurance benefits, are means-tested payments that are payable to people without sufficient contributions to qualify for social insurance benefits. Universal payments, such as Child Benefit and Free Travel, do not depend on either social insurance contributions or means tests.

Traditionally the role of the income maintenance system was a passive one, with responsibility in this area primarily confined to providing income support to people during periods of inability to earn an income. However, over the last decade or so, the Income Maintenance System has taken a more pro-active role in dealing with people's needs. This is particularly so in the case of the unemployed, where various measures have been introduced to support them to return to work. In recent years, these employment support measures have been extended to other groups of social welfare recipients, such as people with disabilities, lone parents etc. The table below shows the total cost of disability related payments for 2002.

Disability payments for 2002 [5]

Payment	No of Recipients	Yearly Cost Million Euros
Disability Benefit	54,590	385 m
Invalidity Pension	52,147	404 m
Injury Benefit	828	12 m
Disablement Benefit	11,612	59 m
Disability Allowance	62,783	408 m
Blind Persons Pension	2,095	14 m
Totals	183,955	1,282 m

Employment/training supports for people with disabilities

Through the range of employment and training supports available, the income maintenance system now aims to encourage and assist people on social welfare disability and illness payments to identify and take up available employment, training and other self-development opportunities, where appropriate. This is achieved through a range of measures such as:

The Back to Work Scheme

Which provides people on long-term illness and disability payments with assistance on a sliding scale for 3 years (or 4 years where they are engaged in self-employment) when they move into full-time employment. In 2002 a total of 808 individuals with a disability were beneficiaries of the Back to Work Allowance Scheme out of a total of 11,526.

The Back to Work Enterprise Scheme

Is similar to the Back to Work Scheme but is aimed at people with a disability who wish to commence self-employment. In 2002 there were 465 beneficiaries with a disability out of a total of 13,510.

Income disregards

In the case of means-tested payments (e.g. Disability Allowance and Blind Person's Pension), for those engaging in rehabilitative employment/self-employment and training. The first 120 euros of income earned is disregarded. Approval must be sought from the Department of Social and Familiy Affairs for the employment to be considered to be rehabilitative. In some situations a letter from the individual's doctor may be required.

Special rules applying to the contributory illness and disability payments

(E.g. Disability Benefit and Invalidity Pension), which encourage recipients to return to work by engaging in employment which is considered to be rehabilitative or therapeutic in nature and occupational retraining.

The Jobs Facilitator Network

Administered by the Department of Social and Family Affairs, which assists people to return to work, training and education by advising them of the options available, encouraging them to take up these options and providing supports, where necessary.

The Family Income Supplement Scheme

Which provides financial support to low income families; and

Exemptions from liability for employer and employee PRSI contributions

In certain instances.

Back to education allowance

This seeks to raise the educational standards of the long-term unemployed in order to help them meet the requirements of the labour market. The scheme allows people return to secondary, vocational or third level education. In 2002 there were 529 beneficiaries with a disability out of a total of 6,860.

These supports allow people with disabilities to access training or attempt to integrate into the labour market while retaining social welfare payments in full or in part. In addition, the associated secondary benefits, such as medical cards, can be retained in many instances. There are about 16,600 people who are ill or disabled availing of these employment support measures. This represents 10% of all of the people on the social welfare illness and disability payments.

Role of insurance and sick pay schemes

In Ireland most workers are covered by the Pay Related Social Insurance (PRSI) scheme as outlined above. This assures all workers of a basic income should they become ill or disabled. Thereafter individual employers and workers may provide or pay for additional income maintenance schemes to cover the contingency of long term illness and absence of work. Most employers would have short term sickness schemes. Entitlement to occupational pensions due to long term illness or disability is varied. As soon as the worker is absent from work the employer has little mandatory obligations. Inability to perform the duties of the job that the person was hired to do due to illness or disability are not seen as reasons for unfair dismissals under Irish Employment Legislation. The Law of Torts and the adversarial system of proving negligence in cases where the worker is trying to prove negligence in order to gain compensation mitigates against the early return to work of injured and disabled workers.

The Income Protection Schemes are mainly provided by private insurance companies. The main thrust of these schemes is to ensure compliance with the terms of the scheme. There is little emphasis on rehabilitation. Often the beneficiaries are wary of engaging in rehabilitation and retraining in case their entitlement is jeopardised. This is an area that requires further research and examination. At a broad level the major employer representatives are supportive of employing people with disabilities. There is no legally enforceable quota scheme in Ireland. The Civil and Public Service has an employment quota of 3% of the workforce. This is being achieved. Monitoring is limited and categorisation of workers as disabled is arbitrary.

Conclusion

Fundamental changes in the Irish model of vocational rehabilitation have taken place since 2000. With the concept of mainstreaming, vocational rehabilitation remains outside the health area and is in a transitional phase; the continuum of care from the hospital to employment requires further development if we are to achieve a seamless service for people with disabilities from the acute phase to return to the community and employment.

The current Irish model of vocational rehabilitation appears to rely on a comprehensive series of measures supporting people with disabilities. Since the change of model in 2000, there has been no published evaluation available of the effectiveness of these measures to date, it is therefore difficult to form any conclusion.

Abbreviations

CCTvs = Close Circuit Televisions
FAS   = Foras Aiseanna Saothair
IBEC   = Irish Business and Employers Confederation
ISME   = Irish Small and Medium Enterprises
SFA   = Small Firms Association
HAS   = Health and Safety Authority
ICTU   = Irish Congress of Trade Unions
PRSI   = Pay Related Social Insurance
ADM   = Area Development Management

References

1. Gilbride D, Stensrud R, Ehlers C, Evans E and Peterson C (2000) Rehabilitation Services. (Statistical Data Included). J. Rehabilitation 66(4) (Oct-Dec): 17-23
2. The Commission on the Status of People with Disabilities – Department of Justice, Equality and Law Reform (1996) Stationery Office: Dublin
3. National Disability Authority Report Towards best Practice in Training and Employment for People with Disabilities 2004
4. Central Statistics Office Irish Household Budget Survey (2002)
5. Annual Report of the Department of Social and Family Affairs 2002, Department of Social and Family Affairs Dublin

Vocational rehabilitation in the Netherlands

F.J.N. Nijhuis, B.A.G. van Lierop and F. Wichers

Introduction

The organisation of social security for workers suffering from disabling conditions caused by illness or disease in the Netherlands has undergone great changes during the past decade. These changes are expected to continue for at least another five years before a new and stable system is established.

Whereas the Netherlands, by the end of the previous century, had almost a million workers suffering from long-term work incapacity as a result of illness or disease, their number has been reduced to 850,000 in 2004 and is expected to dwindle further still in the years to come.

The causes of this reduction should be found mainly in a system modification which has resulted in a higher entry threshold. One of the major factors involved is that responsibility for the reintegration of workers who have dropped out as a result of incapacity for work has been shifted from the public domain to the private market.

This chapter will successively discuss 1) the social security system for those who, as a result of illness or disease, have lost their capacity for work, either partially or entirely; 2) the shift in responsibility from the public domain to the private market; and 3) the methods applied in the new system to realize reintegration.

The social security system

The principle underlying the social security system in the Netherlands has been to insure loss of income-generating capacity as a result of illness or disease.

The causes of illness or disease do not play any role when loss of income is assessed. In the Netherlands, when entitlements to disability benefits are assessed, no distinction is made between "risque professionel" and "risque social". In other words, those who have become incapacitated for work as a result of accidents in the private sphere (sports, hobbies, household activities) have exactly the same rights and are subject to the same regulations as those who have become incapacitated for work as a result of industrial accidents or occupational diseases.

The amount of loss of income is determined by estimating the reduced capacity to earn the same income as could be earned by someone with similar knowledge and skill levels or professional qualifications (theoritical income). This reduced capacity to earn an income is expressed in six categories varying from zero to 100% (0-15, 15-35, 35-50, 50-65, 65-80, >80%) and determines the amount of disability benefit allowed.

When workers have been incapacitated for work for two years, an assessment is made to establish their work incapacity pension. The aim is to assess the worker's disability to work. It must be objectively demonstrated that the disabilities have been caused by illness or disease. The disabilities found are used as a basis to estimate the reduction in the worker's capacity to earn an income as compared to other workers with similar levels of training and education and experience; if a person is still able to realize 50% of his theoritical income, then his work incapacity is reduced by 50%.

Work incapacity is assessed two years after a worker stopped working as a result of a specific illness or disease. During the first two years of work incapacity, the employer is responsible for the employee's reintegration process. The reintegration process may be aimed at achieving placement with the same employer in a specially adapted position or in a different position or it may be aimed at finding a place with a new employer.

The objective of the process is to motivate both employer and employee to realize early employee recovery, either in the employee's previous position, which may be temporarily adapted, or in a different position, either permanently or for the time being.

If employer and/or employee have failed to make sufficient efforts during those two years to find work – in adapted form or otherwise, in a different type of work or in a different position – a financial sanction can be imposed on the employer or the employee.

Employers may take out a reinsurance against the costs of illness and/or work incapacity of their staff during the first two years. This reinsurance on the illness period (up to two years) must be concluded with a private insurance company. When employees receive work incapacity benefits ("WAO benefits") after two years, they are paid by the UWV, a public social fund for the implementation of – statutory – employee insurance schemes.

Summarizing, the implication is that if diseases or disabling conditions cause workers to stop working, their employer will be responsible for their reintegration for a period of two years. At the end of that period, a review is made to establish whether employer and employee have made sufficient reintegration efforts. It is only when the review outcome is positive that the employee may be eligible for disability benefits.

The work incapacity system of the Netherlands will change greatly between now and 2007. Major principles involved in those changes will include:

– Reintegration will be of primary importance.

– Work incapacity insurance will demonstrate a shift towards a complementary and partially privately realized wage addition: everyone will be "obliged" to realize any remaining capacity for work.

It will be a highly restricted group who will receive disability benefits. These benefits are intended exclusively for those people who have lost every chance of returning to work, in whatever form.

Physical examinations will be tightened considerably and employees will receive benefits only if they have lost every capacity to earn an income while their disease results in permanent disabilities.

What are the implications of these developments for vocational rehabilitation in the Netherlands?

The effect of these developments is that reintegration in the Netherlands has turned into a two-track policy.

Firstly, if workers have become incapacitated for work at their jobs, their employer will be responsible for their reintegration for a period of two years. This type of reintegration can be characterized as Disability Management.

Secondly, if an employer-employee relationship no longer exists or has never existed at all – for example, when people have become disabled at an early age or when employees have lost touch with their employer after two years of being incapacitated for work – this is said to be a case of vocational rehabilitation.

Disability Management: principles

Disability Management is understood to be the sum of those activities which are designed to prevent workers from being absent from work (primary prevention), to support their recovery (directing function) and to develop reintegration activities [1]. Disability Management can be seen as a coordinated and coherent strategy aimed at cost-effective prevention and early intervention, both removing the causes of work incapacity and supporting workers to resume work as quickly and adequately as possible. Disability Management focuses on workers suffering from chronic and/or functional disabilities, on restoring individual work and functional capacities, but also on preventing individual capacities from deteriorating. Disability Management is aimed at developing and reinforcing the individual's capabilities and at removing and/or reducing obstacles in the worker's environment which might reduce functional capacities. Essentially, it combines two perspectives: utilizing, encouraging and improving the individual capacity for work of those who have disabilities on the one hand, and the methods used by the organisation to deal with prevention and reintegration on the other. In this approach, the focus is on employees suffering from disabilities and Disability Management activities are designed to learn to cope with disabilities and to reintegrate into the work organisation. Special attention is paid to the continuity of the relationship designed disabled worker and employer. In other words, the aim is to realize early resumption of work within one's own organisation [1]. These views correspond with the prevailing approach in the Netherlands, which was discussed earlier, that reintegration activities should take place as soon as possible, i.e., from day one of being incapacitated for work.

Disability Management: procedure

In Disability Management the focus is on returning to work as soon as possible. The first step in this approach, therefore, is to find or create a temporary workplace where the disabled employee can return to work as early as possible. The underlying assumption is that the disabled worker will carry out other work activities during the time between falling ill and – if possible – 100% recovery. Within the context of Disability Management policy-making, this specific type of early intervention is called "transitional work". Transitional work is started after an average of two weeks following the first day of illness.

Transitional work is designed to support the capacity for work, for example by providing relevant training. It is a provisional measure and it has a hierarchy of work activities in which the focus is on realizing a gradual transition to former work activities within the possibilities which the disabled worker has currently available. Transitional work can be said to exist when several preconditions have been met. Firstly, a thorough assessment should be made to establish both possibilities and impossibilities and the – potential – capacities of the worker involved. Next, job strain, job content and job requirements must be known for a great number of positions in order to realize optimum matching between job and individual. In addition, however, alternative positions may also be developed, knowing their job strain, job content and job requirements. This should be followed by regular monitoring in order to establish any health improvements that have occurred and to readjust work activities to newly developed conditions in order to realize a gradual return to the old position [2].

Several studies have shown that beginning to work or resuming work is one of the major factors to improve health. In this respect, the function of transitional work is twofold. On the one hand, the disabled worker is productive and, on the other hand, his/her recovery is facilitated [2].

In order to get this DM policy started in an organisation, reintegration policies within the organisation should be arranged and coordinated with the requirements of swift interventions. The first step to introduce a DM policy is to appoint a DM committee which will focus particularly on early intervention by using transitional work. Both employees and other interested parties will be on the committee. The DM committee will closely cooperate with both the medical officer and the immediate superior of the disabled worker. In addition, the DM committee also maintains relations with the other actors who have a role to play in early reintegration (family physician, medical specialists, etc.). The main focus will be on the disabled worker, who is invited to participate in all activities undertaken by the DM committee. In most cases the employee is contacted within two weeks after falling ill at most. Employees are invited to have an exploratory interview in which the employee and, possibly, his or her superior can participate in drawing up a first plan of action. In all cases, the plan is submitted to the medical officer, who will need to give his permission to go through with it. If the medical officer feels that the agreed transition work does not present any medical problems to the employee involved, then action can be taken to have it realized.

Thus, Disability Management distinguishes itself from existing reintegration policies by emphasizing – remaining – employee capabilities as well as the collaboration and commitment of the parties involved in order to provide custom-made solutions and to facilitate an early return.

Disability Management: preconditions

Early intervention activities such as those taking place within the context of a Disability Management programme have a chance of success only if the activities are embedded in organisational policy-making and if several specific organisational principles have been met [2].

In the first place, the DM policy principles should be supported throughout the organisation. All the groups that are part of the organisation should take their own responsibilities, based on the same DM philosophy. Thus, this philosophy or approach should be adopted by both higher and middle management, staff support departments (personnel department, Occupational Safety and Health Service) and the workers themselves. Secondly, it is necessary to appoint a Disability Management coordinator who will ensure the collaboration and support of all the parties involved when a worker is in the process of resuming work. Finally, monitoring and assessment are important methods in reintegration policies as they provide some idea of the costs and benefits involved in reintegration. Apart from these three elements, what is also needed is motivation, commitment and flexibility on the part of both workers and managerial staff. Employees should accept that their daily work activities may be changed temporarily while managerial staff should actively think along about alternative work activities which, perhaps temporarily, can be performed by the worker involved. At company level there must be flexibility, for example, in offering flexible working hours, lenient attendance requirements (e.g. teleworking), custom-made positions and tasks and the possibility to create new – temporary – positions.

All these things are then laid down in detailed protocols. After all, they can be incorporated into the company structure only if all the processes, activities and responsibilities are formally laid down in writing. A natural consequence will be that agreements are formalised and that employees make themselves familiar with reintegration.

There is great variation in the implementation of Disability Management programmes. In all cases, however, Disability Management is an inseparable part of the organisation's HRM policy, either as an addition to the existing programme or as an overall concept for reintegration policy-making [1].

Companies which have drawn up these programmes have achieved considerable cost reductions while at the same time improving the position and commitment of their workers – both with and without disabilities [2].

Vocational rehabilitation

Vocational rehabilitation: principles

In a great number of cases, disabled workers have not yet developed relations with an employer or their relation has ceased to exist. These cases include:

Youth who, as a result of congenital or acquired disabilities, are faced with a very high threshold to enter the labour market. Mostly, they are youth with very severe physical or mental handicaps.

Previously employed or self-employed workers who, as a result of disease or disability, have been unable to work for a long time and who have lost their capacity to earn an income which they would have earned, in view of their training and experience, if they did not have their disabilities. In addition, their disease or disability has caused them to break off relations with their employer.

Both categories of disabled workers involve individuals who find themselves at a great distance from the labour market and who want to have a job again, with their disabilities. Typically, they mostly involve workers who have been disabled further still as a result of the social process of work incapacity. One of the effects of curative medical care has been that they tend to be strongly focused on their disabilities, i.e., what they are no longer able to do, rather than on what is left of capabilities that can be developed. Even the opinions of insurance medical officers are based on limitations rather than possibilities. Moreover, the social environment frequently is protective rather than encouraging resumption of work.

Not only the disabled worker and his environment feel trapped by obstacles and disabilities, the employer's ideas, too, are framed in terms of impossibilities, additional supervision, reduced productivity and increased absence risks. Even if studies have shown that these are highly exaggerated, preconceived ideas and stereotypes, this representation still reduces the probability of finding employment [3].

Thus, the vocational rehabilitation process can be characterized as a combination of activities aimed at:

The worker personally. In view of the preceding disabling process it is necessary to help the worker to boost both his or her confidence and self-direction (empowerment).

Achieving the best possible match between job and individual, using training, education and work adaptations.

Linking disabilities to positions available at the labour market. In a number of cases, depending on the possibilities left, it may be practical to investigate regular positions, with or without special adaptations. Or, if this is not possible, it will be necessary to find a job in a protected environment, perhaps even under permanent supervision (supported employment).

Activities focused on both the prospective employer and prospective colleagues which are designed to remove any prejudices and to create an adequate working environment that presents as few obstacles as possible [4].

The objective of vocational rehabilitation can be characterized as follows. Based on an assessment of the capabilities of potential trainees, training and support activities are initiated which should result in improved opportunities in the labour market and which should lead to increased individual effectiveness in finding more adequate ways of dealing with the social and individual problems which persons suffering from disabilities may have to face [5].

Vocational rehabilitation: procedure

In order to realize a successful reintegration path, even if it has a difficult target population, it is based on a process model of labour integration (Fig. 1).

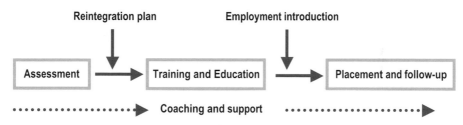

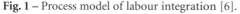

Fig. 1 – Process model of labour integration [6].

The process model of labour integration entails all those activities which are designed to analyse the starting position of disabled workers and to use this analysis as a basis for developing a custom-made plan of reintegration and mediation.

The first phase in this process is a comprehensive assessment to investigate the individual's possibilities. Next, these qualities or characteristics are compared with the demands made by employment. In doing so it is necessary to take as a starting-point the remaining capacities and the possibilities that have developing potential (potential capacities) rather than the disabilities that are currently present. It is on the basis of this assessment that a personal route plan is developed, taking into account work-related social and professional skills. More specifically, the disabled workers will be taught skills that are required in order to deal adequately with both their social environment and their work situation, if the latter exists. Finally, the workers will get support in terms of finding them employment in order to apply the knowledge and skills acquired.

In cases where it is impossible to find regular employment and the worker is forced to rely on permanent support then the method of supported employment is applied. The aim of this method, which is used mainly to help individuals suffering from psychiatric disorders or mental disabilities, is to find the disabled worker a regular employment position in which the individual is trained and supported on the job.

The method of job coaching has five steps:

– To explore the wishes and capabilities of the individual involved (assessment).

– To find an appropriate employment position (job finding). This requires relevant knowledge of the local labour market as well as a thorough understanding of positions and work processes. Having good relations with an employer in this case is a prerequisite. Also, the job finder must be able to estimate the capabilities of the individual involved in relation to the positions available.

– To analyse job activities and workplace (job analysis). The coach must be able to analyse jobs in order to establish whether those jobs, with or without any special adaptations, are suitable for the disabled worker involved.

– To bring together job and individual (job matching) in order to realize the best possible match between the individual's capabilities and the requirements made by the job.

– To coach the worker on the job with the intention of achieving long-term placement (job coaching). This includes "training on the job", i.e. teaching required knowledge and skills. In addition, it may also be one of the tasks of a job coach to educate the individual worker's environment. Depending on the needs of both the disabled worker and the company involved, a long-term coaching plan is then developed.

The difference between the two methods described is found mainly in how they see relations with the employer and with the job. In the method described first, skills are initially taught which are designed to minimize current limitations in a new job. In the second method, more active matching initially takes place between a person's disabilities and job requirements.

Vocational rehabilitation: preconditions

The process of vocational rehabilitation cannot really be successful until a number of preconditions has been met. The first one is that the professionals who are expected to build the process are able to do this properly. This requires a thorough understanding of assessment methods: the professional must be able to make adequate estimates of an individual's capabilities or else to gather the required knowledge through other agencies.

Secondly, the professional must be able to motivate disabled workers (counselling skills), making sure that they will make a choice in relation to their capacity for work. It is also important that there is a growing understanding of how people can be motivated to start working again following a long invalidation process.

Thirdly, the professional involved must be able to coach disabled workers in making decisions about how they wish their capacity for work to be developed (counselling skills).

Finally, they should also allow for the specific problems involved. It is well-known that the total population of disabled workers is highly varied, both in terms of the nature of their disabilities and their social and demographic backgrounds. The implication is that different custom-made change strategies must be developed for the various target populations in order to bring them back to work. In addition to relevant knowledge about specific target groups, this also requires expertise in the disabilities caused by specific diseases or handicaps.

The matching process

Reintegration as described here can be seen as a continuous matching process between the employee and the job. The steps to be made can be found in Figure 2. It is possible that the health status and the related disabilities can develop in a positive way (increase of health status through training), but also in a negative way (decrease in health status). Therefore the model should be regarded as a continuous matching process.

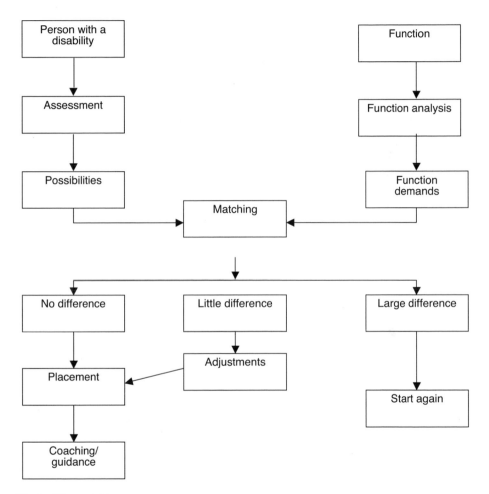

Fig. 2 – The matching process.

As mentioned before, this matching process will only reach a high quality level when making use of a good assessment. A good assessment tool kit should make it possible to provide the user with answers on the remaining capacities and the possibilities for development of an employee. This assessment tool kit should also provide the user with an indication of the employee related demands of the workplace.

In practice, these assessments will mostly be carried out when evaluating the capacities and possibilities of an employee with a specific health problems and/or specific health related diagnosis (e.g. TBI, Diabetes, MS, CAD, etc.).

This implies that evaluations of the physical and psychological capacities of an employee need to be based on a thorough assessment.

If a person is not able to return to his/her former job after sick leave, an estimation needs to be made about his/her specific interests and capacities with respect to specific elements of jobs. This estimation should lead to a concrete idea about future labour related activities.

In many cases, the occupational health service and its professionals are perfectly capable of making decisions about the possibilities. Also these occupational health services are capable of deciding on the necessary adjustments and/or adaptations in the future labour position as well as other labour related activities necessary for reintegration of the worker into the workplace.

If more complex situations play a role, e.g. a more severe disability, an organisation can be advised about how to (re)integrate this employee. The advice should be based on a thorough assessment in relation to the function and demands of the workplace. A tailor-made approach should be used when working with people with severe disabilities.

Practical implementation of reintegration care

Now that the privatisation of social security has been increasing, it can be concluded that public government agencies have lost many of their tasks to support incapacitated or unemployed workers. In contrast, a great number of private organisations have been established to achieve specific parts of the reintegration objective for those same subcategories of unemployed and/or incapacitated workers. Although some 700 reintegration agencies were initially established, ten years later about 300 of them are left. Whereas reintegration agencies were focused primarily on those workers who no longer had any relationship with an employer – or never had one at all – the increased reintegration obligations of employers have produced a considerable shift in attention toward coaching workers who have stopped working or who are at risk of having to stop working as a result of health complaints or diseases.

Consequently, the reintegration agencies have now taken a competitive position against the occupational safety and health services, whose primary task was to provide workers with support and counselling in order to achieve "long-term" employment.

References

1. Akabas SH, Gates LB, Galvin DE (1992) Disability management. A complete system to reduce costs, increase productivity, meet employees needs and ensure legal compliance, New York: Amacom
2. Shrey DE (1997) Worksite disability management and industrial rehabilitation: an overview. In: Shrey DE & Lacerte M (Eds), Principles and practices of disability management in industry. Boca Raton: CRC Press, p 3-53

3. VeermanTJ, Cavé M (1993) Werkgevers over herintredende WAO'ers en hun ziekteverzuim; meningen en selectiebeleid van werkgevers geïnventariseerd. Den Haag: Ministerie van Sociale Zaken en Werkgelegenheid
4. Rubin SE, Roessler RT (1999) Foundations of the vocational rehabilitation process
5. Van Lierop BAG (2001) Reïntegratie na scholing. Elsevier Bedrijfsinformatie BV, Den Haag
6. Van Lierop BAG, Nijhuis FJN (2000) Assessment, education and placement: an integrated approach to vocational rehabilitation. International Journal of Rehabilitation Research 23: 261-9

Vocational rehabilitation: the Spanish model

A. Cuxart

Purpose and characteristics of vocational rehabilitation

The primary objective of vocational rehabilitation is to enable persons with a disability – whether caused by a disease or an accident – to hold a regular job position in a public or private company where they can work and interact with other employees who have no disability, with an employment contract that provides the same salary and professional rights as the other employees. Vocational rehabilitation is used in a wide range of disabling diseases, such as spinal cord injury, stroke, traumatic brain injury, arthritis, multiple sclerosis, congenital or orthopaedic difficulties, cumulative trauma or chronic pain disorders, developmental and learning disorders, mental disorders and occupational accidents and diseases.

Rehabilitation as a comprehensive medical speciality should be managed in active co-operation with the individuals affected, in order to enhance their personal, social and occupational integration. The ideal approach taken with disability policies should move toward the use of proactive actions rather than obsolete protective methods. For instance, policies on rights (for residual abilities) versus compensation policies (payments, favourable discrimination for functional losses, financial benefits), training versus adaptation, mutual benefits versus one-way benefits, self-assessment versus expert assessment, analysis of the person versus analysis of the disability, positive outlook versus negative outlook, analysis on the basis of gender, race, ethnic origin, economic level, age, etc., versus analysis on the basis of handicaps and disabilities.

According to a survey on disabilities, impairments and health status [1] conducted by the *Instituto Nacional de Estadística* (INE, National Statistics Institute) of Spain in 1999, more than 3.5 million individuals in Spain have some degree of disability. This figure represents 9% of the population, with women accounting for more than half (58%) of all disabled persons in Spain. The same survey estimated that 25.8% of all individuals of working age (16 to 64 years) have some kind of disability. The problem clearly has far-reaching consequences for the economy, workforce and social health, and is causing growing concern among the persons affected and those with political or professional responsibility in the field. For the first time, a collective effort to conduct an objective analysis of the problem and seek the best solutions is evident.

Legislative history

The history of vocational rehabilitation in Spain dates back to 1887 with the founding of the *Asilo de Inválidos para el Trabajo* (Handicapped Workers Asylum). In 1922 this organisation became the Professional Work Re-education Institute for the Disabled, and in 1933 the National Re-education Institute for the Disabled. Its objective was to provide retraining and vocational re-education for disabled workers. Although the organisation has had various names and functions throughout its history, it still remains to the present day [2].

With the precedent set in Bismark's Germany where labour laws were created in 1884, the Occupational Accident Act was passed in Spain in 1900 to protect persons disabled in their jobs. In 1903 the Regulation for certifying occupational disabilities was created. This was followed by the *Instituto Nacional de Previsión* (INP, National Welfare Institute) in 1908, and the *Retiro Obrero y el Plan de Seguros* (Work Retirement and Insurance Plan) of the INP in 1919. These measures provided specific benefits such as indemnities, pensions, insurance, disability certification systems, etc., to individuals who had experienced an occupational accident.

Wars and conflicts in Europe, including World War I and II, led to the appearance of large numbers of war-related disabilities, and significant efforts were made in the field of rehabilitation, including the founding of the early rehabilitation services. This was particularly evident after World War II. The goal of rehabilitation was physical and functional recovery of the patients and the possibility to return to work. In Spain, the first rehabilitation service was created in 1933 under the name of *Instituto de Rehabilitación del Inválido* (Invalid Rehabilitation Institute).

In its Universal Declaration of Human Rights (1948), the United Nations (UN) devoted several of its articles to the disabled, stating that they have a right to work, social services, education and an adequate standard of living. In 1955 the U.N. approved an international rehabilitation programme for the physically disabled. In keeping with these guidelines, the *Lucha Sanitaria Nacional contra la Invalidez* (National Health Struggle against Disabilities) was founded in Spain in 1949 [3]. In 1961 an insurance programme was established for persons with occupational diseases or major disabilities, and for children who were orphaned as a result of occupational accidents or diseases. Since 1970 the disabled worker has been recognised and theoretically protected in the job market with a law establishing that 2% of all job positions in companies with 50 or more workers were to be reserved for disabled persons; incentives were provided for the Social Security payments. However, the law was not actually implemented. The Labour Relations Act of 1976 established the special nature of jobs held by the disabled, but the administration regulated the centres providing protected work opportunities more for the subsidies they might receive than to satisfy their technical and staffing needs. No provisions were made for personnel or for the technical, commercial and business assistance needed to carry out their activities. These places were occupational workshops rather than work centres. The laws were founded on paternalistic, benefit-based concepts and were fragmented and biased to these ends. Moreover, the various ministry departments regulated their own areas of responsibility without relating to the other departments and without any overview of the problem as a whole.

The definitive change came when the Spanish Constitution [4] was passed by the Cortes on 31 October 1978 and ratified by the Spanish people in a referendum held on 6 December 1978. In one of the preamble sections, the Constitution states its intent to "promote the progress of culture and of the economy to ensure a dignified quality of life for all." Section III devotes two articles to the protection of the disabled:

– Article 41, in general terms, states that the public authorities are obliged to "maintain a public Social Security system for all citizens guaranteeing adequate social assistance and benefits in situations of hardship";

– Article 49, in more specific terms, indicates that "the public authorities shall carry out a policy of preventive care, treatment, rehabilitation and integration of the physically, sensorially and mentally handicapped by giving them the specialised care they require, and affording them special protection for the enjoyment of the rights granted by this Part to all citizens".

The ratification of the Spanish Constitution also led to the restoration of the Autonomous Governments, starting with the historic autonomous areas (Catalonia, Basque Country and Galicia) and later extending this empowerment to the remaining regions of the country. This has involved a gradual transferral of powers for certain areas such as health, social affairs, transit, etc., as well as occasional differences in the application of some laws.

Based on Article 49 of the Spanish Constitution, the Social Integration Act of Disabled Persons (LISMI) was passed in 1982 to further advance the constitutional rights. This law was the first step toward addressing the assistance provided to the disabled in a specific, definite manner with a focus on rehabilitation and integration, and without paternalistic bias. In terms of management and funding, the Spanish government has undertaken an administrative reorganisation of its overall assistance plan for persons with a psychological, physical or sensory disability. Government funding for full assistance to the disabled is contemplated in the General Budgets of the Spanish government and in the budgets pertaining to the autonomous communities and local authorities.

The law regulates several occupational systems: 1) the system of regular jobs in both public and private companies, 2) protected jobs for individuals unable to work under the usual conditions, whether temporarily or permanently, and who will be employed at special job centres, and 3) occupational therapy centres not directly integrated in the job market, but offering an intermediate step for rejoining the work force in the event that the person has a temporary disability.

Two key documents have been issued since the LISMI was passed:

1. Plan of Emergency Measures for the Promotion of Employment for Disabled Persons, endorsed in 1996 by the *Consejo Español de Representantes de Minusválidos* (CERMI, Spanish Council of Representatives of the Disabled).

2. Action Plan for Individuals with a Disability for 1997-2000, drawn up and co-ordinated by the *Instituto de Migraciones y Servicios Sociales* (IMSERSO, Migration and Social Services Institute), approved by all the autonomous communities and social organizations, and ratified by the Spanish government in 1996. This document contains the results from various previous reports written ten years after the LISMI was passed [5, 6] and shows that there were still many gaps in the available assistance to this population, particularly with regard to rehabilitation, job creation, and implementation of a state policy for the prevention of disabilities. As a result of these previous reports, in 1991 the Ministry of Social Affairs agreed to prepare a preliminary Action Plan for Individuals with a Disability that was undertaken in December 1992 by IMSERSO. The plan has two key objectives: to achieve maximum autonomy and independence among this group, as well as greater, more active participation in the job market and in society. Its efforts focus on five areas: 1) the promotion of health and the prevention of disabilities; 2) full health care and rehabilitation; 3) integration in schools and special education; 4) participation and integration in the job market; and 5) community integration and an independent life [7]. The section on participation and integration in the job market discusses vocational rehabilitation, job creation and job protection policies. The priority objectives of the programme are to ensure that disabled persons have access to high-quality jobs and to promote a coherent support and adaptation system that guarantees their financial independence. This plan also addresses the need to promote transport, communication, architectural and urban accessibility as an essential factor in assisting disabled persons to join the work force and integrate in society. In this case, the IMSERSO and the *Confederación Coordinadora Estatal de Minusválidos Físicos de España* (COCEMFE, State Co-ordinator Confederation of the Physically Handicapped in Spain) and the *Organización Nacional de Ciegos de España* (ONCE, Spanish National Organisation of the Blind) have combined their efforts. The plan is funded by the General Budgets of the Spanish government, as well as by contributions from local corporations. In 1997, final budget allocations amounted to 5,984,393.76 euros (997 million old pesetas).

In November 2000, the Executive Committee of the CERMI approved "an employment plan for persons with disabilities for the 21st century" which addresses the Plan of Emergency Measures on behalf of Employment for Disabled Persons of 1997, for the purposes of improving their working conditions in the early 21st century. An agreement between the Spanish government and the CERMI in 1997 has been completed and developed almost in its entirety, although several major issues are still pending. These include, for instance, support for partially protected employment through working enclaves in ordinary companies, the DISCAP programme to promote extensive creation of jobs in standard working environments, and enhancement of CERMI's participation in organisations that design and implement policies which affect the hiring and training of individuals with a disability. This plan is part of a new socio-political context defined by several factors:

– new political context in Europe, resulting from the entry in force of the Treaty of Amsterdam, which contains a non-discrimination clause on behalf of the disabled (Art. 13), along with approval of an EU Council Directive to promote equal treatment in employment, and a European Strategy for Employment, whereby the common guidelines on employment provide a general framework for co-ordinating the employment policies of the Member States;

– related to the above, a new plan of Structural Funds for 2000-2006 with major allocations of loans from the European Regional Development Fund (ERDF) and European Social Fund (ESF) to support training and employment programmes;

– improved job market for the general population in Spain;

– acceleration of social and technological changes in connection with the information society;

– consolidation and unification of the association movement with the creation of CERMIs in the autonomous communities;

– decentralisation of active job market policies, transferring them from the *Instituto Nacional de Empleo* (INEM, National Employment Institute) to the autonomous communities;

– growing role of the social stakeholders (labour unions and business organisations) in the management of continuous training.

General agreement signed by the ONCE and the government in 1999, whereby ONCE agrees to create 20,000 jobs and provide 40,000 training activities for disabled persons during 1999-2008.

One of the most important measures in promoting vocational integration is to encourage the creation of specialised services in the Public Employment Offices under the auspices of the INEM (or the autonomous communities, if such powers have been transferred). The provision of complete, high-quality services with vocational rehabilitation and counselling that targets the adaptation of job positions should be guaranteed in these services, an effort that requires co-operation with the IMSERSO and the respective organisations of each autonomous community [8].

Financial benefits

The financial benefits in Spain for sick leave and for disabilities due to occupational diseases or accidents are regulated by the General Social Security Act (LGSS) and are further advanced through the Social Security system itself and its collaborating entities (occupational accident and disease insurance programmes of the Social Security system) and the official agencies of the autonomous communities to which these powers have been transferred.

Occupational accident and disease insurance programmes of the Social Security are considered to be those that are duly authorised by the Ministry of Labour and Social

Affairs and which have been founded as non-profit organisations for this purpose. These programmes are regulated by Section 4 of the LGSS, with the Ministry of Labour and Social Affairs holding the authority for management and protection.

The joint collaboration with the Social Security system includes co-operative efforts to manage the contingencies related to occupational accidents and diseases, the performance of prevention activities, functional and professional recovery, and other efforts provided for in the LGSS, as well as co-operative efforts to manage the financial benefits for the occupationally disabled due to common contingencies. The benefits for which an employee is eligible in the event of an occupational accident or disease include the following: a) medical and surgical treatment, pharmaceutical prescriptions, and in general any kind of diagnostic or therapeutic technique deemed medically necessary; b) orthopaedic devices, prostheses, walking aids, wheelchairs, etc.; c) plastic surgery and surgical repairs; d) functional rehabilitation; e) vocational counselling and training for job reintegration; and f) therapy required for non-vocational recovery when the severity of the injury makes vocational recovery impossible [9].

There are two types of financial benefits: pensions for temporary disability or persons undergoing physiotherapy, and indemnities (e.g., lump-sum or pension, as applicable) when the worker has a non-disabling injury, or when a permanent disability (partial, total, absolute or major disability) has been certified.

In the event of sick leave taken because of an occupational accident or disease, the benefits are paid from the day after sick leave is started, and the employer is responsible for paying the full salary. When the sick leave is taken because of an ordinary illness or non-occupational accident, that is, *incapacidad laboral transitoria* (ILT, temporary work disability), the Social Security system pays the full benefits for a maximum period of 12 months, except for benefits provided for the 4th to 15th day, which are paid by the employer. These Social Security benefits can also be renewed for an additional 6 months.

In the case of pensions for *permanent disability*, there are two types of benefits: *contributory* and *non-contributory*. A *contributory* benefit is the benefit received when the disabled worker has paid contributions to the Social Security system. For the *contributory modality*, a permanent disability is considered to exist when the worker has undergone the prescribed treatment and has received a medical discharge, but still retains severe anatomical or functional deficits that can be objectively assessed and are predicted to persist indefinitely, and that decrease or impede the person's ability to work. A permanent disability is also considered to exist when the disability remains after the temporary disability has ended upon completion of the maximum period of 18 months. Any *permanent disability*, regardless of cause, is classified as a function of the percent reduction of the individual's capacity to work. This is assessed according to a list of diseases, approved by law, as follows: a) partial permanent disability; b) complete permanent disability; c) absolute permanent disability; and d) major disability.

The classification into different disability grades is determined as a function of the percent reduction in the legally established capacity to work, also taking into account the incidence of reduction in the capacity to work in the individual's former profession. The financial benefit for *partial permanent disability* for the individual's former profession consists in a lump sum and the right to return to work. The financial benefit for *complete permanent disability* consists in a lifetime pension that can, as an exception, be replaced with a lump-sum indemnity if the beneficiary is under 60 years of age. If the beneficiary is likely to encounter difficulties for being hired in another vocation because of a lack of general or specialized training or because of the social situation and job market at his or her place of residence, the pension can be increased by the percentage set forth by law. The financial benefit for *absolute permanent disability* consists in a lifetime pension. For *major disability*, a lifetime pension is awarded, along with a 50% increase for remuneration paid to the caregiver. If a person is classified as having a major disability and requires institutionalisation, this 50% increase is used to pay this kind of care [10].

Non-contributory benefits are understood to mean the pension received by a disabled worker who has never made payments to the Social Security system. These amounts are small. Persons eligible for the *non-contributory modality* are those over 18 years and under 65 years of age who have resided in Spain and for at least five years, who have insufficient income or no earnings, and who are affected by a disability or chronic disease classified as 65% or more.

Organisation and access to vocational rehabilitation

Generally speaking, individuals who have had a disease or accident that usually requires rehabilitation therapy account for 25% of all hospital admissions. A large percentage of these individuals should take part in vocational rehabilitation programmes because they are of working age. Nevertheless, the number of disabled individuals enrolled in vocational rehabilitation programmes is still low. The reasons for this situation include the "subsidy culture" that still exists among many disabled persons and workers who have had an occupational accident, as well as the limited presence of multidisciplinary teams specialised in vocational rehabilitation within the public healthcare system for the various disabling conditions.

The concept of comprehensive, integrated rehabilitation goes beyond the scope of any specific sector, although partial vocational approaches and planning efforts between independent services with little co-ordination still have significant weight. The organisation of, and access to vocational rehabilitation in Spain has been evolving in line with the legislative changes.

Rehabilitation efforts can fall under various ministries (Health, Education, Labour, Social Affairs). The responsibilities are divided between the central government and the autonomous communities, however. The basic problem lies in interconnecting hospital services for acute patients with other health resources (primary care, convalescent centres) and other structures that offer definitive rehabilitation, such as early care, special education, vocational rehabilitation and community integration. Despite progress in this area, much work remains to be done in order to achieve rehabilitation therapy programmes with a holistic approach toward the patient and with special attention to maintaining continuous care.

In the case of occupational accidents and diseases, the patient is usually cared for at the occupational insurance hospitals and is then enrolled in the vocational retraining programme at the same hospital, while also participating in the rehabilitation therapy plan. This programme includes the social worker, the vocational counsellor and the representatives of the company where the injured person works, and often involves vocational re-adaptation or training courses if the employee must acquire a new profession. Such an approach calls for the active co-operation and explicit interest of the injured person in rejoining the work force. At the time of hospital discharge, the patients undertake the vocational rehabilitation plan on an outpatient basis until they are able to return to the workplace.

For conditions not related to the person's job, vocational reintegration is regulated by Spanish law through two legal standards, the LGSS and the LISMI, as detailed above in the section on legislative history.

Most disabled persons, regardless of the cause for their disability, are attended in the National Health Service acute hospitals and primary healthcare services by multidisciplinary rehabilitation teams responsible for prescribing the therapy plan and determining the indication for prostheses, orthopaedic devices, walking aids, wheelchairs, etc. This healthcare level has no multidisciplinary team for vocational assessment and counselling, and one of the difficulties is interlinking patient care at these levels with the various outpatient vocational assessment and counselling teams assigned to the care centres for the disabled. The vocational assessment and counselling teams are either in private organisations or within the public system, in which case they are included in the social services or, depending on the autonomous community, are under the auspices of the Department of Health and Social Affairs. Vocational training is provided on the basis of reports issued by the multidisciplinary teams and takes into consideration the previous training, existing employment opportunities, motivation, aptitudes and preferences of the disabled person. Vocational training may include general preliminary training and may be taught at special centres or companies. When carried out at companies, a formal vocational training contract (internship) is required.

Vocational assessment and counselling teams in the public system are composed of a physician, psychologist and social worker. Assessment by this team can classify the disabled person as *non-productive* or *productive*, with the latter implying the possibility of an employment contract. For *non-productive* individuals, there are specialised care centres all over Spain for severely disabled persons that also provide healthcare services and there are occupational centres for moderately disabled persons that provide occupational therapy services. Catalonia also has occupational integration services for disabled persons who are eligible for the occupational centres or special work centres and who are awaiting a vacancy.

In the *productive* category, including those with a mild disability who are capable of productive work, the approach taken is usually the open (ordinary) job market. Additional measures include efforts to foster employment, for instance, subsidies, bonuses and fiscal measures for the employers (provided permanent employment contracts are signed), as well as mandatory measures in which certain companies (those employing over 50 workers) must reserve 2% of their jobs for the disabled. The job integration services and the aided-work programmes are intended to promote hiring in the job market. These job integration services are teams that work within private organisations, private endeavours and with government funding, and which have the goal of placing disabled persons in companies with ordinary jobs. In Spain these teams can be located on the premises of private organisations. In Catalonia the ECOM Federation has pioneered the creation of a job integration service network in conjunction with local organisations. These services are housed in public buildings (city halls, county boards), and the staff is composed of a job counsellor (psychologist), employment expert (labour law specialist), staff intern, job trainer, and administrative assistant. The aided-work programmes, which fall under the auspices of the Labour Department, are involved primarily in the promotion of training courses, after which the disabled person can be hired by an ordinary company or by a specialized job centre. These centres represent another job opportunity for disabled persons classified as productive, i.e. those with a mild disability who are working. At least 70% of the workers in these companies are disabled persons. The company receives 9,000 euros per disabled worker if 70% to 90% of the workforce is composed of disabled employees, and 12,000 euros if more than 90% are disabled.

Finally, Spain also has *Centros de Recuperación de Minusválidos Físicos* (CRMF, Recuperation Centres for the Physically Handicapped) that fall under the jurisdiction of the IMSERSO. Their main objective is to offer these physically and/or sensorially disabled persons of working age all the training and counselling they need to obtain employment. These centres teach vocational training courses in the fields of computer-aided design, jewellery, carpentry, electricity, book-binding, shoe repair, electronics, computer repair and data processing. IMSERSO has five CRMF centres in Albacete, San Fernando (Cádiz), Lardero (La Rioja), Salamanca and Madrid [11].

In short, although vocational rehabilitation in Spain has improved significantly in the last 25 years, there is still a need for further progress in various areas. Particular efforts must be made to co-ordinate the various assistance-providing services and enhance the National Health Service teams, within a political will to defend the public system. Such efforts do not produce optimum results in the short-term. The process is rather one of continued interaction that involves educational integration and promoting a competitive culture on the part of the disabled, a willingness to overcome prejudices on the part of employers (both public and private), removal of architectural barriers, transport and communication facilities for the disabled, and adaptation of job positions.

References

1. Fundación ONCE (1999) Encuesta sobre discapacidades, deficiencias y estado de salud. Avance de resultados. Datos básicos. Madrid: Ministerio de Trabajo y Asuntos Sociales
2. Serrano E (1963) Discurso de apertura al IV Congreso Nacional de la Sociedad Española de rehabilitación. Acta Fisioterápica Ibérica VIII(2): 19-24
3. Palacios J (1989) Historia del CPEE de Reeducación de Inválidos. Madrid: MEC-CPEE. Reeducación de Inválidos: 51-83

4. Constitución Española (1978) Comisión Organizadora Actos Conmemorativos del 25 Aniversario de la Constitución Española. Boletín Oficial del Estado, Ministerio de la Presidencia

5. Comentarios a la LISMI (1992) Madrid: Documentos del Real Patronato de Prevención y Atención a Personas con Minusvalía

6. 10 anys de la Llei d'integració social dels minusvàlids (LISMI) a Catalunya: present i futur. Informes tècnics sobre l'aplicació de la LISMI a Catalunya (1992). Generalitat de Catalunya. Departament de Benestar Social

7. MA Alonso, C Martín, B Palomino (2003) Plan de acción para las personas con discapacidad: revisión de un anteproyecto. In: JC Miangolarra (dir) Rehabilitación Clínica Integral. Masson SA, Barcelona, p71

8. Un plan de empleo para las personas con discapacidad en el siglo XXI (2000) Colección CERMI. Ministerio de Asuntos Sociales, Instituto de Migraciones y Servicios Sociales, Madrid.

9. JL Castellá (2002) Aseguramiento y prevención de los riesgos laborales. In: Salud Laboral. Masson SA, Barcelona, p152-7

10. Real Decreto Legislativo 1/1994, 20 Junio (1994) Up date 11.07.03. BOE, Madrid.

11. RE Legarreta (2003) Derecho al Trabajo de las Personas con Discapacidad. Real Patronato sobre Discapacidad. Ministerio de Trabajo y Asuntos Sociales, Madrid

Vocational rehabilitation: the Swedish model

J. Ekholm and K. Schüldt Ekholm

Vocational rehabilitation in Sweden – the problem

Absence due to sickness is much higher in Sweden, Norway and the Netherlands than in Denmark, Finland, Germany, France and the United Kingdom [1]. Also, it varies much more over time in the first mentioned three countries. However, differences in composition of the labour force between the countries influence the sick leave situation. Underlying differences in the composition of the labour force (gender, age, types of industries, number of part-time workers, and employment conditions) explain about one fifth of the differences of the rate of sick leave in Sweden and the average of the countries with the lowest rate in the above-mentioned study of European countries [1]. Age seems to be the most important factor in Sweden, where a comparatively high share of employees has reached an age at which the risk of being ill is higher. Although these factors are important, the main part of the differences between the countries remains to be explained. One interesting area is the differences between countries in design of the system for financial compensation. An example is that generous compensation from public systems, as well as through occupational agreements, could lead to a higher rate of sickness absence, but other differences may also play a role [1].

Another – but related – problem in Sweden is the high rate of disability pension. This means that a period of long-term sick leave often ends with a decision by the national insurance office to grant a disability pension – and not with a decision to provide vocational (or medical-plus-vocational) rehabilitation aiming at resuming working life [2, 3]. Even the government considers this to be a major Swedish economic problem, leading to a too small proportion of the population gainfully employed in relation to the proportion living on disability allowance. The efficiency of the system for vocational rehabilitation is of great importance here. The effectiveness of the various rehabilitation programmes provided is one important aspect, the skill in co-operation of the different rehabilitation actors is another, and also important is the proportion of long-term sick leavers who actually receives a vocational rehabilitation measure from the public system [4, 5].

Who is responsible
for vocational rehabilitation in Sweden?
How is the vocational rehabilitation organised?

Main bodies involved in rehabilitation aiming at resuming working life

There are several actors in the area of vocational rehabilitation. Below follows a description of the main organisations with some kind of official responsibility for vocational rehabilitation; the employers, the health and medical service, the national insurance office, employment offices, and social services [6]. In addition, the patient/client has responsibilities, e.g. for actively participating in rehabilitation measures granted, and to a certain extent the patient, are supposed to be involved in the selection of rehabilitation measures.

The employer

According to Swedish law, employers have extensive responsibility for the working environment of the employees. The employer shall take into account the particular qualifications of the employee for the work task, by adapting working conditions or by taking appropriate actions. The employer must ensure that there exist within the company programmes for adaptation and rehabilitation. Large companies often have staff assigned for this work, but the resources of small companies vary.

In principle, the employer has responsibility for ascertaining and investigating needs of vocational rehabilitation, for the actions to be brought about, and for the financing of those actions. A governmental investigation [7] has observed that this responsibility is not clearly perceived by all employers. In reality the national social insurance office has been pressing on for the investigations to be carried through and for changes to occur.

An employer must initiate a rehabilitation investigation when: (i) an employee is on sick leave more than 4 weeks; (ii) an employee has repeated short term sick leaves; (iii) when the insured person (the employee) wants it [6].

Public organisations

The responsibility for rehabilitation in public institutions is divided into four parallel sectors: the public health and medical service of the county councils, the social service of the municipalities, the employability offices of the state, and the national social insurance system.

The health and medical service

The public health and medical service is, in addition to regular medical examination and treatment, responsible for medical rehabilitation and should occur at least to some extent in all levels of the medical service system: specialist rehabilitation is found in some 30 public clinical departments of rehabilitation medicine located in the various counties. The goal of rehabilitation of the public medical service is to restore functioning as far as possible in all aspects, analysing function in terms of impairments, activity limitations and participation restriction taking into account environmental factors according to the principles of International Classification of Functioning, Disability and Health – ICF [8].

The boundary line between medical rehabilitation and vocational rehabilitation is somewhat blurred because the national insurance system with its health insurance has the responsibility (and public resources) for the "working-life-oriented" rehabilitation. Thus it has become a matter of how the definitions are made with respect to "rehabilitation medicine" and "working-life-oriented" rehabilitation [7]. In reality, most of the county-based bigger clinical departments of rehabilitation medicine run particular programmes aiming at returning to working life and programmes for assessing working capacity, these run in parallel to or in combination with rehabilitation programmes for other purposes. Many of these activities are at least partly financed by the national health insurance and the county councils finance the other parts.

The social services

The Social Services of a municipality is responsible for the residents' potential to live in the society, irrespective of reason for the problems. Support of various kinds including economic support is given. By tradition, the Social Services also have particular responsibility for drug and alcohol addicts and people with chronic psychiatric disease and social problems. Even if rehabilitation is not explicitly a responsibility for Social Services, rehabilitation aimed at some kind of working situation is often a goal in the planning, since it can end dependence on allowances from the Social Services [6].

The employment office

An employment office is responsible for rehabilitation of the unemployed. Their main task is to help healthy people get jobs. However, the major employment offices have special units – employability institutes – for the additional task of supporting unemployed people with moderate or light disability to find, obtain, and maintain a job. The activities of these offices include the testing of working capacity, guidance about job seeking, and organising opportunities to be a trainee or apprentice, or other training situations. Even if the normal labour market is the normal long-term goal, an employment office also has the option of placing a person in sheltered employment [6].

The task of Samhall AB, which is a big governmentally owned company with units spread all over the country, is to provide meaningful jobs which will develop potential for persons seeking a job through the employment office or its employability institutes, and who have been unable to get a job on the normal labour market due to disability related to physical, psychiatric, intellectual, or abuse problems. The group of companies provides adapted work places [6].

The National Insurance office

In addition to supplying insured persons with a variety of allowances, the National Insurance Office is responsible for the co-operation between the various rehabilitation actors. Other responsibilities are to initiate rehabilitation measures and supervise over other vocational rehabilitation actors. The National Insurance Office has a great number of local offices and has responsibility for the decision as to whether the person receives a sickness allowance, rehabilitation allowance, or disability pension, using doctors' certificates and other medical reports as a basis. The National Insurance Office may purchase rehabilitation services to enable a sick leaver to resume work. Such services may include investigations of functioning or measures aiming at facilitating return to working life (e.g. education or measures to increase function or minimize disability) [6].

How is the access to the vocational rehabilitation organized?

In principle, all persons in the country between 18 and 65 years of age are covered by the national health insurance (with only a few exceptions) and all manpower with sick leave has the possibility (but not the right) to receive vocational rehabilitation. The request for vocational rehabilitation can come from different sources, most often from the patient's physician. The doctor's certificate form allows the insurance office of easily informing about a need of vocational rehabilitation for resuming work. The employer, the patient, or an officer of the insurance office can also suggest that vocational rehabilitation is needed. In principle the employer has to initiate a request for rehabilitation (but in reality this does not regularly occur at present). If the person is unemployed the insurance office performs this function. If the local national insurance office approves the rehabilitation need of the patient, and economic resources exist, the next step is that a plan for rehabilitation is prepared at the insurance office. The proportion of patients with rehabilitation needs who receives a vocational rehabilitation measure varies over time and places, depending on the current economic resources and a sufficiency of staff to find and purchase the rehabilitation measures. At present, about one fifth of the patients who are in need of vocational rehabilitation receive it, at least in some measure [4, 5, 7]. That proportion can, of course, be altered depending on political decisions and/or state of the market [9].

Accident and health insurance companies and reimbursements of clients

The private accident insurance provides economic protection after acute injury and invalidity. In principle it adds to the public insurance system, and may cover costs for medical care, medicaments, damage to cloth or spectacles, compensation for pain and suffering, scars and deformities, medical and economic invalidity or costs for a funeral.

This kind of insurance can be taken out individually or collectively, e.g. at the work place. Four criteria must be fulfilled for an injury to be defined as an accident. It must be an injury that has occurred involuntarily as a consequence of a sudden external event. Trouble as a consequence of overload, e.g. heavy lifting, is not regarded as injury due to accident [10].

Private health insurance schemes are supplementary to the public insurance system, and give reimbursement commensurate with the reduction of the working capacity that it has led to a doctor's certificate of illness, granted temporary disability pension or permanent disability pension. Since morbidity increases with age, the cost of insurance premium markedly increases too. At a great age it is often not economically worthwhile to take out a health insurance. The insurance companies usually have the age of 59 years as the upper limit for taking out a health insurance [11].

Organisation of financial compensation for loss of earnings in case of accidents or illness

In the case of falling ill, or having an accident, the patient reports to the employer and to the regional social insurance office (of the national insurance system). The first week of sick leave is certified by the patient him/herself. On the 8th day a doctor's certificate must be available at the public regional social insurance office for the sick leave to be continued. At present, the employer pays sickness benefit the first 2 weeks, (except the first day that is not paid at all) and 15% of full sickness allowance until it is finalized. The (public) national health insurance pays 85% from the third week and on, and in principle, the sickness allowance is unlimited in time in Sweden. Part-time sick listing is possible with 25%, 50%, 75% and full. Self-employed persons, too, can use the national health insurance at varying levels of compensations related to their payment.

The level of benefit from the national health insurance may vary due to varying political decisions and is at present 80% of the salary up to a ceiling (maximum salary 494 euros per week). The benefit is taxed. During the first two weeks sickness payment from the employer, it may be at the same level as the public payment, but is more often set by agreements concluded between employer and employee.

Organization of disability pensions in case of accidents or illness

Usually after some time (e.g. one year) the regional social insurance office suggests a change from sickness allowance to temporary disability pension. The patient's physician is contacted to give an opinion on the patient's working capacity. The regional social insurance office then decides about granting temporary disability pension and the number of years (one or two) until the next assessment. During this period of time rehabilitation measures are supposed to take place [9].

At the next assessment working capacity is evaluated again. If full working capacity is not achieved the regional social insurance office decides once more whether it will be continued temporary disability pension or a move to permanent disability pension. Permanent disability pension can be at different levels – 25%, 50%, 75% and full pension. The payment is substantially lower than that for sickness allowance. The level of both temporary and permanent disability pension is calculated in a way similar to that for old age pension depending on, for example, the total number of years of gainful employment[9].

References

1. Socialdepartementet (the Ministry of Health and Social Affairs) (2003) Den svenska sjukan II – regelverk och försäkringsmedicinska bedömningar i åtta länder. (in Swedish with English summary) (The Swedish disease II - rules and regulations and assessments of working capacity in eight countries). (Group of authors: Mikaelsson B, Ekholm J, Kärrholm J, Murray R, Sandberg T, Söderberg J, Nyman K) Governmental report. Socialdepatementet Ds 2003: 63, www.regeringen.se/propositioner/sou/pdf/remiss.pdf
2. Selander J (1999) Unemployed sick-leavers and vocational rehabilitation. PhD Thesis. Karolinska Institutet (Section of Rehabilitation Medicine, Dept. of Public Health Sciences) Stockholm, Sweden
3. Marnetoft S-U (2000) Vocational Rehabilitation of unemployed sick-listed people in a Swedish rural area. PhD Thesis. Karolinska Institutet (Section of Rehabilitation Medicine, Dept. of Public Health Sciences) Stockholm, Sweden
4. Marnetoft S-U, Selander J, Bergroth A, Ekholm J (1997) The unemployed sick-listed and their vocational rehabilitation. Internat J of Rehabil Research 20: 245-53
5. Selander J, Marnetoft S-U, Bergroth A and Ekholm J (1998) The process of vocational rehabilitation for employed and unemployed people on sick-leave: employed vs unemployed people in Stockholm compared with circumstances in rural Jämtland, Sweden. Scand J Rehabil Med 30: 55-60
6. Ekholm J (2002) Försäkringsmedicin och rehabilitering (Insurance Medicine and Rehabilitation) In: Järvholm B, Olofsson C (eds): Försäkringsmedicin (Insurance Medicine). Studentlitteratur, Lund, 2002 (in Swedish)
7. SOU, Socialdepartementet (2002) Rehabilitering till arbete. En reform med individen i centrum (Rehabilitation to work. A reform with the individual in the centre) (In Swedish). SOU 2000: 78. Fritzes, Stockholm
8. WHO (2001) International Classification of Functioning, Disability and Health – ICF. WHO, Geneva
9. Olofsson C & Mikaelsson B (2002) Regelverk och administrativa processer (Rules and regulations and administrative processes) In: Järvholm B, Olofsson C (eds): Försäkringsmedicin (Insurance Medicine). Studentlitteratur, Lund, 2002 (in Swedish)
10. Netz P (2002) Olycksfalls- och trafikförsäkring. (Accident and trafic insurance) In: Järvholm B, Olofsson C (eds): Försäkringsmedicin (Insurance Medicine). Studentlitteratur, Lund, 2002 (in Swedish)
11. Perman E (2002) Privat försäkring – nyteckning (Private insurance - taking out an insurance) In: Järvholm B, Olofsson C (eds): Försäkringsmedicin (Insurance Medicine). Studentlitteratur, Lund, 2002 (in Swedish)

Vocational rehabilitation: the Swiss model

M.-F. Fournier-Buchs and C. Gobelet

Introduction [1]

Since the end of the 19th century and in line with its European neighbours, Switzerland has devoted itself to setting up a system of social security. In 1890, the Federal Constitution was completed with an article authorizing the Confederation to pass legislation on sickness and accident insurance. Since then, Switzerland's safety net of social security has developed in a piecemeal way over a long period at the mercy of economic crises and their financial risks, which accounts for the lack of harmony in the benefits of the various insurance schemes and makes coordination between the different systems indispensable.

In a statement for the Federal Assembly in 1919, the Federal Council proposed the creation of Federal Disability Insurance (DI), linked to Insurance for Old-Age and Survivors (OASI). Faced by financial difficulties, Switzerland chose to focus its social efforts on Old-Age and Survivors' Insurance (OASI: came into force in 1948) rather than on Disability Insurance, which was enacted in 1960 [2].

Before the introduction of DI, one section of the active population had already been eligible for Accident Insurance (from 1918), although the armed forces had obtained benefits since 1902 (Federal Military Insurance: FMI), as had some employees in the public or private sector affiliated with a pension fund. Compulsory Accident Insurance for everyone was only introduced in 1984.

Since it came into force in 1960, DI gives priority to the principle of "Rehabilitation before Pension". Legislators also had to clarify the boundaries between DI and the other branches of social insurance. In principle, DI is not intended to cover the benefits that are normally the responsibility of health, accident and unemployment insurance but should cover the real risk of disability.

The Swiss insurance framework

Accidents and health are governed by two laws: the Accident Insurance Law and the Health Insurance Law.

Every Swiss worker is compulsorily insured by his employer against accidents and their consequences. The main Swiss accident insurer is Suva (Swiss National Accident Insurance Fund), which insures all construction workers and manual workers in general. Numerous private companies as well as mutual insurance companies provide the rest of the Swiss population with accident insurance cover.

Where health insurance is concerned, each inhabitant is insured by around 69 different mutual insurance companies or groups.

The armed forces are covered for health and accident insurance by federal military insurance, which is directly dependent on and financed by the Confederation.

The disabling consequences of an accident are paid for by accident insurance whereas disability as the result of a disease is the responsibility of disability insurance (DI), financed by compulsory advance deductions from salaries, as is unemployment insurance.

At present, the various social insurances are in charge of the following benefits:

Disability insurance: vocational rehabilitation measures, technical and assistive devices, disability allowances, daily benefits during rehabilitation, pensions in cases of disability as a consequence of disease. Financing is based on advance direct deductions from the wages of every worker.

Health insurance (compulsory): medical and pharmaceutical expenses, medical care, maternity, hospitalisation, medical prescribed spa, supplementary cover against accidents, complementary insurance, optional daily benefits. Health insurance does not cover any benefits for vocational rehabilitation. Financing is by personal contributions whereby employers can participate.

Accident and occupational disease insurance (compulsory): medical, pharmaceutical and hospital costs, medically prescribed health spa stays, technical and assistive devices and daily benefits until possibility to return to work or until the start of a disability pension (but not during rehabilitation measures provided under DI), disability pension following an accident or an occupational disease (possibly concurrent with a DI pension but not in excess of a maximal fixed compensation), integrity compensation, disability allowance. It is financed by employers by means of advance deduction from wages or by individual contributions.

Military insurance: medical, pharmaceutical and hospital costs, technical and assistive devices, disability allowance, rehabilitation measures, daily benefits while unable to work and during rehabilitation, disability pension if due to illness or accident sustained during a period of military service, integrity compensation. Financed by the Confederation.

Unemployment insurance: reintegration measures, unemployment benefits. Finance by advance deductions from wages.

The diversity of these intervening parties is coordinated by the Federal Law on the general part of the social security law, which:

– defines the principles, ideas and the institutions of the social security law;
– standardizes procedures and regulates the judiciary organization within the field of social security;
– harmonizes social security benefits, and regulates the right of social security to press claims against third parties.

Close coordination between the various sectors is essential and cooperation between insurers is imperative, at the risk of being penalized if some insurees are refused benefits to which they are entitled.

The parameters of vocational rehabilitation

Disability insurance is responsible for vocational rehabilitation both in terms of financial aspects and practical implementation by centres for vocational rehabilitation funded by DI.

Epidemiological aspects

The statistics published by Suva [3], which insures 1,8000,000 employees, recorded 446,335 accident cases in 2002, 187,587 of which were occupational accidents and diseases and 245,011 were non-occupational accidents (leisure time, vehicle, domestic) while the total number of unemployed in Switzerland who suffered accidents amounted to 12,023.

Since 1990, accident prevalence has changed, with non-occupational accidents increasing to the figure mentioned above in 2002. 0.7% of accidents result in disability and 3,061 new disability pensions were allocated by the Suva in 2002. The total benefits paid out to accident victims in 2002 amounted to 3,1492 billion CHF for lost earnings and 1,3145 billion CHF for pensions.

During the last years, an increase of 7% to 9% in the benefits was paid out. Among the prevailing factors in this rise from 7% to 9% was the increase in average age of the insurees, which caused a rise in the cost of healing and a rise in life expectancy. This meant that disability pensions would be paid for a longer period of time.

A marked increase in mental complications is one of the factors that make the course of an accident more serious. Unfortunately, there is no data at national level for the various accident insurance companies and the figures given above only cover 50% of all employees in Switzerland.

Any analysis of the consequences of disease is far more difficult due to the lack of national data on the 69 mutual insurance companies or groups that cover health insurance.

The annual statistics for 2001 for disability insurance [4], which is responsible for all the disability pension due to disease show that expenditure amounted to 9,500 billion CHF, of which 5,500 billion CHF were allocated to pensions, 300 million CHF to daily benefits, 200 million CHF to disability allowances and 1,400 billion CHF to individual rehabilitation and training measures.

DI insurance has 7.5 million insurees, of which 4.2 million pay contributions. In 2001 485,000 received benefits (285,000 men and 200,000 women). Thus the probability of receiving disability benefits in 2001 was 7.4%. This probability is relative to age and gender and, for men, rises on a graduated scale from 3% for those aged between 20 and 24 to more than 20% for those aged between 60 and 64.

It should also be pointed out that the likelihood of receiving DI benefits has risen from 5.5% to 7.4% during the course of the last decade.

When all the disability pension benefits (after accidents and diseases) paid out in Switzerland by the various authorities are taken into account, they add up to about CHF 13 billions, which roughly corresponds to 1/3 of the health budget.

This gives a better idea of the financial impact that the disability can have on Federal finances and of the need to develop structured rehabilitation measures to enable all those with a disability to return, at least part-time, to an active working life.

Rehabilitation and the law on disability insurance (DI) [2, 6, 7]

Since its enactment in 1960, the law on disability insurance laid down a basic principle: *rehabilitation before pension*. A series of measures have been formed around this postulate, the purpose of which is to allow persons afflicted by diseases or accidents to regain, safeguard or improve their earning capacity.

As with any insurance system, certain conditions should be met first in order to receive benefits.

Article 8 of the law on the general part of the Social Security Law* (which came into force on 01.01.03) [4], article around which all the law on disability insurance revolves, *states that inability to earn (or disability) amounts to the permanent or long-term impossibility of pursuing gainful employment on the entire job market as a result of health impairment or disabilities and after exhausting all rehabilitation attempts and opportunities.*

The main point of this idea of disability is the causal link between severity of the disease or the accident and the loss of earning ability. With the term *ability to earn*, the law on disability insurance means the ability of a person to obtain an income from an activity adapted to his or her state of health that exists in a so-called balanced job market (cf. paragraph below about self-rehabilitation). The confusion between *disability* and *loss of integrity* is encountered very frequently; sometimes, patients are heard to say "I've paid my contributions, I'm ill, I'm therefore entitled to compensation for the loss of my health". While this may be true within the framework of the law on accident insurance (loss of integrity compensation), this is not the case with the law on disability insurance.

Evaluation of residual occupational capacity

Disability insurance has set specific structures in place that enable claimants' state of health and residual occupational capacity to be analysed.

---

* The Federal Law about the general part of the Social Security Law (ATSG/LPGA) coordinates the law on social security by defining the principles, ideas and the institutions of the Social Security Law; by standardizing procedures and regulating the judiciary organization within the field of social security; by harmonizing social security benefits; by regulating the right of social security to press claims against third parties.

State of health is determined by a general practitioner (GP) and, in cases of doubt, claimants are referred by the disability insurance's office to a medical evaluation centre specifically approved by disability insurance (COMAI: DI's medical observation centre) or to an acknowledged expert. At the end of the check-up, either COMAI or the expert submits a report to the disability insurance office stating the claimant's residual occupational capacity.

Vocational evaluation and, if necessary, vocational rehabilitation is carried out in the DI's occupational observation centres (COPAI) where a claimant's skills are observed and his/her immediate occupational capacity. The DI can also delegate this task to clinics that are specialised in vocational rehabilitation or to private institutions that operate in the same field. These institutions are similarly approached when handicapped people have to be reintegrated into the working market.

Inability to work and inability to earn

There are other ideas that give rise to confusion, in particular those relating to an *inability to work* and to an *inability to earn*. Both of these are the result of health impairment but, where the former is concerned, a patient is partially or completely no longer fit for work in his/her regular activities or sector while, with the latter, a patient is partially or completely no longer capable of carrying out any gainful activities whatsoever, since there is nothing in the job market that is adapted to his or her state of health. Whereas inability to work is determined by the doctor, inability to earn is a matter for disability insurance.

Example

Following an accident, a paraplegic who was previously employed as an office worker will not receive any disability pension if the former job can be resumed once his/her health has been stabilized with full-day presence and a 90% workload. Since the former activity is considered suitable, the loss of ability to earn is 10%, in other words, disability of 10% does not entitle a claimant either to a disability pension or to retraining via the intermediary of DI. On the other hand, this person will receive a one-off cash benefit from accident insurance as integrity compensation and a 10% pension in accordance with the law on accident insurance.

Residual capacity in a modified occupational activity

Once an *impaired state of health* has been clearly established at medical level, the question now arises of *residual capacity in a modified occupational activity*. In order to determine this, the DI office, in line with legislation, consults the general practitioner or the specialists or even the occupational or the company physician who is in charge of the patient.

In this case, the DI office asks them to point out what the *functional limitations* are as a result of the deficiencies or impairments.

If the DI office considers the information provided by the GP or other referred physicians to be insufficient, it can request an analysis by its own medical service or practical observation in specialized institutions or even an expert medical opinion. Pursuing the principle of rehabilitation before pension, the DI office will then investigate whether rehabilitation measures (medical, vocational, technical and assistive devices, etc.) will safeguard a person's ability to earn or even improve it.

Self-rehabilitation, prerequisites with the aim of vocational rehabilitation

No insuree has a right to vocational rehabilitation for no matter what condition. The insurance system not only involves rights but also obligations. Thus, having impaired health and having to change one's job is not sufficient for an automatic right to vocational rehabilitation provided by DI.

Insurees are obliged to cooperate and to do everything possible to reduce the damage sustained. Where jobs are concerned, this means that they must do their utmost to return to occupational activity, without training, to ensure that any loss of earnings is kept to a minimum thereby avoiding the need for the payment of a pension: as a result, the term *self-rehabilitation* is used. If it is impossible to find a job that safeguards a person's ability to earn in a so-called balanced job market (abstract idea that postulates a job market where there is a balance between supply and demand for work and where the range of possible jobs is sufficiently extensive), the DI office will look into the possibility of *initial training* for insurees who have never had any gainful employment or *reclassification* for insurees who have had gainful employment.

In order to qualify for reclassification measures, the *loss of earnings must be a minimum of 20%* between what the insuree's wage was without health impairment and what he/she could obtain without any training and taking into account the functional limitations following health impairment.

Example

An unskilled construction worker suffers chronic low back pain following an operation for a discal herniation. According to his physician, he has long-term 100% inability to work in his normal job (bricklaying) but 0% inability in a suitable job that does not involve carrying heavy loads, that saves him having to work in positions that are painful for his back and allows him to alternate between sitting and standing.

Prior to his operation, this insuree's annual wage was 57,000 CHF. If occupations suitable for his residual capabilities are considered and which are open to him on the job market (assembly work in the field of small-scale industrial production, quality control for various goods, surveillance jobs, small goods delivery, etc.), an annual wage of around 52,000 CHF can be earned, this income being calculated on the basis of statistical surveys that establish the average wages for unqualified employees on the current Swiss job market. The drop in annual wage of 5,000 CHF corresponds to an inability to earn of 9%, thus not entitling him to either a pension (a minimum of 40% loss of earnings is required for entitlement to a quarter of the DI pension) or to retraining (a minimum of 20% loss of earnings is required for entitlement).

Vocational measures can be requested right away from DI from the point in time when it becomes evident in medical terms that a change of occupational activity is essential due to permanent or long-term health impairment. In fact, it is unnecessary to wait for a full year of partial or total inability to work (qualifying period) as is the case when applying for a pension. *It is important for the general practitioner to be familiar with this so that the rehabilitation measures offered by DI can be activated as quickly as possible so that they have the greatest effect.*

Example

A qualified baker develops asthma because of an allergy to flour. Once all the tests have been conducted, a diagnosis made and even the decision taken on inability due to occupational disease, the family doctor should urge his patient to submit a request for occupational rehabilitation to DI as quickly as possible. There is no reason to sit out a whole year of inability to work, which is the minimum legal period for entitlement to disability pension benefits other than vocational rehabilitation.

What distinguishes the baker from the unskilled manual worker mentioned above is their levels of vocational training. In contrast to the manual worker, the baker has a Federal Certificate of Proficiency (FCP). In a case like this, even if the DI office concludes that the baker is less than 20% disabled (theoretical payability), he can be considered for vocational retraining based on the fact that, in contrast to the unskilled manual worker whose income has peaked, the baker has both career and salary prospects and his loss of income is therefore potentially more important (= principal of so-called equivalence).

Legal constraints and vocational training

With regard to the choice of retraining within the framework of vocational rehabilitation, several fundamental principles indicate the route to be taken:

To reduce the claim, the law on disability insurance provides for *simple and appropriate measures*, the aim being to safeguard a person's ability to earn. Such measures are not necessarily the best possible ones, particularly from the standpoint of the insuree and his doctor.

In connection with the choice of a new occupational area, the idea of equivalence plays a central role. DI will permit an insuree to obtain new occupational qualifications to the level of his own prior to health impairment (FCP/FCP) but not, in principle, to a higher level (vocational college if previously FCP) unless this is the only way to safeguard his ability to earn.

The principle of the *sustainability and success of the measure*, the point of which is for the vocational rehabilitation measures taken to have an effect over a certain length of time with a minimum of success at the level of gainful activity. For example, DI will not consider a 3-year training scheme for an insuree who is five years away from his old-age pension.

The principle of *proportionality*: this aims at a reasonable balance between the expenses incurred by the measures and the foreseeable result of the latter. This principle is closely linked to the foregoing one.

In this way, the qualified baker who has an FCP can go in for training at the expense of DI, the aim being to obtain a new FCP in any field whatsoever that avoids contact with the allergen and dependent on his skills and interests.

Job placement assistance

What route is left to disabled patients who fail to cross the threshold that gives them the right to vocational rehabilitation?

For unskilled insurees whose loss of income does not amount to 20%, *the DI's job placement service can be consulted to obtain help from DI experts at the DI office in finding a suitable job*: the preparation of job applications, help in finding work and in editing advertisements, the preparation of job interviews, setting up work experience placements or periods for learning basics. Like all the benefits offered by the DI, this right is subject to restrictions. According to a recent court ruling, an insuree who is, in principle, fit to work 100% in a suitable activity does not have the right to assistance from the DI office in finding work unless hampered in looking for a job by his health impairment (blindness, deafness, mobility disorders, behavioural difficulties, etc.). If this is not the case, the unemployment insurance advisors will accompany him in this process.

In cases where the insuree's ability to work in a suitable activity is greater than 80% and less than 100%, he can receive assistance from the DI office's job placement service. However, the DI office is not obliged to place suitable work at the disposal of the insuree.

Example

The construction worker who was operated on for a slipped disc will not benefit from the DI office's job placement assistance service if his ability to work in a suitable activity is 100% (loss of earnings of 9% in the example quoted above). On the other hand, if the need to take frequent breaks (more frequently than what is generally provided for, i.e. 2 quarter-hour breaks per day) reduces his ability to work to 80% in comparison with a normal employee, he could be assisted in his job-finding process by a rehabilitation advisor. In this connection, it is not the rate of disability that is the determining factor but the rate of ability to work in the suitable job.

Some data

In 2001, 375,000 individual measures were granted by the DI [4] for 301,000 beneficiaries. Preliminary investigation measures at specialist offices external to DI (COMAI, experts) affected 166,000 people at a cost of CHF 85 millions (measures intended to verify the right to a DI pension).

One hundred and three thousand people benefited from medical rehabilitation measures at a cost of CHF 492 millions (average of CHF 4,769 per case). Vocational rehabilitation and training measures (the most expensive on a per-case basis) affected 13,000 people at an average cost of 21,298 CHF per case.

Concerning the results of vocational rehabilitation measures between 70,2% and 71,9% of the measures carried out between 1997 and 2000 were still effective two years later. In 1997, the number of vocational measures was 4,577.

Conclusion

During the period of inability to work, the chances of work resumption and long-term reintegration are considerably increased if insurance institutions intercede at an early stage in the form of vocational rehabilitation measures. For this to take place and given the complexity of the Swiss insurance system, inter-institutional cooperation (disability insurance, unemployment insurance and social assistance) is absolutely vital since, if these rehabilitation measures fail and for all that the inability to earn is greater than 40%, disability insurance will be obliged to pay out disability pensions pro rata based on the degree of disability.

References

1. Viscomi A (2003) L'assurance invalidité, cours 2ᵉ cycle AEAS, January/February
2. Federal law on disability insurance (LAI) of 09 June 1959
3. Suva statistics 2002 Swiss National Accident Insurance Fund. CP. 6002 Lucerne
4. 2002 social security statistics. Federal Social Insurance Office, Berne
5. Federal law on the general part of the social security law (ATSG/LPGA) of 6 October 2000
6. Circular concerning occupational rehabilitation measures (CMRP), valid from 1st January 2004
7. Fournier Buchs M-F, Rivier G (2003) De la prise en charge médicale à la réadaptation professionnelle. Revue médicale de la Suisse romande 123: 617-20

Composition, mise en page et impression : Imprimerie BARNÉOUD
B.P. 44 - 53960 BONCHAMP-LÈS-LAVAL
Dépôt légal : septembre 2005 - N° d'imprimeur : 508086
Imprimé en France